Innovations in
HOSPITAL
ARCHITECTURE

Innovations in
HOSPITAL
ARCHITECTURE

Stephen Verderber

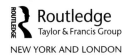

Routledge
Taylor & Francis Group

NEW YORK AND LONDON

First published 2010
by Routledge
270 Madison Avenue, New York, NY10016

Simultaneously published in the UK by Routledge
2 Park Square, Milton Park, Abingdon, Oxon, OX14 4RN

Routledge is an imprint of the Taylor & Francis Group, an informa business

Designed and typeset by Alex Lazarou
Printed and bound in India by the Replika Press Pvt. Ltd., Sonepat, Haryana

British Library Cataloguing in Publication Data
A catalogue record for this book is available from the British Library

Library of Congress Cataloging-in-Publication Data
Verderber, Stephen.
Innovations in hospital architecture / Stephen Verderber.
   p. ; cm.
   Includes bibliographical references.
   1. Hospital architecture. 2. Health facilities–Design and construction. I. Title.
[DNLM: 1. Hospital Design and Construction–trends. 2. Architecture as Topic–trends.
WX 140 V483i 2010]
RA967.V474 2010
725'.51047–dc22

                                                            2009035054

ISBN10: 0-415-77795-X (hbk)
ISBN10: 0-203-85575-2 (ebk)

ISBN13: 978-0-415-77795-7 (hbk)
ISBN13: 978-0-203-85575-1 (ebk)

The very first requirement of a hospital is that it shall cause neither human nor ecological harm

Contents

Illustration credits

CHAPTER 2

2.1, 2.8, 2.12, 2.36	Collection of John Currie
2.2	Drawing: E. Boehringer, Gebruden Mann Verlag, Berlin.
2.3	École Nationale Supérieure des Beaux Art, World Atlas of Architecture
2.4–2.7	Photos: Alexander Verderber
2.9	Courtesy of E.T. Archive, London. Barnes and Noble Books, New York
2.10	A.J. Ochsner and M.J. Sturm
2.11, 2.15	Photo courtesy of Florence Nightingale Archives, London
2.13	Photo: Alexander Verderber
2.14	Photo: Grace Goldin
2.16	Photo: Alexander Verderber
2.17	Photo: Courtesy of National Library of Medicine, Washington, D.C.
2.18	John Thompson and Grace Goldin
2.19	Photo courtesy of Oskar Diethelm Library
2.20	Drawing: Jacob Weidenmann
2.21	Source unknown
2.22	Courtesy of State Historical Society of Missouri, Columbia
2.23	Photo: Loring Bullard
2.24	Photo: Charlotte Boles

2.25–2.31	Photos courtesy United States Army Medical Library, Washington, D.C.
2.32	Photo: The Crippled Children's Hospital School, Memphis, Tennessee
2.33	Source unknown
2.34	Drawing: Richard E. Schmidt
2.35	Photo: Suomen Ilmakuva Oy, Helsinki
2.37a-b	Diagrams: Stephen Verderber
2.38	Photo: Stephen Verderber
2.39	Photo: Alexander Verderber

CHAPTER 3

3.1	Burger/Grunstra Architects/Planners, Alkmaar, the Netherlands. Photo: R. Hoekstra
3.2	Drawing: Burger/Gunstra Architects/Planners
3.3–3.6	Eric Gutmorgeth, Architect, Innsbruck, Austria
3.7–3.9	Photos: Odell Associates, Charlotte, North Carolina
3.10–3.12	Photos: NBBJ Seattle, Washington
3.13	Photo: Office of João de Gama Filueiras, São Paulo, Brazil
3.14	Photo: Wang Yan/Zhong Lu Architects, Shanghai, China (Borong Chen)
3.15–3.16	NBBJ Seattle, Washington
3.17	Clemson University Graduate Program in Architecture+Health, South Carolina

CHAPTER 4

4.1–4.2	Photos: Courtesy of National Library of Medicine, Washington, D.C.
4.3	Photo: David Allison
4.4	Photo: HPP Laage & Partners, Stuttgart, Germany
4.5–4.7	Photos: NBBJ Photography, Seattle, Washington
4.8	Drawing: NBBJ Seattle, Washington
4.9–4.14	Photos: Perkins + Will, Minneapolis, Minnesota
4.15	Drawing: Perkins + Will, Minneapolis, Minnesota
4.16–4.21	Clemson University Graduate Program in Architecture+Health, South Carolina
4.22	Photo: Stephen Verderber
4.23–4.24	Photos: Hitoshi Abe Atelier, Tokyo, Japan/Los Angeles, California
4.25	Photo: J. Buwalda

4.26	Drawing: Burger Grunstra Architects/Planners
4.27	Photo: RRP Architects+Engineers, Munich, Germany

CHAPTER 5

5.1–5.2	Photos: RMJM Hillier, Philadelphia, Pennsylvania. Charity Hospital Archives, New Orleans
5.3	Drawing: RMJM Hillier, Philadelphia
5.4	Photo: Stephen Verderber
5.5–5.9	Renderings: RMJM Hillier, Philadelphia

CHAPTER 6

6.1	Diagram: Stephen Verderber

CHAPTER 7

7.1–7.6	Drawings: Stephen Verderber
7.7	Photo: Paul Toman
7.8	Drawing: Kroeker/Lilly Architects/Piskwepag Design, Inc., Halifax, Nova Scotia
7.9	Photo: Kahler Slater Architects, Inc., Madison, Wisconsin
7.10	Drawing: Stephen Verderber
7.11	Photo: Maggi-Moreno Maag/Studio Altieri S.P.A., Thiene, Italy
7.12	Drawing: Stephen Verderber
7.13	Photo: Dieter Leistner, Würzburg, Germany/ Angela Fritsch Architekten
7.14	Drawing: Stephen Verderber
7.15	Photo: Tom Arban Photography
7.16	Photo: Jeffrey Totaro/RTKL Associates, Inc.
7.17	Drawing: Stephen Verderber
7.18	Photo: Dana Wheelock Photography
7.19	Drawing: Stephen Verderber
7.20	Photo: Behnisch & Partners, Stuttgart, Germany
7.21	Photo: Linus Lintner Fotografie/SEHW Architects, Berlin, Germany
7.22	Photo: NBBJ Photography, Seattle, Washington
7.23	Photo: KMD, San Francisco, California
7.24	Photo: Paul Ott Photography
7.25	Drawing: Fasch & Fuchs/Lukas Schumacher
7.26	Photo: Eckert & Eckert Photography
7.27–7.32	Drawings: Stephen Verderber

Acknowledgements

The story behind *Innovations in Hospital Architecture* begins with an informal meeting with my editor, Caroline Mallinder, at the 2005 annual conference of the North American organization of university-based schools of architecture. We were in the publisher's exhibit area going over some details of my then-forthcoming book, *Innovations in Hospice Architecture* (London: Taylor & Francis, 2005). I brought up the idea of a parallel, or companion book, this time focused on recent developments in hospital architecture. We agreed, with a handshake, to pursue it. I was to begin work on it later that year. Little did I know that day just how much everything would change a few short months later.

In the frantic hours leading up to Hurricane Katrina's landfall in the early hours of Monday 29 August, my wife, Kindy, me, and our two teenagers, E. Leigh and Alexander, were hurriedly moving valuables, carpets, furniture, and anything else we could lift out of harm's way in our home in the Uptown section of New Orleans, where we had lived for twenty years. At Tulane University that morning, where I taught, my research assistant and I frantically burned CDs and DVDs of my current work, the few materials I would take with me in a suitcase to Texas, our evacuation destination. Before dawn the next morning we set out for Houston, along with a half million others who appeared to have made the same decision to flee to the west. What would normally have been a five-hour car trip ended up taking fourteen through a circuitous path of backroads across Louisiana and Texas. Katrina was by that time bearing down on New Orleans as a Category 5 monster storm. It was billed as the Big One.

To make a long story short, our home flooded and we ended up as evacuees in Austin, Texas until Christmas that year. My verbal agreement with Caroline in March suddenly seemed like a million years ago. I was focused on finding a place for us to *live*, immediately. With no home to go back to, our house uninhabitable, and our jobs in a weird sort of animated suspension, family needs were elemental. Of course, we were by no means alone in being involuntarily forced to cope with the aftermath of this catastrophe. In retrospect, the sudden dislocation was very difficult but, according to the old adage, we made the best of a bad situation. With the children in a new school (St. Stephen's Episcopal), and the family in a rented house, we persevered. Having thoroughly been shaken by Katrina and the Diaspora, I now shifted focus 180 degrees, and began work on what would become a book, *Delirious New Orleans: Manifesto for an Extraordinary American City* (Austin: University of Texas Press, 2009). The School of Architecture at the University of Texas at Austin provided a safe haven.

Meanwhile, what was to come of the verbal agreement Caroline and I had struck. Katrina abruptly set in motion an entirely new set of life events. Like every single New Orleanian, I suspect that everything in my life from here on will be categorized as either having occurred pre-Katrina, or post-Katrina. Global climate change, combined with most of New Orleans being below sea level, made the eventual decision less difficult. In 2007 I joined the faculty at Clemson University, as the third faculty team member in its prestigious Graduate Program in Architecture + Health. Its director, David Allison, and I had become colleagues over the years. Our paths crossed at a number of conferences and meetings. It was a good decision. The post-Katrina period of upheaval for my family would continue even after we arrived in South Carolina. As for this book, I remained unable to focus on it with any reasonable clarity until the start of 2008. Perhaps the unplanned hiatus of nearly two and a half years away from the project had been a blessing in disguise. The field of healthcare design was moving fast in the 2005–2008 period.

Hospital design, as a subfield within the professional practice of architecture, certainly has not enjoyed the same reputation for cutting edge aesthetic innovation compared to other building types such as museums, residential design, schools, libraries, or the ambitious buildings built by Olympic Games host cities. A hospital is a highly complex, often contradictory, building type. How can such a large place be made to look and feel like someone's home? What might carbon neutrality have to do with a hospital, since it requires so much energy to operate? Internationally, however, bonafide aesthetic and tectonic innovations have occurred in the past decade that refute such misperceptions. There is no longer any reason (or excuse) whatsoever for a hospital to be any less aesthetically or technically interesting, or any less 'sustainable' compared to any other building type. This fact was a source of inspiration for this book.

This book is about the first decade of the new century (2000–2010). At first, it seemed impossible to think that any single book could capture even a small portion of everything that happened in hospital architecture in this decade, let alone in the broader field of healthcare architecture. The present book picks up where my first book, *Healthcare Architecture in an Era of Radical Transformation* (London and New Haven: Yale University Press, 2000) left off. It spanned the period 1965–2000 with regard to international developments in the field, purposefully embracing the spectrum of building types and trends in healthcare architecture. The buildings, writings, and research of many colleagues since then shaped the present book. Notable among these was *Sustainable Healthcare Architecture* (2008) by Robin Guenther and Gail Vittori. The efforts by so many architects to bring the hospital up to the forefront and an equivalent level with other sustainable design initiatives globally has been most impressive and a notable achievement.

This book would not have been possible without the support of the students and faculty in the Graduate Program in Architecture + Health at Clemson University. I have had the privilege to work with David Allison and Dina Battisto, and Keith Green, Peter Laurence, Rob Miller, Ted Cavanaugh, Jose Caban, many other numerous faculty members in architecture, as well as Chip Eagan, the Interim Dean of the College of Art, Architecture, and Humanities. All have been instrumental. Thanks to the generous financial support for this project provided by Clemson University, through a University Research Grant (URG), and from the McMahon Fund for Excellence in Architecture, housed in the School of Architecture. A special debt of gratitude is owed to Katherine Yohman, for her most able assistance in constructing and managing the database of case studies over a period of many months, and to Lindsay Todd, for her extraordinary assistance in assembling, refining and managing the book's total image database, her adroitness in digging through the literature, and for her strong commitment to the field. They were a source of positive energy, skill, and inspiration throughout, and especially for staying focused from start to completion. Thanks also to Christine DeVerneil and to Lin Zhang for their research work and translational contributions, Lindsay and Christine made significant contributions to Chapter 4. All are M.Arch candidates in Architecture + Health at Clemson. Thanks also to Esther Kaufman for her accounting and logistical support, and to the outstanding staff of the Art and Architecture Library at Clemson. Thanks to Alex Hollingsworth, Katherine Morton, and Georgina Johnson at Routledge/ Taylor & Francis for their support, experience, and encouragement (and to Caroline Mallinder, who retired in 2007).

It continues to be an honor to meet colleagues from so many places so deeply interested in and committed to architecture for health. In particular, I am indebted to my colleagues in the *Global University Programs in Healthcare Architecture* organization, a productive confederation of university educator-researcher-practitioners devoted to advancing graduate level education in this area. Through this organization I have been able to extend the horizon line far beyond the United States. Many thanks also to the dozens of architectural firms from around the world who contributed their work. It would not have been possible without their efforts.

There are too many contributors to list by name and yet it remains perplexing, even troublesome, that so few university level programs at this time offer a specialized degree concentration in this area of research and/or professional education. It is especially worrisome given the fact that healthcare is certain to remain an important career track in architecture in the coming years in the face of explosive global population growth and continued environmental and ecological challenges. It is hoped that this book might aid in the creation of additional university level degree and certificate programs worldwide. Interdisciplinary programs centered on the planning, design, and management of environments for healthcare are also urgently needed to bridge the planning and design disciplines, including industrial design, with the social sciences, public health, medicine, nursing, the engineering professions, and healthcare policy.

My wife, and our two children, now 18 and 21 respectively, my students, and my mother continue to be a source of guidance, support and great inspiration.

Stephen Verderber
GREENVILLE, SOUTH CAROLINA
2009

PART 1

Background

Introduction

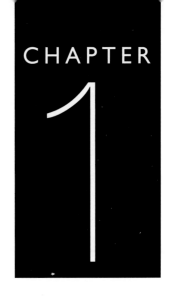

This book has been a decade in the making. When *Healthcare Architecture in an Era of Radical Transformation* was published in 2000 I did not expect it would take ten years to produce its sequel. The idea behind that book was to capture events in the final third of the twentieth century. For a few years thereafter I thought about expanding that book with additional chapters but eventually decided it best to leave well enough alone. It made little sense to extend a book about the last century into the new one. The date of its publication had been fortuitous, and anyway, the field continued to move forward at breakneck speed. In retrospect it was worthwhile to wait long enough for a companion volume to cover the first decade of the new century.

No one has ever accused me of being an apologist for the architecture of most hospitals. I do greatly admire what happens inside them, however. They are marvels of technology, of human accomplishment, and they represent the highest aspirations of the human spirit. But a hospital is not an island. I recall an essay I was assigned to read while an undergraduate in the late 1970s titled 'A city is not a tree' (1964), authored by an upstart named Christopher Alexander. In it, it was argued that cities are systems of interdependent subsystems. No one aspect is entirely autonomous of any other. All the parts must work together, or at least relatively well together – transportation systems, buildings, parks, commercial, educational, and civic places, and most importantly the simple, nondescript everyday places and events in our everyday lives. This was an abstract notion to me – weren't trees a part of systems as well? Were they not a part of an ecosystem? Later, I would come to appreciate more fully Alexander's thesis, especially when it was expanded into the seminal book *A Pattern Language: Towns, Buildings, Construction*, first published in 1977. Some years later, after having chosen to specialize in the field of architecture and health, I came to realize the far deeper meaning of his thesis although not until only relatively recently would it re-resonate within me with intense force. This happened after I witnessed the destruction caused by Hurricane Katrina in 2005. It was stunning to see at first hand what took hundreds of years to build and nurture, in the case of New Orleans (founded in 1718), could be taken away in a matter of hours. The interdependences are fragile between the myriad subsystems of a city even in normal times but especially in the aftermath of an urban catastrophe.[1]

It is a painfully slow, arduous, and costly process to rebuild a city. It is an equally painful process to rebuild a city's healthcare with the stakes now higher. A hospital/medical center can no longer think of itself as an island, or for whatever reasons exempt from its urban ecological context. It must now also demonstrate leadership in environmental stewardship from the building and campus scale to the intermediate scale of its neighborhood, to the scale of the city, region, and entire planet. It functions within a delicate urban ecosystem. In broader terms, the promotion of human health remains its core mission but with ecological health no less integral to the total equation. To 'Do no harm' now denotes far more than it did a century or even a mere decade ago: *a hospital must cause neither human nor ecological harm*. A hospital is not an island.

Challenges to human health and wellness

The global healthcare landscape is becoming flat. New trends spread from region to region faster than ever before. Medical procedures once unique to a particular country are now performed on every continent. The United States is by no means a paragon in terms of the health of its citizens. Every nation has lessons to learn and worth sharing with other nations. For decades patients have traveled to London from Cape Town for neurosurgery. Telemedicine now makes it possible for a surgeon in Boston to synchronously assist in an experimental surgical procedure being performed in Lima, Peru. Healthcare is becoming transnational, jumping across borders with more and more regularity. This poses many legal and cultural challenges but both trends are likely to continue. In the U.S. nearly 47 million people (including 8.1 million children) did not have health insurance in 2009. The U.S. however spends the most per capita on healthcare in the world, representing 18 percent of the nation's total gross domestic product. This figure rose to $2.6 trillion in 2009, averaging to about $8,000.00 for every person. This is unlikely to decrease in the near future, as healthcare is something that people tend to want more of, not less. The demand for healthcare is elastic. Hospitals in the U.S. are the direct recipients of one-third of all total U.S. fiscal expenditures. Healthcare should not be tied to if someone has a job; it should be portable and travel with them wherever they go. We insure every car on the road; don't all people deserve the same?

Despite high expenditures for health, the U.S. lags behind many developed nations who spend far less per capita on healthcare.[2] Hospitals charge and receive differing amounts for the services they render based on the third party reimbursor. Charges are often presented as 'list price' for hospital services, set at a rate to cover other patients who lack insurance, as well as institutional overheads, administration, and debt. The system is breaking apart, overwhelmingly skewed toward after-the-fact sickness care versus preemptive wellness care and prevention. It is an unsustainable system and certainly no model for the world to emulate, in its present form. This problem will become further exacerbated by a projected population increase in the U.S. of 135 million over the next 40 years. In the next decade if no structural changes are made to the system 9 million more Americans will lose their health insurance.[3] Meanwhile, the mad dash to embrace the all-private-room hospital in the U.S. (and elsewhere to a growing extent) is to its critics a classic exercise in being out of synch with funding realities, carbon neutrality, and the escalating cost of construction.

It is axiomatic that architects follow the money. That is, they tend to gravitate to clients most able and willing to pay for something (of quality, one hopes). What defines quality? Is it justifiable to narrowly define quality in a work of architecture for health primarily in terms of its aesthetic/formal attributes? Mainly for the wealthiest patients? The plight of healthcare availability for underserved minorities is worsening in most parts of the world. There simply is not enough money to go around for each and every newly built hospital or clinic to be of publishable quality in terms of its so-called aesthetic integrity. It is highly doubtful whether the residents in the East End of London, in the Lawndale community on Chicago's South Side, in the barrios of Caracas, or in the slums of Mumbai care much about whether their local storefront or neighborhood clinic is published somewhere in a glossy architecture magazine or book. In most cases, and for a litany of reasons, this is unachievable anyway. The first and foremost priority must continue to remain clear: to promote and advance the health and well-being of all individuals and populations everywhere in an ecologically responsible manner.

On the other hand, it makes equally little sense to define a high quality work of architecture for health in purely functional or non-aesthetic terms, either: that is, on only whether its design results in a higher level of patient safety and fewer medical errors without any concern for its attractiveness, aesthetics, or visual amenity. Perhaps a clinic's miniscule construction budget allowed for few if any high-end aesthetic amenities. Do its staff and patients really care about how it looks as long as it succeeds in this regard? The fact remains that an aesthetically undistinguished design may yield positive health outcomes although its chances for publication in a professional media outlet are slim to none. Everyone knows that the world has more than its share of less-than-beautiful hospitals, and these alone could fill up many volumes.

A third option appears to be by far the better course of action: strive to achieve both at once. This is the challenge – to first and foremost promote community health through design and ecological responsibility. It should in and of itself be rewarding to provide Architecture (with a capital A) to those who would otherwise never be touched by it in their lives. There is no longer a place for mutual exclusivity in global architecture for health in this regard. Embrace diversity. Embrace user constituencies of all classes and income levels. Embrace racial diversity. Embrace the medically underserved in *your* community. Provide paid professional services as well as pro bono services to these individuals and groups. Become a leader in your community beyond your role as an architect, engineer, landscape architect, or whatever. We can all be lifelong students as well as teachers in this regard, current trends in healthcare architecture notwithstanding. A real danger exists that the nascent but growing evidence-based research and design movement discussed in the following chapters will be unable to overcome the digital divide that isolates the haves from the have-nots. Internet access will remain inaccessible to the poorest, most remote patients. What good to these would-be patients is it for their local hospital to be noise-free, aesthetically superior, afford a high level of privacy, be safe of medical and staff errors, and so on, if they lack access to it?[4]

Challenges to ecological health and wellness

One hears talk constantly about 'sustainability' but what does it really mean? The arguments are compelling but architects need to acquire a much better operative understanding of their work in the context of environmental ecology, an expanded knowledge of material ecologies and their effects, the capabilities and culpabilities of high technology as a fix-anything panacea for any problem, the social ramifications of technology, and a greater knowledge of environmental history. Architects tend to narrowly think of sustainability in solely an ecological context, or in economic terms. Rarely do they/we think of it in holistic terms, including supply–demand tensions over the earth's limited, highly pressed resources. But clean air and water,

a livable climate, and a healthy standard of living are not the only endangered elements in our social order we seek to sustain. Broader realms include community, psychological health, meaningful work, intellectual openness, individual and social empowerment, a sense of heritage and history, cultural diversity, art, and music. These dimensions of everyday life are interrelated.[5] Poor healthcare policy inevitably damages not only humans but also local cultural traditions.[6] Sometimes sustainable goals come into direct conflict, as when green development inadvertently jeopardizes historic preservation and conservation, or catalyzes cultural, racial, or social conflict.[7] Architecture, as a blend of the humanities and the sciences, can provide an ideal forum from which adjacent disciplines can learn and from which we can in turn learn much.

Environmental critic Richard Heinberg, in his recent book *Powerdown*, points out that hydrocarbons have been both the greatest blessing and the greatest curse our species has ever encountered. Coal, oil, and natural gas have given us the Industrial Revolution but have also brought global warming, pollution, habitat destruction, and modern industrial-scale warfare. It is a deeply intertwined set of benefits and costs and this is what makes our dependency on fossil fuels so problematic.[8] Engineers, trained as problem solvers, have a tendency to respond to the crisis in isolation from its holistic and ecological contexts. It is oversimplified to a simple cause–effect problem: if we are running out of oil, the solution is simply to discover a new energy source capable of substituting for fossil fuels. The reality is that unless humanity pulls back its demands on the earth's life support systems a new energy source will make little difference. When viewed as an ecological and cultural problem, and not merely as an engineering or architectural problem, it is critical to focus concurrently on reducing population pressures on the planet, to slow the rate of resource depletion, reduce the rate of habitat destruction and remain cognizant of valued local cultural traditions. Heinberg also argues it is much more than a simple supply–demand relationship:

Much of our usage of energy goes to facilitate the extraction, transformation, and use of other sources – metals, soils, water, and so on. Without an accompanying demand-side response, merely increasing the supply of energy to our species will mean the continued depletion of other resources, more competition for dwindling resources, and an eventual crash. It is our reluctance as a species to undertake demand-side solutions to the ecological dilemma – and not merely our inability to find a suitable substitute for oil … we are in deep trouble, and it is essential that we understand the nature of the trouble we are in.[9]

The alternative in the decades ahead will be increased competition for the remaining resources and this will lead to countless global and regional conflicts (this theme is reprised in Chapter 6). Julia Whitty writes:

The Antarctic as recently as 2001 was thought invulnerable in the 21st century, but it is leaking at the seams. It is well known by now that that since 2000 atmospheric carbon dioxide levels have increased 35 percent faster than expected, despite the pledges of 100 nations to rein them in. The polar seas are defying the laws of expectation, warming, in places, a staggering nine degrees Fahrenheit since 1995, opening the door for non-native plants and animals to cross the polar thresholds and claim new waters for themselves. This bodes poorly for penguins and people alike.[10]

What has happened is that the private healthcare industry and governmental healthcare systems have to think and act *systemically* on two fronts: first is the challenge within the healthcare sciences to become a paragon of ecological stewardship, second is the challenge to become a paragon of ecological stewardship in society. Grim forecasts of the future are not meant to shock and discourage but should be seen as a call to action.[11] It is naive to think that any single profession can solve these problems alone (another theme reprised in Chapter 6). Of course, architects and other designers are beginning to make some progress but these actions remain in the very early stages with the overarching goal to greatly reduce carbon dioxide emissions and repair the earth.[12] But these efforts alone will not suffice unless we act in consort to curb demand as well. We, in other words, have to think far beyond our relatively narrow role as a designer, engineer, physician, healthcare administrator, and the like, to work collaboratively on multiple fronts.[13] The actions of architects in the past decade represent a promising start but this is only a very small step compared to the enormity of the challenge that lies ahead. The *Intergovernmental Panel on Climate Change* (IPCC) has since 2001 issued a series of reports on the state of global climate change. It has illustrated the effects using maps of each region and continent, with particularly 'hot spots' tagged. It

would be informative if the IPCC were to issue a similar report on those hospitals in greatest risk of harm due to rising seas, drought, and related, increasingly severe weather occurrences.[14]

The *Green Guide for Healthcare* had 159 registered projects at the start of 2009, representing 39 million square feet of new construction in 36 U.S. states, 5 Canadian provinces, and 7 other countries. There were 22,000 registrants with 500 new registrants per month. As of January 2009 there were 35 'Leadership Through Energy Efficient Environmental Design' (LEED) certified healthcare projects, the largest being the 328-bed Prentice Women's Hospital in Chicago (LEED Silver Certification). The Dell Children's Hospital in Texas was the first LEED Platinum-Certified project in the U.S. (2009).[15] Meanwhile, critics maintain that the LEED program is flawed, costly, and will soon be eclipsed.[16] The *Whole Building Design Guide* published a primer on the subject of green healthcare facilities. It provides definitions, a list of organizations, and literature references on the subject.[17] In Australia the *Green Star* system is growing, and in the U.K., the Commission for Architecture and the Built Environment (CABE) is gaining momentum, including its section on architecture for health. Many other countries are currently establishing similar certification programs in 'green' architecture. The goal is carbon neutrality, and walkable, pedestrian-scaled, regenerative strategies centered on new construction as much as adaptive reuse, preservation, and increasing social capital through thoughtful environmental design. The ill-fated Las Gaviotas rural hospital in Columbia, and a clinic in Bhopal, India, that is built on a brownfield site and cultivates its own food on site, are but two visionary examples.

All this became even more daunting due to the global economic recession that began in 2008. The gridlocking of international financial systems has made banks reluctant to lend. Private investors are finding it difficult to finance new construction or renovation projects. This is causing a harmful impact on new capital investment in healthcare facilities in many countries. Construction activity in rapidly expanding places such as Dubai has come to a crashing halt; large construction projects sit uncompleted in cities around the globe. It is part of a global *reset* process, albeit a painful resetting. The dovetail effect of runaway speculation, poor lending practices on the part of financial institutions and governments, and excessive consumer debt were three main factors that fueled this debacle. Hospitals are among the institutions suffering from the global economic malaise and many are reacting by laying off staff, limiting certain services, and delaying or cancelling construction projects.[18]

On a larger scale, the sprawl epidemic that has run unchecked in the U.S. for nearly thirty years has been curtailed due to the widespread economic downturn. Is this the beginning of the end of the American dream?[19] The global economic contraction/reset that began in 2008 may yield a spectacular moment of global consciousness, as an unforgettable reminder that all 6.7 billion of us are in this together.[20] It can result in more rational thinking about how and where we live and work and this equally applies to how and where we receive healthcare and what those places are like as the healthcare landscape becomes ever more flattened in the coming years.

Three broad underlying trends, or movements, define this book's underlying narrative: first, human and ecological sustainability, second, formal and aesthetic advances/new residentialism/functional deconstruction, and third, evidence-based research and design. Another way to visualize this conceptual structure is to think of three overlapping circles, with one defined as formal and aesthetic advances, another as human and ecological sustainability, and a third as evidence-based research and design. The space at the center of the overlapping circles represents the core thesis insofar as an in-between condition constituting a fourth condition, one of fluidity and synthesis, holding the most promise for the future viability of the hospital as a building type. Each chapter addresses this fourth condition in relation to the other three.

Chapter 2 is an excursion through the annals of architectural history as a means to perhaps shed some new light on the naturalistic, that is sustainable, dimensions of healing environments as they evolved through the centuries. This, to some, may appear as little more than an exercise in revisionist history, but it can be instructive to look back at past building types, such as the Kirkbride asylums of the late nineteenth century in the U.S. to see and reappraise their extensive use of narrow, linear building footprints as a means to draw natural daylight and fresh air into the interior. Six epochs are presented, each representative of the ontology of environments for healthcare through the millennia, from the cave infirmaries of the earliest Neolithic settlements, to the city-states of ancient Greece, to the church-ward infirmaries predominant during the medieval period, to the advent of the palace hospitals of the Renaissance, to the wickedly institutional insane asylums of the seventeenth and eighteenth centuries, to the humanist revivalism of the Nightingale wards of the late nineteenth and early twentieth centuries, to the International Style modernist 'machine hospitals' predominate in the post-World War II period, to the advent of postmodernism and subsequent developments up to the present. The purpose of this discussion is to illustrate the reality that history does in fact tend to repeat itself.

In Chapter 3, the focus shifts to the functions of site, landscape, and nature in contemporary architecture for health. The prior discussion serves as the backdrop for the discussion of the ways in which major figures from the twentieth century, such as Frank Lloyd Wright, R.M. Schindler, and Alvar Aalto, made extensive use of transparency and organic expressionism in an attempt to dematerialize the rigid compositional and planar barriers that characterized neoclassicism. Prior to modernism, the walls of hospitals were massive; load-bearing stone edifices with minimally sized apertures for windows and transitional spaces. This leads to an intriguing area of research, biophilia, and its relationship to the making of a nature-attuned architecture for health. Its intended and unintended commonalties with anthropomorphism and organic formal languages are shown. A new term, *theraserialization*, is introduced, and is defined as the transparent and semi-transparent layering, and/or superimposition, of interior and exterior space in such a way that a serialized continuum is achieved. This concept holds much promise in extending far beyond the narrow, by now almost quaint term *healing garden*, to become something much more potent.

In Chapter 4, recent advances in the patient care unit (PCU) and the inpatient room are examined. The focus is on aesthetic, functional, and experiential aspects of the patient care experience and that of the patient's family. Case studies illustrate recent innovations, such as the Adopt-a-Room prototype in Minneapolis, the growing dominance of the all-private-room hospital, the rise of the single-handed PCU (where the bed is oriented identically in every patient room), to recent innovations in nursing care. This facet includes the shift away from highly centralized nursing stations to decentralized workstations that involve fixed and mobile 'stations' throughout the PCU, with caregivers who, through the use of advanced wireless technology, now enter and retrieve data entirely digitally. The patient safety movement is discussed in terms of its implications for PCU and patient room design. And finally, the American near-obsession with the all-private-room PCU is critically reconsidered, particularly in light of the high cost of construction, advances in infection control protocols, construction, and operational funding mechanisms, and cross-cultural differences.

In Chapter 5, covariances between historic preservation and conservation, sustainable urban and building design, and innovative practices in the delivery of healthcare are examined. A case study serves as a vehicle to explore the sustainability (as well as drawbacks) of restoring and rebuilding anew from within a historic 1938 art deco hospital in the heart of post-Katrina New Orleans. This venerable institution, Charity Hospital, dating from 1737, was flooded in Hurricane Katrina in 2005 (and remains shuttered as of 2010). An underling theme throughout this chapter is why it so often is that so-called 'old' hospitals are routinely dismissed as obsolete, unsustainable, and unwieldy without the benefit of their administrators having commissioned any due diligence analysis of the potential for reuse (or a new use other than as a hospital). This pitched battle between a misguided governmental healthcare bureaucracy and a grass-roots community-led movement to rescind the decision to build a new replacement facility is recounted. It is hoped that this saga will be seen as a cautionary tale for others globally.

In Chapter 6, nine prognostications are postulated on the future of an ecohumanist architecture for health. These are rendered against a backdrop of global events with some probability of having a transformative influence on architecture for health between now and 2050, including the rise of nanotechnology, environmental robotics in the home and workplace, holography, cures for diseases such as cancer, virtual reality and the role of nature in healing, and spinal cord regeneration. On the other side of the coin, the challenges of the end of oil and natural gas, regional conflicts over scarce water, soil, scarce cultivatable oil, overpopulation and food shortages, human cloning, and air that is contaminated in cities are likely to trigger regional and global conflagrations between now and 2050. How will the built environment for healthcare respond? It is concluded that environmentalism fused with humanism – ecohumanism – will be required, denoting an equal concern for human well-being and ecological well-being.

In Chapter 7, a compendium of 100 planning and design considerations is presented. These center on seven aspects of the architecture of the hospital and medical centers – issues of site planning and community context, public and semi-public spaces on the campus and within the facility, the planning and design of the patient care unit and the inpatient room, diagnostic/treatment and trauma units, outpatient clinics and services, the influence of theraserialization and landscape upon healing and wellness, and holistic considerations in the administration of the total healing environment. These considerations are reinforced with examples. They are presented in relation to six 24/7 subtypes – acute care hospitals, rehabilitation

hospitals, childrens' hospitals, psychiatric hospitals, heart and related specialty institutions, and women's hospitals. This compendium is not to be construed as some sort of set-in-stone lexicon or any sort of prescriptive formula for a 'successful' project. Rather, they are ideas, meant to prod, question, and test the status quo. It is hoped they might be of some usefulness to planners, designers, engineers, product manufacturers, clients, healthcare providers, health policy specialists, government agencies, private philanthropic organizations, and interested individuals.

In Chapter 8, 28 case studies are presented. These are grouped into five types – autonomous community-based hospitals, children's hospitals, rehabilitation and elderly care centers and hospitals, regional medical center campuses, and unbuilt projects. All of the case studies were completed within the past five years with the exception of the four unbuilt projects. These four are the proposed ER One post-disaster trauma center for Washington D.C., the CORE Hospital prototype in Europe, a German firm's competition entry for six medical center campuses in India (Apex Prototypes), and a proposal for an International Red Cross Transportable Trauma Center. Fifty or more case studies could easily have been included and it was very hard to settle on this set. The one quality they all have in common is a quest for innovation, in extending beyond convention, and challenging the status quo.

This book is global in scope but much of it is based, for better or worse, on my life and experience in the United States. Additional efforts are needed that are transnational in scope such as the book *The Architecture of Hospitals* (2005), an edited volume of the proceedings of a conference held in the Netherlands in April 2005.[21] The present book could easily have been twice as long and, in fact, even expanded into a series, as a multi-volume set, with each volume devoted to a different sub-type, i.e. psychiatric hospitals, childrens' hospitals, rehabilitation hospitals, mainstream acute care hospitals, and specialized critical and tertiary care hospitals. Additionally, a separate volume is overdue on recent global architectural innovations in the architecture of veterinary hospitals. Finally, it is rare if not virtually impossible for any one hospital to 'succeed' in every respect (site planning, aesthetics, person–nature congruence, regenerative capacity, internal functionality, and so on). Yet *every* project featured in this book excels in one or more ways, and in many. In the final analysis it can stand as no more than a broad survey of developments at this moment in the architecture of hospitals in all their diverse, fascinating, complex, and at times maddeningly idiosyncratic manifestations.

Architecture for health: a brief history of sustainability

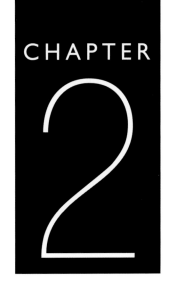

Since the mid-nineteenth century, architecture and health, as a specialized area, has slowly evolved, rising to a place of recognized professional stature and relevancy. Its autonomy exists within the profession of architecture and within the community of professions beyond architecture, namely, medicine, public health, and the allied health sciences. Relevancy and autonomy, it may be reasoned, correspondingly carry greater stature, legitimacy, and prestige than one or the other alone. By re-reading – reappraising – the past in order to better understand the present in this specialized area of research and practice, reflective investigation and critical discourse can be advanced. Critical discourse is surprisingly limited on the role of historical precedent in relation to a sustainable architecture for healthcare. Much can be learned, however, from history. The present situation is problematic in light of the enormous capital investment countries around the globe expend annually. This warrants discussion of a subset of landmark breakthroughs in the history of architecture, health, and sustainable planning and design.

By comparison, a century ago the medical and legal professions had already successfully adopted a model of critical inquiry and precedent-based research as a means to establish their positions. As these disciplines achieved this, they elevated themselves to their present positions of visibility and prestige. It is arguable that this could not have occurred without a critical, and continual, re-reading and reappraisal of their respective histories. Acquiring an historical perspective can therefore help to make sense of recent developments and foster engagement in paradigmatic discourse. The following discussion focuses on six aspects of the relationship between the built environment, human health, and sustainability. Each is viewed as a pattern, or healing agent, and is assumed here as of intrinsic therapeutic amenity for the patient. These patterns in healthcare settings were viewed by the Ancients as of therapeutic value but were lost by the Middle Ages, were later rediscovered in the mid-nineteenth century by Florence Nightingale and her contemporaries, only to be dismissed once again in the mid-twentieth century, and rediscovered again, recently. These six patterns are:

- *Natural ventilation* – the provision of natural ventilation and its transmission to interior spaces in settings for healthcare, as opposed to hermetically sealed care settings with windows that are non-operable and thereby sever contact with the outdoors.

- *Natural daylight and view* – the provision of natural light and its transmission to interior spaces in healthcare settings, as opposed to care settings that do not provide meaningful views to the exterior, or are poorly sited and therefore preclude the transmission of daylight into the building envelope.
- *Water and sanitation* – the provision of water as a therapeutic and aesthetic amenity and as a means to achieve personal hygiene and public health, as opposed to unsanitary care settings devoid of clean water for personal, aesthetic, or related civic uses.
- *Landscape, building configuration and site planning* – the provision of site planning and building form principles attuned with the therapeutic amenity in nature and in natural landscapes, including gardens, and walkable, pedestrian-scaled communities, as opposed to care settings that preclude connections to nature, consume excessive non-renewable resources, or contribute to unsustainable suburban sprawl.
- *Conservation of historic resources* – the provision of principles and protocols to identify, restore and adapt historically significant buildings, landscapes, and civic places for new functions compatible with personal health and public health, versus the senseless destruction of buildings and excessive consumption of nonrenewable natural resources.
- *Local building materials and self-sufficiency* – the provision of healthcare environments built with locally available materials, methods of construction, and with land resources allowing these places to achieve relative autonomy in terms of the on-site production of food, clothing, and the means of daily life, versus overdependence on geographically far-flung sources.

Collectively, these six determinants provide a discursive framework. They are drawn from history, are transactional, and dialectical. They speak to the relationship between nature, healing environments, and human health. They manifest and co-mingle at various times and in various ways and function individually and collectively at key intervals in history. Key 'moments' are cited at those intervals where some degree of symbiosis is achieved between any subset of two or more of these dimensions of a given healing environment. They are then placed in the context of a broader set of six chronological patterns, or *waves* (not always denoting periods of advancement) in the history of architecture and human health – the Ancient, the Medieval, the Renaissance, the Nightingale movement, the modern megahospital, and the sustainable healthscape. Within each wave, the functions of culture and society are shown to function as a backdrop to architecture, health, and environmental sustainability through the centuries. An attempt to portray these waves visually is presented (in Figure 2.37a–b at the end of this chapter). Unfortunately, due to limitations of space this chronology can provide little more than an introduction, a primer of sorts, on a fascinating, extensive, and at times highly complex, contradictory subject.[1]

The Ancient

From earliest times, the cave functioned as a refuge for the care and treatment of the sick and dying. In the earliest Neolithic settlements, a sick house was set aside for the care of the ill as it was gradually considered acceptable practice to separate these individuals from the mainstream community. Immediate family members, however, provided most care, in this 'home' setting. Throughout Europe the sickhouse and the deathhouse evolved as the repository for the disenfranchised, indigent, insane, and terminally ill. In these buildings, patterns of segregation and discrimination dominated the landscape.

Early hospitals in the Middle East and in Asian urban centers were advanced in comparison to their European counterparts. Early on, healing environments in Japan and in the Far East distinguished between sacred and secular settings. Similarly, Chinese healing environments centered on the home, with the private dwelling as the principal care setting where, in multigenerational settings, younger family members cared for the aged within the household. The earliest known formal hospitals, later to have a profound impact on European hospital architecture, were in the Middle East in Iraq, Iran, Egypt, and Turkey.[2]

In the West, Hippocrates was the first to systematically distinguish medicine as existing apart from philosophy. Hippocrates argued that the rationalist physician must possess a strong understanding of the influence of environmental determinants upon human health. The occurrence of sickness and disease, in his view, was in large part due to the influence of climatic and environmental factors.[3] He saw it particularly essential to possess knowledge of the four seasons, fresh water supplies, site orientation strategies for cities and towns, and the impact of prevailing winds, relative to their impact on human health:

First, he [physician-healer] must consider the effect of each of the seasons of the year and the differences between them. Secondly, he must study the warm and the cold winds, both those which are common to every country and those peculiar to a particular locality. Lastly, the effect of water on health must not be forgotten … when a physician comes to a district previously unknown to him, he should consider both its situation and its aspect to the winds. The effect of any town upon the health of its population varies according as it faces north or south, east or west. This is of the greatest importance. Similarly, the nature of the water supply must be considered; is it marshy and soft, hard when it flows from high and rocky ground, or salty with a hardness which is permanent? Then think of the soil, whether it is bare and waterless or thickly covered with vegetation and well-watered; whether in a hollow and stifling, or exposed and cold … a physician who understands (these factors) well … will not fail in observing what diseases are important in a given locality … (and would) know what epidemics to expect, both in the summer and in the winter.[4]

Hippocrates linked site planning and microclimate conditions with health outcomes and the propensity for illness in a manner linked to astronomy, requiring knowledge of the seasonal rising and falling of the stars. With regard to the health-promoting properties of water, Hippocrates argued the purest water comes from the highest ground and hills. It is cool in summer and warm in winter because it comes from very deep springs, and he considered rainwater to be health promoting when allowed to mix with fresh air and sunlight. On the influence of the natural environment on sustainable wellness attributes, he wrote:

The chief controlling factors, then, are the variability of the weather, the type of soil and the sort of water … as a general rule, the constitutions and the habits of a people follow the nature of the land where they live. Where the soil is rich, soft, and well-watered and where surface water is drunk, which is warm in summer and cold in winter, and where the seasons are favorable, you will find the people … incapable of great effort. In addition, such people are, for the most part, cowards … but if the land is bare, waterless and rough, swept by the winter gales and burnt by the summer sun, you will find there

a people hard and spare, their joints showing … they are wakeful, headstrong and self-willed.[5]

Places considered most desirable were therefore those where health promoting, i.e. health sustaining, determinants were considered the most favorable. These places also posed a challenge yet in a way that helped to build up resistance to disease. By contrast, places that did not possess these properties were classified as ill suited for habitation. They were viewed as countertherapeutic to nature and to the maintenance of healthy citizens.

The era of rational medicine would not emerge until Rome in the first century AD. Yet it had been the ancient Greeks who first evolved rational systems of medicine free from superstition and a blind belief in the supernatural.[6] In addition to causing disease and death, the ancient Greek gods also possessed curative powers. Religious-based medicine became firmly established in ancient Greece, not unlike in Egypt centuries earlier. The sick turned to a range of gods with initially Apollo the most powerful. But he was subsequently 'eclipsed' by his son Asclepieus, who had been transformed in the fifth century BC into a major god. At the Asclepieion at Cos, by the late fourth century BC, the influence of Hippocrates' teachings was influencing the work of the physician-healers although within a curious amalgam of the supernatural with the rational.

The Hippocratic theory of the four humours, with subsequent addenda through the centuries, was visually depicted as a series of concentric rings with the four seasons at the center. Spring is diametric to autumn, summer is diametric to winter in this diagram, where:

Each of the four humours is associated with a particular season and with two of the primary opposites. Blood, phlegm, black bile, and yellow bile are held to predominate in turn according to season. Blood, the dominant humour in spring, is like that season, characterized by qualities hot and moist. In similar fashion, yellow bile, like summer, is hot and dry. Black bile, like autumn, is cold and dry, and phlegm, like winter, is cold and moist. This symmetry … [is] later embraced in the four main organs of the body [and in] the four ages of man.[7]

The stoa had evolved as the principal commercial building type in the five Greek city-states. Built in the fifth century BC the linear double hall at the Asclepieion of Epidauros, in Athens, expropriated the stoa type as a patient care setting. The left side of the hall was

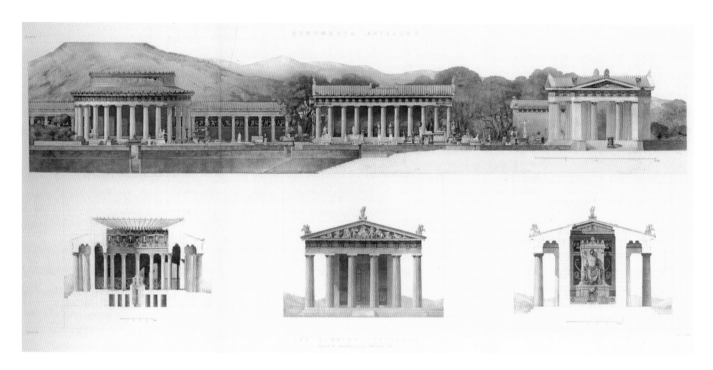

2.1   The Temple of Asclepius at Epidauros, 5th century BC

2.2   Pergamon, plan of Asclepiad and sanctuary complex at
Epidauros, 5th century BC

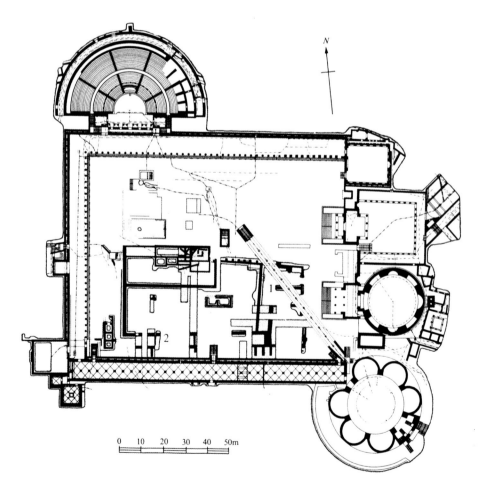

built directly on the ground. The right side of the hall rested upon a full basement. Patients could see the temple through the portico from their beds in the long open hall. They also could experience natural ventilation and daylight, as the beds were deployed along the inner wall for the entire length of the hall. Its dimensions were 24 foot deep by 108 foot in length and completely enclosed on three sides and open to the south. The southern exposure was articulated structurally by a row of columns – a portico – a device directly taken from the porticos of the commercial stoas in the town center – and always oriented toward the sun. This was done to allow the maximum amount of daylight to transmit into the interior. In the winter months, animal hides or textiles were used to screen out inclement weather (Figure 2.1).

In Athena and at Pergamon, the Asclepia were typically built on the lower slope of the hillsides, nearest to the water source. The most divine temple was situated at the top of the mountain, closest to the gods. Residential and commercial zones were situated in between. Fresh water was supplied by natural springs adjacent to the Asclepieion, or via natural gravitational flow from a higher topographic point on the hillside. Latrines were provided for patients and the wastes were transported off the site, usually to a different water source than that from which potable water was drawn.

The latrines at Pergamon (now Turkey) date from the Hellenistic period, second century AD. Pergamon had relatively sophisticated bathing facilities for patients, including a combination of large tubs and mud baths, with waters drawn from a nearby sacred spring. The degree of architectural and site-planning sophistication at Pergamon is evidenced by the creation of a courtyard with stoa-cum-infirmary treatment halls on three sides.[8] A circular terrace and a corresponding circular interior hallway, with windows, afforded southern exposure. Awnings most likely screened the circular opening at the top of the dome. Little is known if in winter this opening was closed off entirely from the elements. A heated subflooring system provided heat in the treatment building during the winter months (Figure 2.2).

The natural environment became a central component of care settings. By contemporary standards ancient Greek treatment was not strikingly different from wellness care, with an emphasis on a regimen of communality with nature and the outdoors, involving exercise, respite, water, vegetation, sunlight, improvements in nutrition, and immersion in landscape. The medical theories behind such treatment regimens became a topic of increasing debate during this period as care up to this time was largely based upon the

unyielding belief in the Greek gods and the supernatural. Asclepia were places for inpatient nursing and wellness treatment, including bed rest, medications, bathing regimens, nutrition regimens, and therapeutic exercise.[9] The typical treatment regimen was for the caregiver to interpret the patient's dreams and then prescribe a treatment regimen accordingly. Treatment might have consisted of horseback riding, or bathing every afternoon for a week, or reading beneath a beautiful tree in a garden.

The Romans

Pliny and other pioneering Roman physicians strived for a synthesis between Greek influences and the growing acceptance of surgery. Yet for this predilection he was soon nicknamed the 'executioner' (carnifex) and his profession became the object of great misunderstanding and scorn by the public. However, by the first century AD Greek medicine was accepted practice in Rome. In AD 162 Galen arrived in Rome, and his writings, highly influenced by Plato, Aristotle, and the Stoics, as well as Hippocrates, came to be seen as the foundation of medical philosophy through the Dark Ages up to the Renaissance. The successful physician had to master the natural sciences in order to understand human physiology, anatomy, and pathology. He had to be versed in logic, able to analyze proofs, and to avoid fallacies, and be well trained in ethics.

Vitruvius told the story of the town of Old Salpia in Apulia. Year after year of sicknesses had plagued its citizens until finally the Roman Senate voted to relocate the entire town in a healthier seaside location four miles from the old town, as written by Vitruvius, in Book I, 'The Site of a City'.[10] Vitruvius wrote of the therapeutic amenity of 'favorable winds' and also the threat of disease caused by unfavorable (contaminated) winds. In Book VI Chapter 1, 'On Climate as Determining the Style of the House', he called for local climate to be a major factor in building design. Regional variations were to be expressed in building size, roof forms, composition, materials, and fenestration, in Vitruvius Book VI.[11] Significant Roman contributions to medicine were centered for the most part on public health advancements. Innovative public works projects consisted of advanced sanitary systems, the construction of a network of massive aqueducts across the empire, the invention of indoor plumbing, and the invention of the first military hospital, the valetudinarium.[12] Across

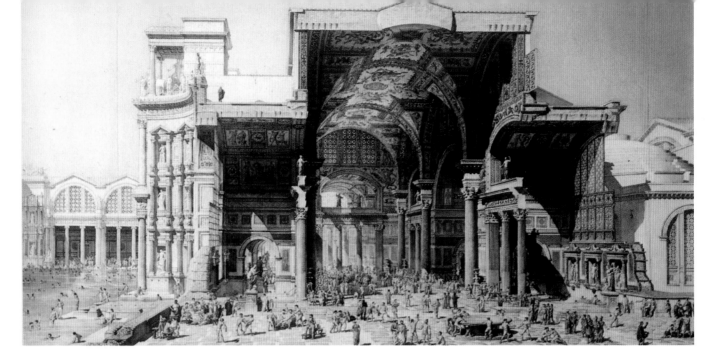

2.3 Great Baths of Diocletian, Rome, constructed AD 298–306

the Roman Empire, *valetudinariums* were constructed to stabilize, repair, and return soldiers to battle-ready status as quickly as possible. These early hospitals functioned reasonably well in support of the growing military requirements of the Empire.

While the *valetudinarium* itself cannot by any means be held up as exemplary in history as an example of a sustainable building type for healthcare, it does merit some attention in this regard. First, the construction of these institutions, built on the fringes of the Empire as well as near cities, was based on floor plans replicated across a wide geographic area. Each facility variant provided a series of inpatient rooms deployed along double-loaded corridors, with natural ventilation provided by a clerestory that ran down the center of the corridor. The four sides (corridors) yielded an open-air courtyard at the center. It was these clerestories that allowed for the warm air to pass upward and out through the window openings placed at specific intervals along the interconnected hallways. These openings could draw stale air out from the inpatient rooms, each of which was provided with a small square window of its own as a source of some light and natural ventilation.[13]

Roman *thermae*

An additional medicinally based public health innovation of the Romans perhaps remains of most interest and relevance with regards to the present movement towards a sustainable architecture for health – the Roman Bath. A network of highly sophisticated public baths was built across the Empire. As new regions came under the jurisdiction of Rome, work was initiated soon after on a local public bathhouse complex. These baths incorporated all the aforementioned innovations, including indoor planning, the transport and handling of fresh water as well and the removal of waste water, use of locally available construction materials, and various new techniques in building construction.

The terms *balnea* or *thermae* were used by the ancient Romans to describe these buildings and bath complexes. *Thermae* (based on the Greek adjective *thermos*) meant natural hot springs or bathing places with warm water. Later, the term was applied to the large-scale complexes that proliferated across the Empire, and these eclipsed Greek precursors (bath houses and public gyms). Most Roman cities had at least one, if not many such buildings. Baths were extremely important places in Roman society, as patrons stayed there for several hours at a time and some patrons went there on a daily basis.

One or more slaves accompanied wealthier Romans to the local bathing complex. Upon paying a fee, they would enter a changing area to disrobe and place sandals on their feet to protect them from the heated floors. After bathing, the patrons exercised, engaging in such wellness activities as running, weight lifting, wrestling and swimming. After exercising, oil and dirt were scraped off by servants. Roman bath houses were also built at private villas, town houses, and small-scale military installations – also referred to as *thermae*. The baths were nearly always supplied with water from an adjacent river, hot spring, stream or, in some places, a nearby aqueduct. Vitruvius, in *De Architectura*, discussed at length the design and functions of the baths.[14] Pliny made reference to the term *balnea* to denote a public bathing place, and of a *balneum* to denote a private bathing place. Built as civic monuments, public baths were used by everyone, rich or poor, free or slave. The modern equivalent would be a combination library, art gallery, mall, bar/restaurant, gym, and spa. Emperors often built baths to gain favor for themselves or to create a lasting monument to themselves such as in the case of the Great Baths of Diocletian, constructed between AD 298 and AD 306 (Figure 2.3).[15]

The bathing complex adjoining the forum at Pompeii is among the best preserved Roman bath complexes.[16] It comprises a double set of baths, one for males and one for females. There were six separate entrances from the street, and five additional entrances to the male domain. Passing through the entrance the bather encountered a small chamber containing a *latrina* (water closet) and proceeded into

14

a covered portico which ran along three sides of an open courtyard. These together formed the *vestibulum balnearum* (vestibule of the baths). There, servants were poised to assist. This atrium served as an exercise space and as a promenade for visitors. Within this court were the *balneator* and his staff (keeper of the baths), who exacted the *quadrans* paid by each visitor. Also in this courtyard, public announcements were posted, including those for upcoming gladiatorial contests.[17]

A passage led to the *apodyterium*, a room for undressing which everyone had to visit before entering the bathing area(s) proper. The staff who took the clothing were known as *capsarii*.[18] A door led from this space to the *tepidarium* (lukewarm bath) and another door to the *frigidarium* (including a cold plunge pool referred to as a *putron* or *natatorium*). From the *frigidarium* the bather who wished to go through the warm bath and sweating process entered the *tepidarium*. This did not contain water at Pompeii nor at the baths at Hippias, but was merely heated with warm air in order to prepare the body for the great heat of vapor and warm baths, and, upon returning, to prevent a too-sudden transition to the open air. In the baths at Pompeii this chamber also served as an *apodyterium*. The walls contained a number of separate compartments for clothing and personal belongings. These compartments were separated from one another by wall figures called *atlantes* or *telamones*; these projected from the walls, supporting a cornice above.[19] One statue sat on a bronze bench near to the *hycaust* of the adjoining chamber. Sitting and sweating in this space was called *ad flammam sudare*.[20] The patron then moved to the *caldarium* and then to the *laconicum*, which was a chamber still hotter than the *caldarium*, and used simply as a sweating room, having no bath per se. This room was also referred to as a *sudatorium*.[21]

The public baths became the social epicenter of the community, combining the core civic functions of personal hygiene, spiritual worship, social interaction, and wellness in a single location. They were frequently built adjacent to commercial centers and nearby arcades, and were often built near to or atop a renewable fresh water source. Key examples include, besides those at Bath in the UK (discussed below), the baths at Caracalla, from the early third century AD, and the aforementioned baths of Diocletian, both in Rome, from the late third century AD, both of which remain strong reminders of the sheer ingenuity of Roman building technology and elegance. These bath complexes rather elegantly served their core public health functions.[22] The most successful were transcendent, becoming genuine civic centers, and were built with myriad architectural details on their immense wall surfaces. Their impressively scaled structural columns were highly opulent in their ornamentation.

The baths were separated into male and female realms. Fires were tended to as a source of warmth during the winter months, and heat was transferred vis-à-vis innovative sub-floor systems, raised floors, wall cavities, and through clerestories. Similarly, water was heated, cooled, and conveyed through, as mentioned, innovative plumbing systems to a complex series of bathing pools.

Bath, UK

The first shrine at the site of the hot springs was built by the Celts and was dedicated to the goddess *Sulis*, whom the Romans identified with Minerva. The name Sulis continued to be used after the Roman invasion, with the Roman town given the name *Aquae Sulis* (the waters of Sulis). The temple was constructed in AD 60–70 and the bathing complex was expanded incrementally over the next three centuries.[23] In the second century AD the springs were covered with a series of barrel vaults and gradually expanded. During the Roman occupation of Britain, engineers drove oak piles to provide a stable foundation into the mud and lined the spring with an irregular stone chamber sheathed with sheets of lead. By this time the complex at Aquae Sulis included the same five core elements as found at Pompeii: the *caldarium* (hot bath), the *tepidarium* (lukewarm bath), the *frigidarium* (cold bath), the *sudatorium* (a moist steam bath), and the *laconicum* (a dry steam bath-sauna). The Romans' massive stone buildings built around the spring obliterated any evidence of the pre-Roman rituals practiced at the site (Figure 2.4).

The water which bubbles up from the ground at Bath initially falls as rain in the surrounding hills, where it then percolates down through limestone aquifers to a depth of between 2,700 meters (8,858 feet) and 4,400 meters (14,108 feet). There, geothermal energy raises the water temperature to between 64 degrees Celsius (147.2F) and 96 degrees Celsius (204.8F). Under pressure, the heated water rises to the surface along fissures and faults in the limestone. This process is similar to an artificially induced process widely referred to as enhanced geothermal, a process that similarly utilizes high pressures and temperatures deep in the ground.[24]

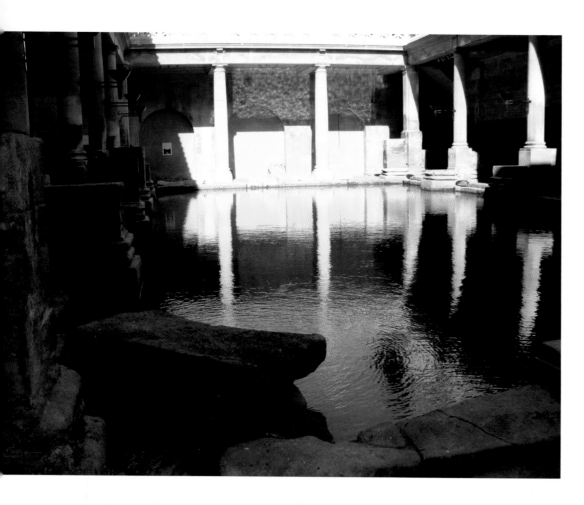

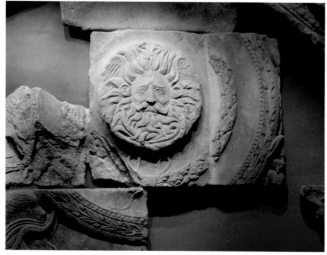

2.4 Roman bathing complex at Aquae Sulis (Bath, England), constructed AD 60–70 and expanded over the following three centuries

2.5 Representation of Roman water/sun god, partial reconstruction of the temple at Aquae Sulis (Bath, England)

image of the water god Oceanus. In the corners of the pediment are *tritons* (half men/half fish), servants of the water god Neptune. In the lower ground at the center is a face helmet in the form of a dolphin's head. Various other elements within the pediment consist of snakes and other objects in nature. The building at the site contained numerous carved stone locks, one of which honored Aesclepius, the god of healing. It was found at the cross bath in 1885. Another stone tablet depicted the goddess Minerva with a Gorgon's head mask affixed across her stomach, also found in the baths in the 1880s.

A model of the Roman baths and Temple of Sulis on exhibit at the site depicts the complex as it would have appeared at its greatest extent in the fourth century AD (Figure 2.6).[26] The *caldarium* floor has been removed in the bathing complex to reveal the plenum space – perhaps the earliest example in the West of *interstitial* space – through which the hot air flowed to evenly heat the entire floor surface. In addition, hollow box flue tiles facilitated the flow of excess hot air from beneath the floor up and out through the walls and eventually out of the building through an ingenious array of roof vents. The spring water flowed through an ingenious plumbing system into the large pool (Figure 2.7).

The temple at Aquae Sulis rested on a podium more than two meters above the surrounding courtyard, approached by a flight of steps. On the temple approach there were four large, fluted Corinthian columns supporting a frieze and decorated pediment above. The pediment (parts of which are displayed in the museum at the site today) is the triangular ornamental section, 7.9 meters (26 feet) wide and 2.4 meters (8 feet) from the apex to the bottom.[25] This pediment featured an ominous image of a Gorgon's head looking outward from a height of 15 meters to all visitor-worshipers (Figure 2.5). Alternate interpretations are that it is a Celtic sun god, or the

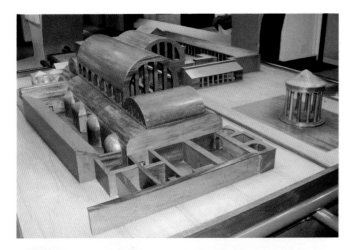

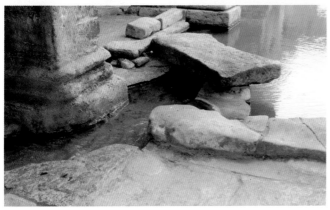

2.6 Scale model of the bathing complex at Aquae Sulis (Bath, England)

2.7 Spring water was provided to the pools at Aquae Sulis by means of an ingenious plumbing system (Bath, England)

The Medieval

With the fall of Rome in the fourth century AD chaos ensued across Europe. Extremely deadly epidemics such as the bubonic plague swept through entire communities in a matter of days, at times killing more than ninety percent of the inhabitants. With the decline of secular city-states the Catholic Church emerged to fill the void in healthcare across Europe from the third through to the late fourteenth centuries. A mainstay of medicinal care throughout this period, bloodletting, was relied upon to treat a vast assortment of ailments, diseases, and sicknesses. The Seven Works of Mercy governed religious-based care for nearly a thousand years. Later, the antecedents of modern scientific surgical procedures would be introduced as a progressive alternative to medieval and strictly faith-based treatment protocol.

In Europe, Christian religious orders provided care through networks of monastic hospitals based on cross-ward plans, and the separation of sacred from secular facilities. Gradually, the rise of the Catholic Church, with its singular emphasis on faith as the means to redemption and salvation (if not recovery, which seldom occurred in

these hellish places), correlated with a diminished belief in nature and landscape as viable aspects of treatment. The virtual disappearance of the belief in and use of nature in this manner in Western health institutions would last until the advent of the first natural spring wellness spa/retreats in the late nineteenth century.

In villages and cities across medieval Europe a feudal social order emerged whereby social misfits, undesirables, the disfigured, the disabled, and the infirm were sentenced to miserable institutions by public decree. In large cities vast institutions de-evolved into hellholes for these outcasts. Physicians and hospital administrators, ironically, first achieved a modicum of autonomy and self-sufficiency in terms of social status and influence at this time. Fortifications were built to protect monastic medical centers. Within the compound were myriad secular structures, all of which supported the function of the sacred space – the open church-wards. Infirmaries and accident rooms were created for those deemed in need of overnight observation.[27]

In the ninth century AD, St. Gall's monastic hospital was constructed in what is now Switzerland. The Cluny monastery was built in France, in 1157. Dozens if not a hundred or more such medical centers were built although the exact number remains unknown. The concept of care centered on the patients hearing mass each day from their bed within the large open ward, as close to the altar as practicable. Single wards were eventually expanded into replicated cross-ward open-plan monastic chapel-wards on a single site. These chapel-wards were places of disease, displacement, illness, and utter misery. The hospice first appeared at this time as an alternative: part inn, part infirmary, providing a counterpoint to the wretched conditions of the chapel-ward. These waystations served capably during the Crusades (as do their contemporary counterparts up to the present day), affording contact with gardens and landscape, and respite for the sick and the dying.[28]

Based on the evidence to date, the only aspect of the monastic hospitals that may be construed as having been sustainable, as defined in the present context, was their self-sufficiency. They were autonomous institutions from the standpoint that all basic necessities of daily life were self-produced versus the reliance of today's hospitals on supplies shipped from sometimes thousands of miles away. This especially pertained to aspects of daily sustenance because they operated farms on site. Similarly, they raised their livestock on site. A major portion of the grounds were therefore devoted to agriculture. These institutions could not have survived otherwise. This autonomy was of critical importance during periods of war

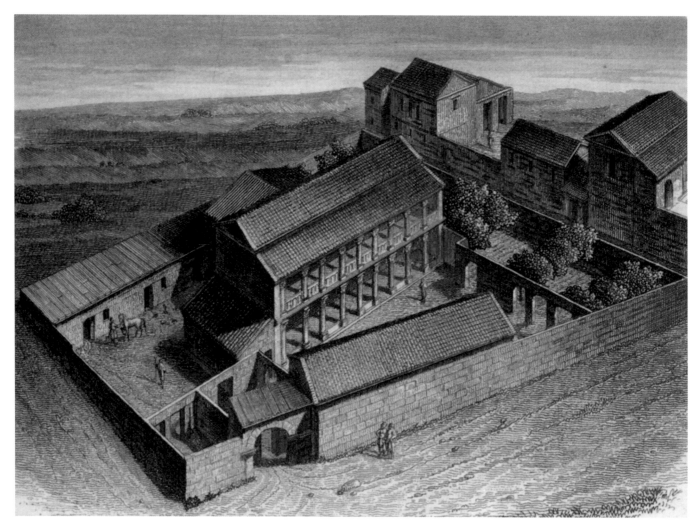

2.8 German illustration of a medieval monastic hospice-hospital complex, circa 1890. Exterior courtyards and terraces were typically used to accommodate those seeking care, with rooms provided in the guesthouse

and social upheaval, which were a constant (Figure 2.8). Later, vast urban plague hospitals, such as the Ospedale Maggiore in Milan, were constructed with public funds and then subjected to severe neglect due to chronic underfinancing. In many cities, including Basel, Paris, and Dublin, large cisterns were constructed to capture rainwater, and many public buildings, including hospitals, built their own cisterns to maintain self-sufficiency in uncertain times such as during wars and famines.

Natural daylight and ventilation were of minimal importance in most cross-ward monastic hospitals, such as the Hôpital des Fontenilles, in Tonnerre, France, which had small drainage holes bored through the stone beneath each window in the open ward, barely visible from the exterior. They were a crude hygienic device, in cold stone buildings such as this, as steam would naturally condense on the inside of the glass and run down to the inner sills, at which point the condensation would drain through the small holes in the stone. Another device was the small cloverleaf-shaped ventilation holes bored into the wooden slats of the ward ceiling. These vented fouled air directly into the attic above. The ceiling was a barrel vault while the attic above had a gabled roof.[29] The infirmary at the

Abbey of Ourscamp, France (1210) had three types of windows: two upper rows for light, both non-operable, but with detailed tracery, and a bottom row of three simple, small operable windows, each with shutters for fresh air. The upper rows were the most *sacred* windows; with the bottom row the *profane* (minimally operable, if at all) windows. Regardless, patients could see out from neither row of apertures.[30] Heating systems were therefore extremely crude, if natural, by contemporary standards. It was often very cold at night in these great stone halls, and with poor heating patients were forced to huddle in their beds, sometimes six per single bed on a bug-infested straw mattress, behind a drawn curtain during the winter.

A new building type, the insane asylum, was developed as the repository for the mentally ill and for social outcasts. Except for large courtyard-centered institutions, the indoor air quality in the typical lunatic asylum during this period was extremely poor; natural light was extremely sparse if present at all. Later, expansive asylums would be built in many places in Europe and North America. Similar to the monastic medical centers in feudal Europe, these asylums were self-sufficient from the standpoint of all food being produced on site. At some places, thousands of acres were devoted exclusively to agricultural production where, with few exceptions, this practice was sustained up until the twentieth century, with these vast land holdings farmed by the inmate-patients. On-site food production is perhaps the early asylum's only enduring contribution to any contemporary interpretation of sustainable site planning principles for healthcare facilities.[31]

The Middle East

In the Muslim Near East the first recorded Islamic institution for the sick was founded by the Caliph al-Walid in 88 AH (AD 707). Later, the Nuri Hospital in Damascus (1154) consisted mostly of outpatient examination-consultation rooms; staff support spaces and a prayer hall were situated around an open-air courtyard. This outpatient hospital had no overnight beds for inpatients. The plan was symmetrical, with male wards to one side and female wards to the other.[32] In Iraq, between AD 786 and AD 809 a free public infirmary was built adjacent to every mosque. In the second half of the twelfth century, Ibn-Jubayr founded more than sixty hospitals, nearly all of which were built around central open air courtyards with porticos to provide shade from the intense desert sun.

In Egypt, one of the most significant early Muslim courtyard hospitals was the Ibn Tulun Hospital in Cairo (AD 878). The opulence of this hospital was surpassed by the Mansuri Hospital in Cairo built four centuries later (AD 1284). Free care was provided. Founded by Qalawin, it was part of a larger complex that included a mausoleum, *madressah*, and specialized departments for ophthalmology. The total area was 2,150 meters and accommodation was provided for 100 inpatients. A large courtyard was at the center with inpatient wards on three adjoining sides and a waiting room on the fourth side. It was part of a large complex, including a school and a mosque. The hospital was 100 meters long with walls 20 meters high. Patients were brought out into the open courtyard, surrounded by porticos, for sunlight and fresh air. Separate treatment spaces were provided for men and women, and a small ward was provided for the insane. However, these individual cells were placed on either side of a second courtyard, one-fourth the size of the central courtyard. This hospital included a pharmacy and a dispensary, a social space, a library, and a small mosque for patients' use. Hospitals in Turkey,

Saudi Arabia, and North Africa were similar to the aforementioned hospitals – hospitals located in urban centers near available water sources, constructed next to or very near canals and rivers.

Nearly every Islamic medieval hospital had a central courtyard, and these were modeled after the Prophet Mohammed's home at Medina. Mohammed's advice against elaborate and costly civic buildings was widely disregarded. These featured heavy enclosing walls with few protected openings, open, spacious courtyards, and atriums oriented to carefully control excessive sunlight penetration and provide shade where needed. Privacy was maintained through elaborate screens and semi-private balconies, which allowed ventilation to pass freely from exterior to interior. This differs from counterpart European hospitals of this period, where exterior courtyards were usually visually cut off completely from adjoining interior spaces and few doors opened directly into them.[33]

Visual surveillance between indoor and outdoor realms in the Islamic medieval hospital was of high priority, especially between the central courtyard and the adjacent wards. The courtyards were often paved with marble, and in some, a stream ran through the middle. Many fountains were provided which drained via gravity into a pool at the center. Due to the desert setting water was a particularly precious therapeutic amenity for the sick and diseased, and a source of special comfort. The earliest hospitals in the Middle East made use of its aesthetic and medicinal benefits. In colder regions the same general plan was adhered to, except a vaulted masonry dome would usually cover the central courtyard. This was similar to conditions at Roman bath complexes located in less temperate climates, such as at Bath.

The first Islamic hospitals were built in Baghdad of sun-dried mud and brick. As the center of culture shifted to Damascus and later to Cairo these simple materials gave way to limestone, granite, and marble. In most respects, Islamic hospitals were well advanced compared to their European counterparts during the Middle Ages. Building techniques and the medical and administrative aspects of these hospitals were also more advanced. It is unclear if these medical centers were as self-sufficient as those in Europe in terms of food production, however. After the thirteenth century these institutions fell into decline as civic centers of daily life and by the twentieth century Western colonial powers had colonized much of the medieval Islamic world. This was usually the case when conquering Western armies built their own hospitals and infirmaries to care for their own. This pattern continues in the early twenty-first century whenever an advanced

Western medical institution building a healthcare campus in this region carelessly falls prey to the (often poorly done) generic transposition of Western architecture carelessly into an Islamic context.[34]

The Renaissance

The Renaissance, which flourished in Italy in the fifteenth and sixteenth centuries, represented a reawakening of interest in classical antiquity and in the idealization of the cultural values embodied in classical thought and governance. The abbot of the earlier medieval medical center had overseen a vast staff of ward superintendents, logistical support assistants such as bookkeepers and dietitians, and ward attendants. The Hippocratic traditions were now to be rediscovered and celebrated. Specifically, the natural environment and landscape, and their therapeutic role in sickness and disease would slowly re-emerge. Hospitals were designed and built principally to emulate the stately palaces of the period. The public hospital would eventually supplant the donor hospital as a place for care for the masses, i.e. a hospital donated as an act of charity by a wealthy philanthropist or private benefactor. Humanism placed 'man' (human) at the center with attendant interest in the workings of the human body and scientifically based medical education, practice, and administration advanced during this period.

For the insane, new techniques were developed to maximize control of the patient-inmate, such as in the seventeenth century at Bethlehem (Bedlam) Hospital in London. Bethlehem Hospital typified the style of neoclassical architecture as expressed in healthcare facilities. Its stately appearance, from the exterior at least, was to convey a noble face (facade) to the world. Within, however, conditions for the patient-inmate were deplorable. The private room, by no means a recent invention having first appeared in private rooms for the influential in early monastic hospitals, essentially was for the benefit of the upper classes. Meanwhile, the lower classes continued to be relegated to immense, unkempt, disease-ridden, hellhole wards. At the palace hospital in Wurtzberg, Germany (1576–1585) and similar institutions built in this period in Italy, England, and France, the chapel diminished in physical size, placement, and importance, paralleling the rising status of organized medicine.[35] Building footprints, however, were usually narrow to allow fresh air and some daylight into the asylum. Window apertures were small.

In terms of the use of nature, the new loges at Bicêtre (1822) had a double row of 10 single patient rooms, dayrooms in the corner pavilions, and a heated corridor along the inboard side. The plan included two large fireplaces, and wood floorboards elevated 18 inches above the paving stones at grade with small holes provided for warm air to circulate. The two rows of rooms opened directly onto a courtyard with a quincunx and flower garden.[36] Advanced (or so-called) care philosophies for the mistreatment of the maladaptive insane were personified by the invention of the straightjacket, first used at St. Thomas' Hospital in London in the eighteenth century. Based on the writings of Jeremy Bentham, among other leading healthcare facility experts, a new prototype developed, the Panopticon Asylum. The Glasgow Asylum (1801–1810) was among the most significant of this new building type although it certainly was not innovative from a contemporary sustainability perspective.[37] In fact, the environmental sustainability of these places, as well as the amenity provided for the patient-inmate, i.e. windows and views, was negligible to non-existent. Nature per se had vastly diminished in importance in Western culture. Large, frequently multiple courtyards dominating the urban palace hospitals of the Renaissance dramatically decreased in size and eventually disappeared entirely from most urban hospitals, so they constantly expanded their footprints on land-starved sites in ever denser and unsanitary urban neighborhoods. Water sanitation standards were equally dismal.

The Nightingale movement:
1860 to World War II

Innovations in environmental sustainability did occur to some extent in the hospitals built in the various colonies ruled by the British Empire during the eighteenth and nineteenth centuries. The political pressure back at home to succeed at war elevated the overseas military hospital to a level of critical importance. This trend would manifest in a period of healthcare architecture dominating a period of approximately 85 years (1860–1945) beginning with the work of Florence Nightingale and ending with World War II (1939–1945). The modern transposition of effective medical and nursing principles into architectural form began with her work. Nightingale was dispatched to the front lines of the Crimean War in Turkey in late 1855 in a last-ditch attempt to reform a failing makeshift barracks hospital. At

2.9 Florence Nightingale tending to the sick and wounded at the makeshift converted barracks-hospital at Scutari, Turkey, 1855

2.10 Prefabricated barracks field hospital built at Renkioi, Turkey, 1855. Designed and built by Isambard Kingdom Brunel, a civil engineer. The site was selected for its seaward slope, its porous, sandy soil, proximity to the sea for water transport and sewage disposal, and nearby natural springs

2.11 Prefabricated steel-clad 'Iron Kitchen' and wood-clad hospital huts at Renkioi, Turkey, 1855

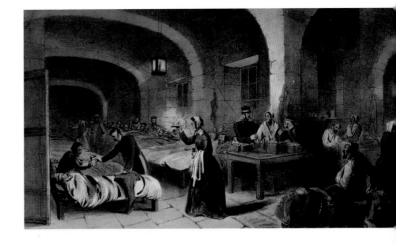

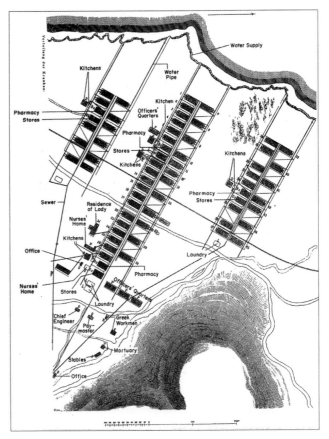

Scutari, in a converted military installation atop a bluff fortification, she encountered a mortality rate unacceptably high. Prior to her arrival nearly 11,000 out of 14,000 troops were housed in the infirmary or deemed too sick for battle. The ensuing scandal caused Parliament to fall. At Scutari, with 38 nurses Nightingale transformed a deplorable facility. She was widely praised back home for this achievement (Figure 2.9).[38]

Meanwhile, an engineer named Brunel designed and constructed an innovative prefabricated barracks hospital at Renkioi, Turkey (1855) in a variant of what would soon become known internationally as the *Nightingale Ward*. A prefabricated patient care ward, housing 50 patients, was designed and pretested in Paddington, England (Figure 2.10). The hospital at Renkioi consisted of a pair of rows of numerous one-level prefabricated wards, built of wood, arrayed along a dual circulation spine. The building components were shipped from England and assembled on site. This facility proved highly successful in terms of reducing patient mortality rates (Figure 2.11).

Upon her return after the war, Nightingale authored two influential books, *Notes on Nursing* (1858),[39] and *Notes on Hospitals* (1859).[40] In *Notes on Nursing*, she stated the five essential points in securing a sustainable, health-promoting environment: pure air, pure water, efficient drainage, cleanliness, and natural daylight. Among Nightingale's many innovations were her provisos for fresh air circulating within a bright, cheerful open ward with no more than 30 patients per ward, in a volume 30 feet wide by 128 feet in length, such as at the Hospital de la Santa Cruz y San Pablo, in Barcelona, Spain (1905–1928), designed by a disciple of the renowned Spanish architect Antonio Gaudi.[41] Her functionally driven planning model was modernist in its expression, interiorly, at least. Wards were typically one level in height. These were replicated on the site, separated by courtyards in between. At one end of the ward was a connecting corridor for people and supplies. These typically had large windows and in temperate climates were sheathed in screens. They efficiently allowed for transport of supplies and people throughout the hospital. Usually, on the opposite end of the ward, a terrace or screened porch provided an opportunity to take patients outdoors in good weather and this would become a key feature of tuberculosis sanitariums in subsequent years, as discussed below.

The interior of the first Nightingale wards were rather utilitarian yet attractive. The plaster walls were unadorned and were painted white in most cases. Later, as in the hospital in Barcelona, a more elaborate interior would become the standard in Nightingale hospitals

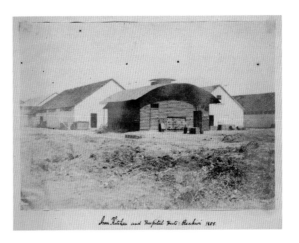

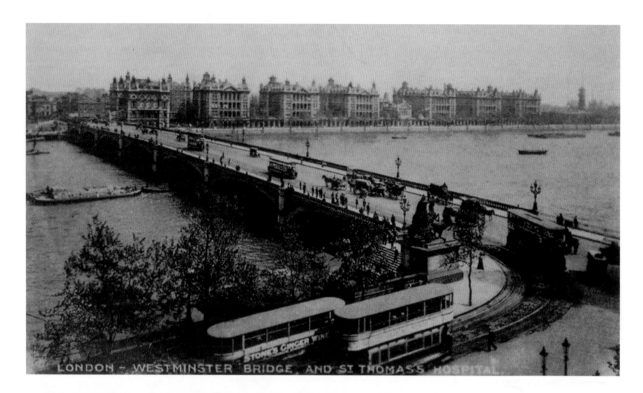

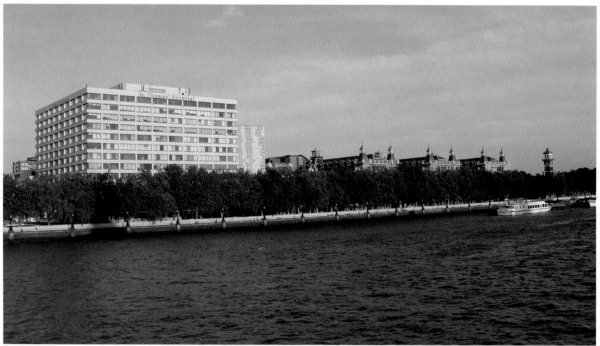

2.12 Westminster Bridge with St. Thomas' Hospital, London, circa 1900. Thomas Currey, Architect

2.13 Thames River and St. Thomas' Hospital, London, 2008

built in urban areas. However, nearly all hospital exteriors in the late nineteenth century continued to be cloaked in the neoclassicism then in vogue. Nightingale's writings, nonetheless, set the standard for sustainability against which the performance – functionally or otherwise – of all hospitals would be judged to a greater extent until the outbreak of World War II.

At St. Thomas's Hospital (1868–1872), a pavilion plan was employed on a long narrow site along the Thames River in London. Seven pavilions were arranged in a linear plan nearly a quarter of a mile in total length (Figure 2.12). The site plan has since been greatly altered (Figure 2.13). The inpatient pavilions were not very different in proportion from what Nightingale advocated at the time (Figure

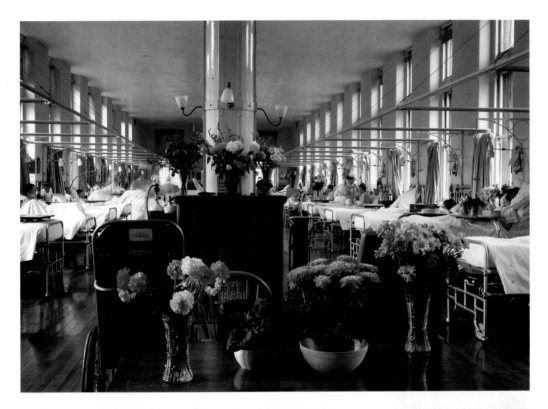

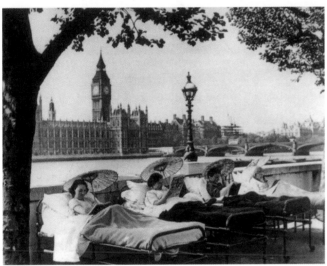

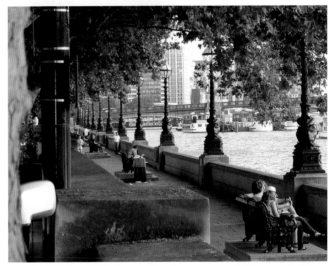

2.14 Interior of inpatient ward, St. Thomas' Hospital, London, 1966. Nightingale was a firm believer in the miasma theory of disease

2.15 Patients convalescing on the outdoor terrace, St. Thomas' Hospital, London, a practice that continued until the late 1930s

2.16 The terrace at St. Thomas' Hospital was devoted to patient use, though in recent years the water's edge has been redeveloped as a public promenade

2.14). The exterior was sheathed in an Italianate skin in a manner sympathetic with Big Ben and the Houses of Parliament, directly across the river from the hospital. The wards were each 28 feet wide and 120 feet in length, as determined by the number of beds, 28, plus the space between beds.[42] A porch was situated at the end of each ward, overlooking the Thames, and, in Grace Goldin's words, 'Fresh air and the lively river traffic do the patient no end of good'.[43] A state-of-the-art steam pipe system for heating was developed, and rooftop cupolas allowed foul air to pass upward and out through an elaborate system of roof vents. Patients convalesced outdoors on the open veranda overlooking the Thames (Figure 2.15). Today, this space is a public promenade (Figure 2.16).

Nightingale's influence was profound in the military hospitals built during this period. This was due as much to her ability to communicate

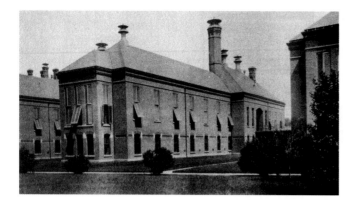

2.17 Inpatient ward, Johns Hopkins Hospital (1877–1885), Baltimore, based on plans developed by John Shaw Billings

2.18 Section, inpatient ward, Johns Hopkins Hospital, Baltimore. Intake of fresh air was by means of small vent openings in the sidewall between every two beds. An aboveground 'basement' level functioned as an air intake reservoir. Outer walls were lined with thousands of 3-inch cast iron pipe coils, producing steam-heated water

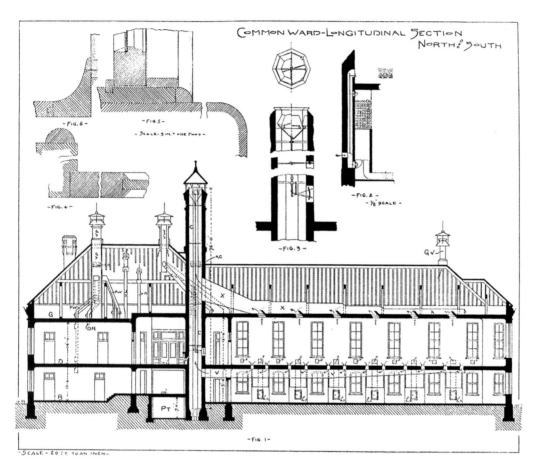

well as to her social position and extraordinary energy. For these attributes she was the most widely quoted hospital reformer of her era. In rapidly expanding cities in America and in Europe, the pavilion plan appeared by 1860 to be the best method to house patients in an attractive campus setting – amid landscaped grounds and a reliance on natural ventilation, daylight, views, and terraces for patient use. However, plans for American urban hospitals were put on hold in 1861 with the outbreak of the Civil War. Regardless, a number of prominent military barracks hospitals built by the Union Army were directly influenced by Nightingale's open ward prototype. These emphasized cleanliness, hygiene, ambiance, and functional efficiency. They were constructed adjacent to a rail line, a body of water, or both. This facilitated the efficient transfer of supplies and soldiers to and from the front lines.

The acceptance of germ theory, namely, the acceptance of disinfection as the principal means to control the spread of diseases, gained a foothold at this time. In the early 1870s John Shaw Billings, probably America's preeminent authority on public health and its symbiotic relationship with hospital architecture, concluded that fresh air and hygiene must be of highest priority in hospital architecture. In 1875 Billings produced a report on military hygiene as well as a model plan for the Johns Hopkins Hospital, to be built a few years later in Baltimore. The Johns Hopkins prototype would emphasize the continual replacement of toxic indoor air with fresh air combined with the disinfection of all hospital spaces, equipment, and patient wounds (Figure 2.17 and Figure 2.18). This was done to rid the interior spaces of disease germs, microzymes, micrococci, biplasm, and germinal matter he referred to as key contributors to hospitalism.[44]

Germ theory, together with Nightingale's columnist advocacy, drew acceptance in new hospitals in the 1870s and 1880s.[45] This theory made common sense, it was scientifically verifiable, and the day-lit, naturally ventilated, narrow open pavilion was ideal for this new understanding of infection and disease control. In the early decades of scientific medicine germ theory accelerated the evolution of holistic, individual, and moral understandings of health and illness.[46] In the next fifty years this advancement would profoundly reshape civilian and military hospitals and transform medicine itself. This new perspective would be immediately put to the test in North America during the Indian Wars waged against Native Americans during the 1870s and 1880s. The U.S. Army constructed military tent hospitals in the western sector as a means to provide medical treatment to wounded soldiers. These facilities carried forward advancements from a decade earlier during the American Civil War (1861–1865).

Kirkbride hospitals

Asylum architecture has been treated as a stepchild within the canon of architecture and health. From medieval hospital-prisons for the insane, to the panopticon of the seventeenth and eighteenth centuries, the asylum as a building type has in general been neglected in the literature. However, numerous sustainable site planning and architectural design principles expressed in late-nineteenth-century asylums offer much insight to present-day architects and others who design environments for mental health treatment. The emergence of psychiatry and the concept of environmental determinism are two advancements that afford particular insights for contemporary expression in sustainable healthcare architecture. The Kirkbride network of asylums in the United States was based on the writings and work of Dr. Thomas S. Kirkbride (1809–1885). He was the superintendent of the private Pennsylvania Hospital for the Insane. When the hospital relocated to a new facility in 1841, Kirkbride was able to introduce many innovations to the treatment regimen and to the architectural treatment milieu.[47]

Prisons and asylums had become virtually indistinguishable by this time and Kirkbride's work, together with the humanitarian contributions of Dorothea Dix (1802–1887) represented a radical break from convention. Dix was a leading crusader for the establishment of state-supported mental asylums, places where the patient was to

be treated with dignity and respect, and not as a creature possessed by demonic forces, as had been the popular stereotype. Through her efforts the first state asylums were constructed. Dix fought for individualized care for all social classes and races. Patients were placed in a rural botanical setting away from the ills of the city. Kirkbride separated patients by severity of illness and advocated the incorporation of natural sunlight and ventilation. Patients partook in normalized lifestyles by exercising outdoors, working, and undergoing classroom and religious instruction.[48]

Kirkbride and his principal architects developed what would become known as the 250-bed linear plan. The 'Kirkbride System' was based on a narrow, stepped, linear building footprint. An overcrowded hospital could be expanded by building a duplicate on the same site, in a reflecting configuration. The central building housed the administration offices, with the superintendent's residence on an upper floor. A water tank was concealed beneath the ornate dome at the center of the roof (Figure 2.19). The left and right wings were symmetrical:

> The wings have been offset to the rear to allow a corridor open to sun and wind at both ends. A corridor of reasonable length, with bay windows in the middle, would permit the economic measure of locating rooms on both sides of it without detriment to light or ventilation … windows can be opened running from floor to ceiling on both sides and on all stories. So sun and air are let into what is ordinarily the darkest corner of a hospital as freely as if the wards were separate buildings and with considerably greater convenience – one has here an all-weather passageway … an ornamental grille guards the windows on the inside and a very pleasant sitting area is created … the far wings being reserved for the excitable. Indeed, in an insufficiently endowed institution … [construction may] begin with [these opposing] far wings and then built toward the center because the first patients to be committed are sure to be the most unmanageable.[49]

Isolation rooms were to be no larger than 8 by 10 feet so not to allow a second bed to be added. Regular private rooms were slightly larger. About one-fourth of the patients were assigned to general wards; the ill and dying were assigned to isolation wards. The wealthy could pay for additional privacy in a VIP room of their own, thereby rendering the Kirkbride asylums feasible and socially

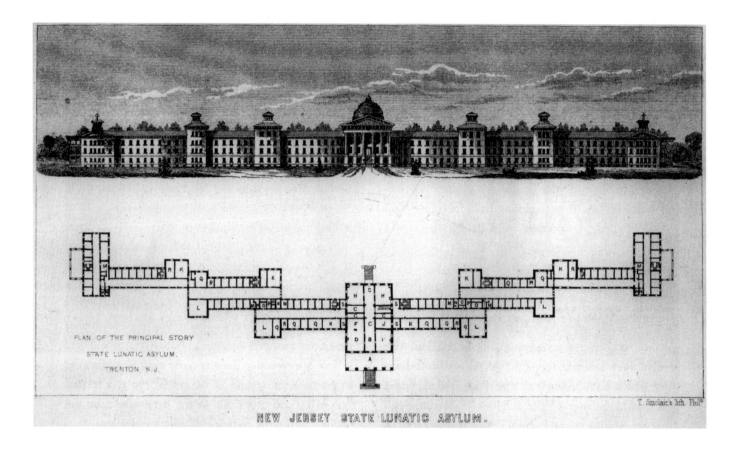

NEW JERSEY STATE LUNATIC ASYLUM.

2.19 New Jersey State Lunatic Asylum, Trenton (1846–1849), J. Notman, Architect. An expansion in 1850 consisted of additional wards added to each end

2.20 Frederick Law Olmstead's landscape plan for the Hartford Retreat (Connecticut) 1860. The campus plan included retreat buildings, barn, icehouse, patients' yard, a superintendent's dwelling, vegetable gardens, an orchard, conservatory, and a museum

acceptable for patients of all classes. African-Americans were always housed apart from other patients.[50] The asylum footprint consisted of a stepped series of elongated single or double loaded corridors that housed males and females in separate wings, on multiple floors, and isolated the most severe cases in autonomous, freestanding structures deployed on the surrounding grounds not unlike a private estate.

On the topic of sustainable site planning and stewardship, Kirkbride wrote:

The building should be in a healthful, pleasant, and fertile district ... the land chosen should be of good quality and easily tilled; the surrounding scenery should be varied and attractive, and the neighborhood should possess numerous objects of an agreeable and interesting character. While the hospital itself should be retired, and its privacy fully secured, the views from it, if possible, should exhibit life in its active forms, and on this account stirring objects at a little distance are desirable ... and [space] for pleasure-grounds, and also for future extensions of the building ... Every hospital for the insane should possess at least one hundred acres of land, to enable it to have the proper amount for farming and gardening purposes ... and

to secure adequate and appropriate means of exercise, labor, and occupation ... for these are now recognized as the most valuable means of treatment ... as much as fifty acres should be appropriated as [patient-only] pleasure-grounds ... several acres of this tract should be in groves of woodland, to furnish shade in summer.[51]

These institutions and their campuses evolved into large, imposing Victorian-era institutions with expansive grounds, including farmland. They were built in rural settings although gradually urban development began to encroach upon the campuses (Figure 2.20). Between 1841 and 1887 thirty-two Kirkbride template state asylums had been built in the United States. Asylum architecture ranged in style from Richardsonian Romanesque to Neo-Gothic.[52]

During this period a number of private asylums were built to appease the whims of the wealthy, able to afford a higher quality of care and accommodation. By 1888, Kirkbride's construction standards for asylums no longer prevailed because politicians had imposed draconian cost-cutting reforms.[53] Additionally, physicians deemed the Kirkbride asylum architecture archaic and obsolete with regard to advancements in psychiatry in the late nineteenth century. This was due as well to chronic underfunding, staff shortages, growing

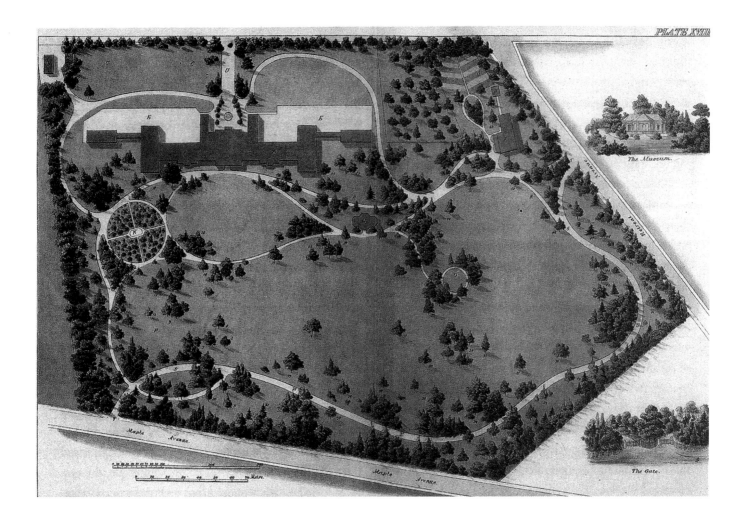

PLATE XVIII

The Museum.

The Gate.

public disenchantment with Kirkbride's notion of the 'curability' of the insane, and the widespread proliferation of foul 'backwards' to house individuals who had to be repeatedly institutionalized.[54]

In late nineteenth century America, the rural Kirkbride asylum expressed to varying degrees Nightingale's five precepts for a sustainable, health-promoting care and treatment setting: fresh air, pure water, efficient drainage, cleanliness, daylight, and view. Kirkbride asylums were innovative and a century ahead of their time from this perspective. In this regard, contemporary architects, planners, interior designers, engineers, and others can glean much insight. The design guidelines put forth by both Nightingale (wards) and Kirkbride (private rooms in most cases) centered on the long, narrow inpatient unit. The narrow footprint (width) of the patient housing unit allowed for abundant light and ventilation, made possible through the use of large operable windows and operable transoms above wood doors. The windowsill heights were no higher than 3 feet above the floor. This allowed for views looking onto the adjoining landscaped grounds. A forced air system based on fans and natural air was developed.[55] The heating and ventilation systems were advanced for their time, yet primitive by today's standards.

The Nightingale and Kirkbride hospitals, beyond this, were typically built of locally available building materials – most transported from within a 25 to 100 mile radius of the construction site. The incorporation of nature within the open patient ward was another innovation that is of importance in contemporary healthcare environments. Flowers, plants, and in some cases pets were an important therapeutic element in the overall inpatient experience. In short, many of these architectural, site planning, and care standards are now a part of the LEED certification criteria for healthcare facilities in the U.S. (see Chapters 7 and 8). At this same time an alternative healthcare movement peaked in the United States – the American mineral springs spa/retreat. This movement expressed both a new American building type and a resort town type rooted in sustainability, stewardship, and the therapeutic benefits of nature in healthfulness and restoration.

The nineteenth century spa movement and sustainability

The American resort tradition was a direct reaction to the deplorable public health conditions gripping U.S. cities by the late nineteenth century. As cities and towns grew in size, toxic pollutants released

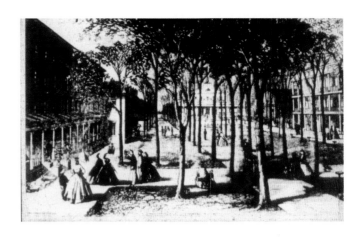

2.21 Union Hall (1860–1864), Saratoga Springs, New York. Shaded outdoor plazas were integral therapeutic adjuncts to the specialized treatment regimen

from industrial sites contaminated the earth and air. Outbreaks of malaria, dysentery, cholera, smallpox, yellow fever, and typhoid fever were common. In the American South, urban residents fled the hot, humid conditions of cities where conditions were ideal for these widespread epidemics to proliferate virtually unchecked. In the antebellum (pre-Civil War) period, mineral springs resorts flourished in Virginia, Arkansas, and elsewhere. Thomas Jefferson's University of Virginia campus became the trademark of nearly every American southern spa.[56] In the North, new resorts and resort towns proliferated in the upstate New York region and along the Atlantic seaboard.

Based on European precedent, the mineral springs spa/retreat was for the well-off middle and upper classes. In time, Americans developed two styles, a northern and a southern style spa. The European spa tradition had begun in the late sixteenth and early seventeenth centuries and blossomed later. Places such as Spa, Vichy, Wiesbaden, and Marienbad developed their unique style of health and pleasure seeking as well as a unique architectural style. In the book *English Spas,* William Addison defined the typical resort as a collection of hotels, boarding houses, music pavilions, gaming rooms, tearooms, bathing and drinking houses, tree-lined promenades, and formal gardens.[57] This complex was typically at the center of a resort town and possessed direct road and rail connections to nearby towns and cities.[58]

American counterparts evolved more slowly, by comparison. In the 1740s when the aforementioned spa at Bath was hosting several thousand English visitors each month and Harrogate and Epsom were, in Henry Lawrence's words, 'dowagers of the British resort circuit', only a handful of mineral springs were being used for medicine and as rural retreats, in the colonies.[59] By the time of the American Revolution (1776) more than a dozen spa/retreats existed in America and as settlement spread inland and cities grew, more were established.

The spa/retreat was based in the therapeutic use of mineral spring water for both drinking and bathing. Water was employed to treat ailments ranging from gout and rheumatism to syphilis and pneumonia. This treatment was affirmed by a growing medical literature and most recipients reported some improvement in their health. However, the therapeutic amenity of the mineral springs spa/retreat was also attributable to the change of scene, immersion in relaxing surroundings, fresh air, exercise, and healthful nutrition. At the very least the water was unpolluted compared to that in the cities. Until the late nineteenth century it was believed that these diseases were the result of bad air and miasmas that occurred due to poorly drained lowlands and crowded tenements. These theories were in part correct though the root source was through mosquitoes that carried malaria and yellow fever in breeding grounds of standing water. Typhoid and cholera spread where shallow aquifers were polluted by toxic sewage. For this reason the fresh air, high elevation, and abundant forests of the mountain resorts became particularly popular as health-promoting environments and with each new annual round of epidemics in the nearby cities these places became ever more popular.[60]

The average length of stay was three weeks, and the entire clientele would change three or four times each summer season. The more fashionable spa/retreats soon became social centers for nearby cities' social elite classes. In time, the America spa/retreats became more like their European precursors although in the South they remained more rural in character and took on the appearance of Americanized Palladian villas. They had wide tiered verandas set behind rows of large white columns in a style that was an amalgam of Palladian and Caribbean influences. This style would come to dominate American southern plantations, with a large main building and a series of smaller 'outbuildings' arrayed on either side. Union Hall in Saratoga Springs, New York was one of these. When the hotel was enlarged in 1864 the courtyard plan was developed more fully. The trees, visible in the illustration of Union Hall, featured prominently (Figure 2.21). By 1886 the U.S. Geological Survey counted 634 spa/retreats from the Atlantic to Pacific coasts.[61]

In the American West, spa/retreats later became more medically based:

By the 1880s, many spas offered ... magnetic baths, mud baths, carbonic acid baths, peat baths, Russian baths, and Turkish baths. Doctors prescribed particular baths for specific ailments at mineral spring sanitariums, and white-frocked attendants assisted bathers. The federal government, recognizing the value of baths in therapeutics, established the Army and Navy General Hospital at Hot Springs (Arkansas) in 1882, where baths were integral to the medical regimen. By this time, the

2.22 The main pool at Sweet Springs (1873–1875), in Saline County, Missouri, was expansive, modeled on the ancient bathing pools at Aquae Sulis (Bath, UK)

2.23 The Hall of Waters (1933–1935) at Excelsior Springs, Missouri, celebrated the virtues of natural mineral springs, and its art deco exterior aptly expressed the era's civic aspirations in public buildings

2.24 In the early twentieth century, the 'Mineral Water Well No. 1 Bath House' (1905–1906) in Carbon, Texas, was typical of the small towns that competed for business in the Texas hill country west of Austin

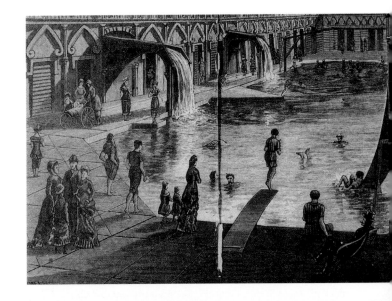

science of bathing for health had even acquired a specialty designation within the field of hydrotherapy and was awarded the awkward name of balneology.[62]

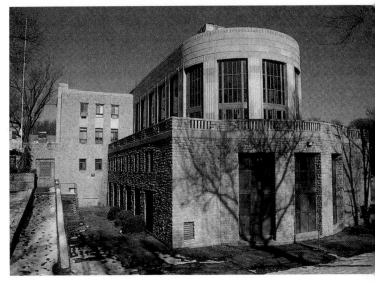

The swimming pools at Sweet Springs, in Saline County, Missouri (1875) were elaborate in scale and amenity, not unlike the extensive Roman bathing complex at Aquae Sulis in Bath, England (Figure 2.22). Another town, Excelsior Springs, Missouri, managed to weather vicissitudes in public and medical opinion on the therapeutic amenity of mineral springs. The town aspired to be America's 'Haven of Health'. Its elaborate Hall of Waters, built in 1935, symbolized a time when the nation's attention had once again turned to the therapeutic possibilities of natural mineral waters (Figure 2.23). It survived due to its proximity to Kansas City and to good roads and rail connections. The town also boasted impressive spa hotels and professionally staffed facilities.[63]

In Texas, about a dozen spa/retreats operated during the height of the movement. These were located in the hill country area west of Austin and in the heavily wooded eastern region of the state. The town of Carbon had its own establishment in the early 1900s. Above the porch, the sign proclaims 'Mineral Water Well No. 1 Bath House' (Figure 2.24).[64] This establishment was far more modest than the baths at either Sweet Springs or Excelsior Springs, and illustrates the diverse types of places available to the general public.

The decline of the American spa/retreat coincided with cures for the urban epidemics that had spawned these precursors to contemporary 'green' wellness healthcare treatment centers. Improvements in public health sanitation and pharmacology in the 1890s cut the death rate significantly. With the diminishing support of medical science, physician belief in the medicinal uses of natural mineral springs declined drastically and by 1927 the number of U.S. spa/retreats fell to only 271. Most of these clung on precariously until the Great Depression of the 1930s when most closed permanently. Five types of mineral-springs-based treatment environments survive to this day: government-operated sanitariums for physical therapy, private camps that are often religious-based, the classic European-based spa/retreat, small hot springs resorts in the American West,[65] and the fashionable resort where horseback riding, tennis, skiing, golf, and swimming have largely supplanted the classical use of mineral spring water.[66]

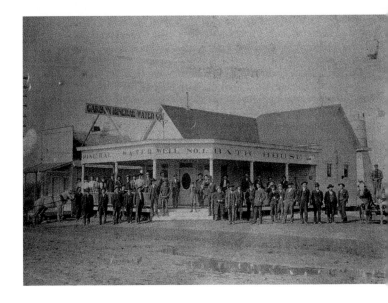

Later, these forgotten places in the everyday landscape would provide the template for lavish upscale resort vacation hotels in the U.S. in Las Vegas, Orlando, Palm Beach, and elsewhere. These include the International Style resorts built in the late twentieth century in the Cayman Islands, Cancun, Bermuda, and the Bahamas. The automobile would have a profound influence on this movement. Hospital campuses built in exurban suburban settings in the past decade have sometimes included freestanding wellness centers that borrow much from the American spa/retreat tradition. These are places for 'outpatient' physical activity and therapeutic treatment based on physical therapy, sports medicine, health-promoting exercise, and nutritional regimens, and in most cases incorporate direct contact with some form of nature or landscape. However, their sustainability quotient revolves around non-invasive treatment regimens for patients versus any premeditated emphasis on carbon neutrality.[67] Regardless, community-based examples such as at Carbon, Texas, provide useful lessons for contemporary healthcare providers and their architects because they represent a viable alternative to far more costly hospital-based care.

The rise of the TB sanitarium

Meanwhile, the rise of tuberculosis during this period was transforming attitudes towards the design of treatment settings. Tuberculosis in humans is a disease caused by several species of bacteria in the genus *mycobacterium*. The symptoms of this disease, fatigue, weight loss, and a persistent cough, can advance to a state of consumption – the emaciated condition of the body. The disease is most commonly transmitted through the inhalation of airborne droplets of *tubercle bacilli*, which can remain suspended in the air for many hours.[68] American sanitariums in the period 1885–1945 were considered among the most progressive treatment settings for tuberculosis in the world. As the principles of bacteriology became known and the epidemiology of tuberculosis understood, the design of outdoor spaces at American sanitariums evolved. Major determinants of facility design included location, the siting and orientation of buildings, building configuration and density, window placement and size, courtyards, balconies, views to landscape, water elements, the organization of paths and roads, and gardens.

Deborah L. McBride writes:

The landscape designs at sanitariums mirrored the changing architecture and structure of sanitariums … the garden styles [can be] broken down into three groups, comparable to those of the rural romantic cemeteries being built at this time. Because of their topography, the earliest American sanitariums had a rugged or rustic character similar to the 'picturesque' style … buildings sited to maximize the views of dramatic landforms and spectacular scenery … This created a passive, reflective relationship to nature, and it reveals the contemporary understanding of humans' reactive, contemplative relationship to the healing process. Views of distant mountains and forests were believed to emotionally stir and physically heal patients as they rested on their porches. Because these institutions stressed rest in the open air, they placed a greater emphasis on providing awe-inspiring views from their balconies and verandas and had fewer facilities for graduated exercise on the grounds than later institutions. The entire landscape was … designed. Later sanitariums had gracefully curved paths and flower beds similar to English gardens … this third style introduced geometric forms such as ovals, squares, and circles to establish formality … the last category of sanitarium landscape design consisted of the … 'lawn style' … characterized by large, manicured lawns, unbroken by plantings or monuments … large lawns reduced construction costs, economized on maintenance, and simplified supervision of patients while they were outdoors … if order were enforced [in daily regimens] … patients could reform their unhealthy habits, and the public health would be protected.[69]

Key examples from this period include the Glockner Sanitarium, in Colorado Springs, Colorado (1877–1880), Winyah Sanitarium, in Asheville, North Carolina, the first in the U.S. (1873–1875) and basically a large manor house, Saranac Lake, in New York (1882–1885), and, later, state sanitariums including the Maryland Tuberculosis Sanitarium, in Sabillasville, Maryland (1911–1913). Various innovations in the landscaping of these facilities for TB treatment remain popular, and include naturally ventilated respite porches, grounds that promote paths of increasing cardiovascular stimulation, and gardens to simulate a homelike ambiance.[70] Innovations in the design of late-nineteenth- and early-twentieth-century public and privately operated sanitariums would parallel numerous innovations in the design and deployment of early-twentieth-century military field hospitals, as discussed below.

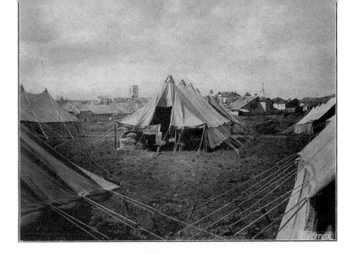

2.25 Mobile Field Hospital No. 353 of the 80th Division, United States Army, as deployed at Bernecourt, France, during the St. Mihiel Operation, 1917. The hospital consisted of twenty tents

2.26 Drawing of a fully deployed Mobile Field Hospital Operating Unit, United States Army, 1917. Note the cross atop the surgical tent

2.27 Mobile field hospitals consisted of as many as forty trucks, with convoys stretched as far as a quarter of a mile during transport

2.28 Interior, Mobile Field Hospital No. 39, United States Army, depicts sparse accommodations in an exceedingly inhospitable environment in terms of terrain, humidity, and temperature levels

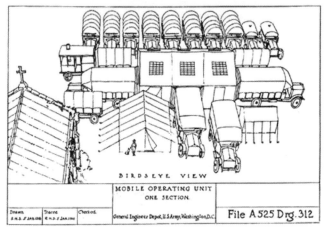

Redeployable military hospitals and sustainability

During World War I (1914–1918), many innovations in transportable military hospitals were introduced in the battlefield.[71] These remain impressive because these structures were highly efficient, mobile, lightweight, and made the maximum use of the minimum amount of materials – all virtues in the current quest for carbon neutral buildings. The lessons learned in the American Civil War (1861–1865) had been incorporated in subsequent military conflicts in later decades. The objective in World War I was to provide the largest number of beds on site in an enclosure that was transportable, erectable, and serviceable in a matter of hours. Soldiers were receiving more severe battle wounds than ever before in history due to the use of increasingly lethal weaponry, including armored tanks, hand grenades, poison gas, and the machine gun. Lessons previously learned on the importance of infection control, natural ventilation, and cleanliness were not lost on the military physicians and their engineers. Field Hospital Number 353 of the 80th Division, United States Army, was deployed at Bernecourt, France, during the St. Mihiel Operation. The installation consisted of twenty tents, each housing a constituent function of the overall hospital (Figure 2.25).

Medical support was categorized into three echelons. The first echelon was the *zone of the advance*, consisting of aid posts, battalion aid stations, dressing stations, and field hospitals. Each division was assigned an infirmary train to care for its wounded. After treatment at the field hospital, the wounded were then transported to the second echelon of medical support, the *line of communications*, consisting of evacuation hospitals, base hospitals, and mobile surgical hospitals. The third echelon was the *service of the interior*, consisting of hospital care provided back home in the U.S. The field hospital section of the division infirmary train operated four field hospitals set up six to eight miles from the Front. Each had a normal capacity of 108 beds, expandable to 162, therefore providing a 432-bed (648-bed expanded) capacity for a division in combat. In addition, dispensaries were operated for routine medical care. The field hospitals were redeployed as the front lines of battle moved.[72]

The hospital was transported to the site via truck convoy, often over unpaved roads and frequently near enemy lines. As many as 40 trucks would be used to transport and deploy a tent hospital, and in this case included a tent designated as a chapel with a cross, as depicted in the accompanying bird's eye rendering of the

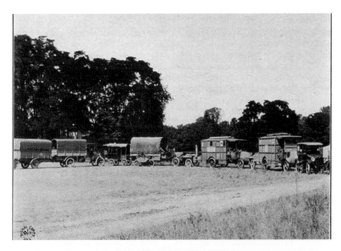

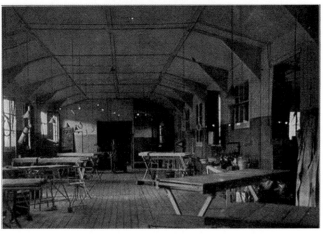

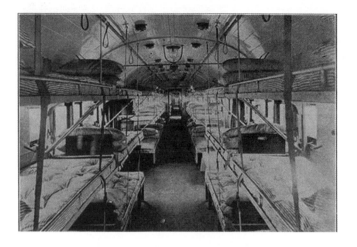

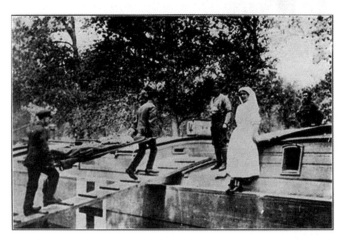

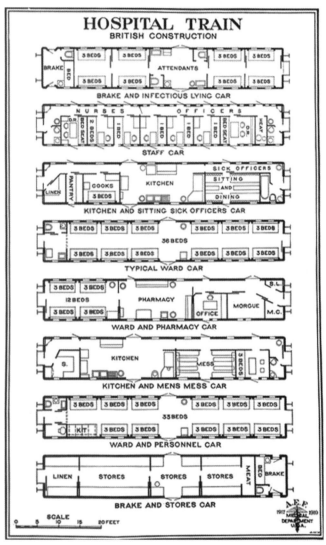

HOSPITAL TRAIN
BRITISH CONSTRUCTION

BRAKE AND INFECTIOUS LYING CAR

STAFF CAR

KITCHEN AND SITTING SICK OFFICERS CAR

TYPICAL WARD CAR

WARD AND PHARMACY CAR

KITCHEN AND MENS MESS CAR

WARD AND PERSONNEL CAR

BRAKE AND STORES CAR

2.29 Interior of British Army hospital infirmary rail car, World War I. Infirmary rail cars contained up to thirty-three beds

2.30 British Army infirmary trains in World War I consisted of eight types of rail cars with each rail car fitted for a specialized function. They consisted of up to fifty rail cars

2.31 World War I hospital barge infirmary, European theater, 1918. Many of these redeployable 'floating hospitals' had been adapted from different pre-war uses

night (Figure 2.27). The interior of Mobile Field Hospital Number 39 of the United States Army depicts spartan accommodations in an environment that was exceedingly difficult to control in terms of humidity or temperature levels. Only a minimal amount of supplies could be stored on site and supply replenishment was usually a risky undertaking (Figure 2.28).

Hospital infirmary trains were another type of transportable hospital used in World War I. These were designed and built by the British and deployed by British and American expeditionary forces. These highly elaborate nomadic facilities could be transported over conventional rail lines to and from the battlefront. The interior of a typical patient ward-rail car contained eleven triple bunks, for a total of thirty-three beds per ward-car (Figure 2.29). Eight types of rail cars collectively constituted this rolling hospital. These consisted of a brake and infectious lying car, a staff car, kitchen and sitting sick officers car, one or more typical patient ward cars, one or more patient ward and pharmacy cars, a kitchen and men's mess hall car, a ward and personnel car, and a brake and supply (stores) car (Figure 2.30). These rolling infirmaries could have as many as fifty rail cars. This mode of transport was less difficult in many cases than being forced to travel over land on the poor roads so common in the combat zone.

Hospital barge infirmaries were also used in Europe during World War I. A number of barges designed as floating infirmaries were deployed vis-à-vis waterways, including canals, rivers and lakes. Other barge infirmaries were converted from a different prior use – usually agricultural or merchant marine – to inpatient wards whereby the patient was carried on a stretcher across a gangplank to topside and then maneuvered to the ward, below deck. These vessels typically had small windows and were most frequently affiliated with larger

mobile surgical unit at the field hospital installation at Bernecourt (Figure 2.26). Ambulances were required to have direct access to the surgical tent-theatres in order to transport the wounded to and from the surgical staging area. The convoys of equipment supply trucks and ambulances could stretch a quarter of a mile and were poised for deployment or redeployment at any time of the day or

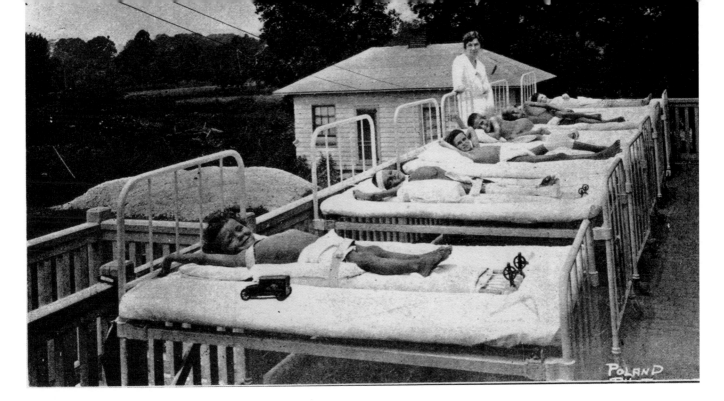

2.32 Outdoor heliotherapy veranda, King's Daughters Home (1918–1920), Memphis, Tennessee. The terrace was next to the ward, accessible via full height French doors

hospital ships. These satellite facilities, whether adapted or built as infirmaries, were deployed to the front lines to transport the sick and injured to either a hospital mothership or to land-based infirmaries away from the front lines (Figure 2.31). This means of providing care and treatment was innovative insofar as it made use of an existing technology and (often) the adaptive use of barges converted to medical use.

Advancements continued in field-based medical care throughout World War II. The Medical Army Surgical Hospital (MASH) first became widely deployed during the Korean War in the early 1950s. In the Vietnam War (1962–1974) the tents that comprised the MASH units in Korea were replaced by inflatable systems known as MUST (Medical Units Self-Contained and Transportable). This system was inflatable and utilized a double-walled fabric membrane system. They were inflated by turbine engine power racks called U-Packs. These supplied heating and cooling, compressed air for the structure as well as hot water. However, while these structures were innovative from a rapidity of response deployment standpoint, they required 2,400 gallons of aviation fuel per 24-hour period, fragments from mortar attacks could collapse them, and they required concrete pads to preclude their 'floating' during torrential rains.[73]

The problematic MUST hospitals were replaced with standardized modules designed to replicate as much as feasible the functional areas of a standard brick and mortar (fixed site) hospital, and the medical technology required to treat the wounded in a combat environment. This system – DEPMED (Deployable Medical Center) – allowed for the design of a mission-specific field hospital.[74] The DEPMED system uses a variant of standard intermodal shipping containers shelters to house critical areas such as laboratories, radiology, pharmacy, sterilization departments, and operating rooms; these rigid container-

like units are combined with TEMPER (Tent, Expandable, Modular, Personnel) units to house patient wards and other support functions. Passageways connect these various modules to collectively function as a full service field hospital. This Compact Support Hospital (CSH) was deployable in a 16-bed to a 256-bed capacity. Flexibility is achieved by linking additional tents together to expand inpatient wards. The CSH differs from the MASH primarily in size and the sophisticated medical diagnostic and treatment equipment it houses. However, DEPMEDs are far less mobile than their MASH predecessors. Due to this limitation, they are not deployed as near to a combat zone as a MASH. The wounded are evacuated swiftly to a CSH for longer-term treatment. The DEPMED field hospitals performed admirably during the Iraq War (2003–).

Early twentieth-century sanitariums and sustainability

By 1920, the hospital was being transformed by the need to provide spaces for heliotherapy. This was due to the rapid spread of tuberculosis. Children's hospitals were beginning to be designed with this facet of care as a major element in the architecture. In response a number of TB sanitariums and hospitals were built in Europe and in North America whose facilities were designed to rely on the use of natural daylight, ventilation, exterior terraces, and balconies in daily treatment. This practice was prevalent in the design of children's TB institutions although institutions for all ages were similarly influenced. Allied healthcare facilities in the U.S. and elsewhere were also designed in this manner. In the case of the

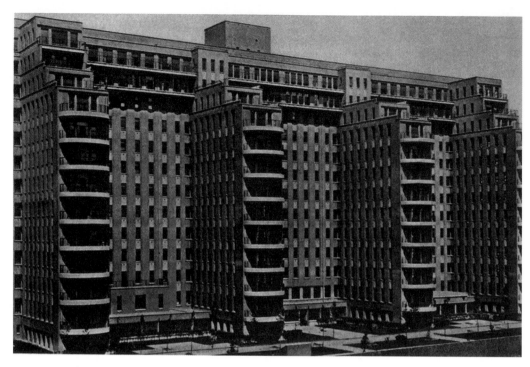

2.33 Hospital Beaujon (1932–1935), Clichy, near Paris. With 1,100 beds in vertically stacked wards, this institution personified the International Style high-rise hospital

King's Daughters Home for Incurables (1918–1920) in Memphis, Tennessee, a large open ward was provided for children with physical and developmental disabilities. By 1920 there were more than 500,000 'crippled' children in the U.S. and progressive healthcare providers believed that exposure to sun and fresh air was highly beneficial. At the King's Daughters Home, an adjoining terrace, fifteen feet in width and running the entire length of the ward, was accessed via large French doors. The patients' beds were rolled out for up to four hours a session, in good weather. The caption beneath the photo read, 'Hours of sun treatment on this special porch for boys make little faces beam and small bodies healthy' (Figure 2.32).[75]

Early skyscraper hospitals and sustainability

In 1905 Chicago surgeon Albert Ochsner presented a radical proposal for a high-rise urban hospital. His presentation, at a meeting of the Association of Hospital Superintendents, proposed that if floors are 'piled' on top of one another, new economies can be yielded in the areas of space, heating, supervision, housekeeping, materials management, and staff travel distances. He presented (in 1907) four diagrams for a prototype 500-bed hospital: as one 10-storey structure on a five-acre lot, as a single 10-storey structure on a city block 500 feet square, as 10 single-level Nightingale pavilions on a five acre lot, and as 10 one-level Nightingale pavilions on a city site 520 by 520 feet. He reasoned that if green public parks were to be the sites for future hospitals then densification would not be an issue. Besides, rising land values dictated that innovative strategies had to be adopted to attain greater urban densities.[76] The invention of

the steel frame in the 1870s and its applications in the great works of the Chicago School of Architecture of the late nineteenth century had allowed for greater building heights and the use of curtain wall technologies. This allowed for formerly massive masonry walls to be transformed into thin exterior cladding systems, or skins. Soon, hospital towers were built in many cities as outmoded facilities were demolished to provide space for this more efficient use of land and capital resources.

The skyscraper hospital came to France with the Hospital Beaujon (1932–1935), opened in Clichy near Paris. Directly inspired by its American precursors, it was hailed as the most innovative hospital in Europe. With 1,100 beds it was a full service institution. Imposing in scale and constructed of steel with a clip-on concrete panel exterior skin, it was boldly designed according to the precepts of the emerging International Style (Figure 2.33). Le Corbusier, the celebrated French architect, was an originator of this new minimalist aesthetic language in architecture. It was an approach that totally rejected the precepts of the 'restrictive' and excessive neoclassicism that had heretofore dominated this building type in the West.[77] The four inpatient ward wings of Hospital Beaujon extended outward from a linear service spine. An exterior solarium was provided at the end of each wing. Each ward housed sixteen beds. Due to the south exposure of the wings every window received sunlight for at least some part of the day. This was also the case for the single rooms, situated in linear groupings between the wards. Support services were provided across the corridor from the nursing station in each ward. Each floor was designed to function as a semi-autonomous infirmary (see Chapter 5).

Vertical 'streets' provided a circulation network for supplies and people. Its elevator core was configured as a semi-detached tower and was positioned at midsection, in plan. A stairway was situated

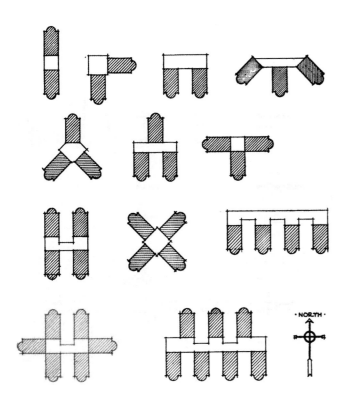

2.34 Numerous 'tapered wing' plan configurations recommended for early-twentieth-century high-rise urban hospitals, as reproduced from the book *The Modern Hospital* (1913)

at the entrance to each inpatient ward. One may assume from this that most vertical trips were made via the staircases, as they were so close in proximity to the wards. This concept of the accessible, aesthetically inviting vertical circulation element has been reprised in green hospitals in recent years as a health promotion device, as a means to promote walking versus always opting to use the elevator.[78] In addition, the thin footprint of the inpatient wings and the thinness of the central treatment and support spine were innovative in terms of the level of natural light and ventilation transmitted to the interior; the stepped back configuration of the top floors housed TB patients and their adjoining roof terraces were used for heliotherapy sessions. Other hospitals of the period included the Westminster Hospital in London (1936–1939) where support services were arrayed vertically from the main level to the top floor, as opposed to the more horizontal, stacked massing of hospitals such as the Hospital Beaujon.

Based on Ochsner's proposal in 1907, American innovations with respect to the densification of the high-rise urban hospital were summarized in 1913 by John A. Hornsby and Richard E. Schmidt. They proposed various configurations for urban hospitals and their inpatient-nursing units (Figure 2.34). Various footprints were recommended based on 'particular conditions, special sites, and individual taste'.[79] By this time U.S. hospitals were being designed with more single rooms and semi-private wards of three to ten beds compared to their large-ward European counterparts. High-rise hospitals of the pre-World War II period first incorporated central air conditioning systems in their adaptation of Nightingale's open ward to modern healthcare facilities. Specialized departments with new architectural requirements, i.e. radiology, appeared and dramatic growth occurred in the urban centers adjacent to where these skyscraper hospitals were constructed.

The hospital's superintendent typically answered to a board of directors in a period of expansionism that occurred in order to keep apace with new medical technologies, expressing a 'bigger is better' attitude. Bed capacity was a key indicator of institutional status among peers. As community hospitals were built in new suburbs, new networks of roads were built outward from the older urban center. The private automobile now made it possible for patients to travel farther distances more expediently for their care, thereby fostering an entirely new type of hospital – the suburban community hospital (see Chapter 7).

A modern masterpiece of sustainable design: Paimio Sanitarium

When it opened, the Paimio Sanitarium (later Hospital), in Paimio, Finland (1927–1929) by the Finnish architect Alvar Aalto, was seen as innovative for its site planning and architectural vocabulary. This tuberculosis sanitarium was conceived as a medical instrument itself. Before the discovery of a definitive antibiotic for TB in 1944, the curative powers of dry, fresh air and sunlight were emphasized to combat this disease. Paimio included sunning balconies where patients could spend hours even in winter months. The hospital's footprint was composed of a series of pavilions connected to a main administration building. These patients' rooms and respite terraces were housed in a linear, single-loaded wing six levels in height with a roof terrace (Figure 2.35). The hospital was designed to foster a communal atmosphere for both staff and patients, who generally remained at the facility for many months. Aalto wrote what amounted

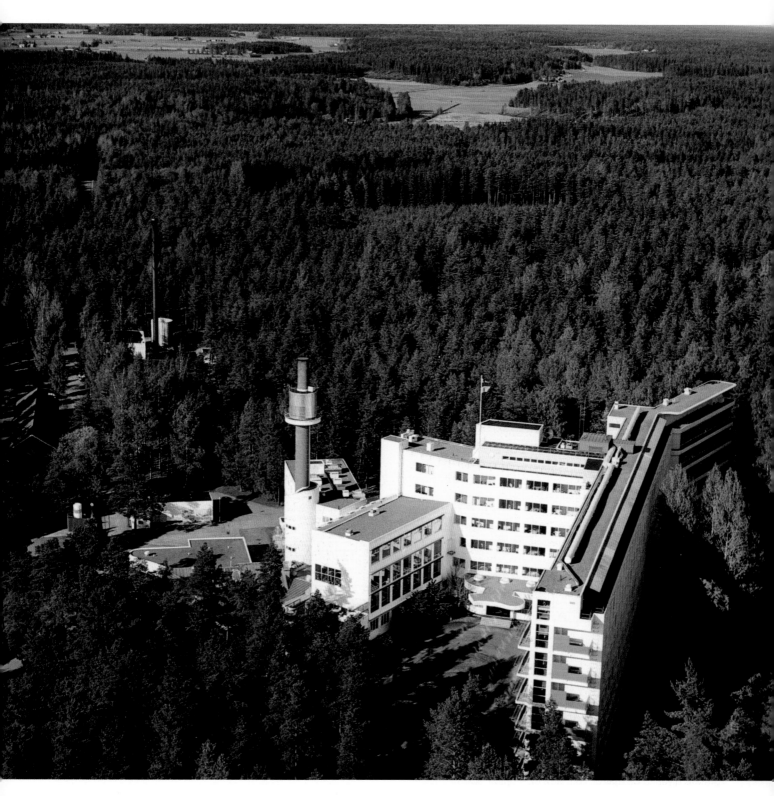

2.35   Ariel view depicting the rural site context of the Paimio Sanatorium
(1927–1929), Paimio, Finland, Alvar Aalto, Architect

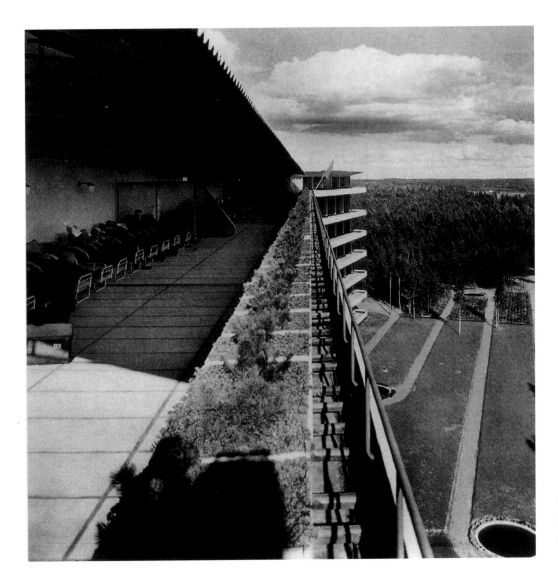

2.36 Respite terraces, Paimio Sanatorium, Finland. An open-air roof garden provided extensive views of the surrounding natural landscape

to a manifesto in his submittal to the design competition held to award the commission for this hospital. He oversaw virtually every aspect of its design and construction.[80]

Built with the collaboration of forty-eight surrounding communities, the hospital today remains situated amid a forest. The sense of respite, and the views from within, has been of therapeutic value to patients for eighty years. A series of interconnected, linear wings is bisected with vertical circulation elements. Aalto paid almost excessive attention to harnessing and directing light, given Finland's proximity to the Arctic Circle and TB's reliance on the powers of heliotherapy. Great care was given to window design, view orientation, aperture size and placement, their operability, and the amount of sunlight transmitted to the interior reaches of the patient room. Windows were double-glazed and in three parts: between the double panes were placed a heating element that warms the air as it flows through the exterior.

The ceilings contain radiant heat panels so that, as Aalto wrote, 'a weak patient lying in bed does not receive the strongest radiation directly, instead he is in the medium strength radiant sector'.[81] Wall panels of varying materials and thicknesses, and noise reduction measures, were pioneered. Public realms were similarly bathed in sunlight, with views of the surrounding landscape.

At Paimio, respite terraces were of two types: one accommodating 24 patients adjoining each ward, and a large terrace seating 120 on the roof, combined with a roof garden (Figure 2.36) that allowed for seating or strolling not unlike at the Royal Sea Bathing Infirmary, in Margate, Kent, England (1878–1882), built fifty years earlier. Covered sunbathing balconies were also provided for the resident staff. It is both a serene and exhilarating atmosphere. In the 1960s it was converted from a TB treatment facility to the Paimio Hospital. Perhaps the most remarkable aspect of this place was that it was built at all in the era of the pre-World War II urban skyscraper hospital. Paimio is just as relevant today as when it opened and remains a major influence on the emerging sustainable healthcare architecture movement. Unfortunately, the successes of this hospital, from a sustainable design perspective, would be eclipsed in subsequent decades in the era of massively overscaled, resource-hungry medical centers.

The unsustainable megahospital: 1945–2000

The suburban community hospital was a post-World War II phenomenon. It contributed greatly to the phenomena we refer to today as *suburban sprawl*. The proliferation of the suburban hospital as a type was necessitated by the growing dependency on the automobile. Previously, hospitals were typically located in older, walkable neighborhoods and were accessible by streetcar, bus, or train. As cities grew denser, residents fled to outlying areas, and the urban hospital in the 'old neighborhood' was confronted with a difficult dilemma: should it stay and reinvent itself on its original site, or should it follow the outward migration of its patients and staff to these new communities? By building anew, hospitals that opted to relocate typically built on open land, adjacent to high volume traffic arteries, with the facility surrounded by a sea of asphalt. The evolution of the suburban hospital differed little in this regard from the rise of the suburban shopping mall in the 1950s and 1960s. It too was built on open land and was surrounded by hundreds of parking spaces. The low density that characterized their surrounding communities was in sharp relief set against the high density of the neighborhood left behind. Often, the abandoned hospital in the inner urban neighborhood was sold for redevelopment, then demolished.[82]

On the gravitational pull away from the city center, in an earlier discussion of this issue, I described how:

[m]any urban medical centers were faced with the choice of remaining in their present location or moving out to the booming suburbs, which needed schools, libraries, and roads in addition to new health facilities … for decades, the relationship between the (old) neighborhood and the voluntary hospital had been awkward, yet the community had usually accepted the 'manifest destiny' of the institution. Now, the hospital had

to weigh, on the one hand, land constraints and pressures for expansion against … its avowed mission to serve its traditional core constituency … was the institution to build upward, or outward?[83]

Most boards of directors, administrators, their major donors, master planners, and architects considered virtually every possible factor under the sun except the harm caused by being a contributor to suburban sprawl and its unintended and in most cases unforeseen negative consequences. For the institution, at the external level it was all about staffing, public relations, recruitment, patient referrals, and what would happen to the patients left behind without their longtime neighborhood hospital. Internal justifications typically centered on the overcrowded conditions within the hospital, the lack of parking, rising crime in the neighborhood due to changing demographics, and the lack of incentives to stay (not) put forth by local politicians. In this era of rampant hyper expansionism, the old rules seemed no longer to apply.

In the process, the loss of the neighborhood hospital, not unlike the loss of a beloved church, would have a transformative effect on the physical appearance, social cohesiveness, and collective memory of the place and the residents left behind. By 2000, the entire premise of suburbia and its civic institutions – including the suburban medical center – was being thoroughly reexamined as unsustainable in the wake of rising energy costs. A growing body of scientific data pointed to the deleterious health consequences of the unchecked sprawl that had by then engulfed the everyday landscape. Its unhealthful outcomes included an increase in stress, cardiovascular disease, obesity, and hypertension.[84] As for those care providers who elected to remain in their longtime 'old neighborhood' locations, an entirely new set of problems arose: how do we expand without obliterating the surrounding neighborhood? Through the use of eminent domain powers, many urban U.S. hospitals elected in the 1950s, 1960s and 1970s to destroy their surrounding residential neighborhood in the name of institutional advancement and as a grand gesture in ecological anti-stewardship. In the end, unfortunately, this quest for expansion became highly contradictory to any notion of land conservation or historic preservation. The harmful consequences of this 'anything goes' strategy would from then on place the hospital firmly at the center of the contemporary movement in unsustainable environmental design for health.

The search for alternatives

The aforementioned timeline is re-presented at this point in the discussion to provide an overview of the key events in history that were discussed above and to illustrate the five major waves, or epochs, in architecture for health across the millennia. This is meant as a guide and therefore should not be construed as definitive. Events and building types with 'green' attributes are indicated in green type (Figure 2.37a–b). This timeline spans from the earliest Neolithic settlements up to 2010. One thing that has become apparent is that many of the thousands of hospitals demolished worldwide in decades past would now at the very least be worthy of a reconsideration and reappraisal of their relative merits. The high cost of replacement facilities, their rock-solid construction, and prime locations, often in redeveloping neighborhoods, would warrant high ratings in any due diligence analysis of their reuse potential (see Chapter 5).

Since 2000, noteworthy case studies of adaptively transformed (and spared from destruction) former hospitals to sustainable new uses are numerous and include the former Naval Hospital in Chelsea, New York, converted to 750 residences (2001), Bradley Hospital, in Bay City, Michigan, converted to 180 apartments for the aged (2003), the former New England Hospital for Women and Children, in Roxbury, Massachusetts, converted to a substance abuse treatment center (2004), the Maine Eye and Ear Infirmary, in Portland, Maine, adapted to 36 residential units (2005), the former City Infirmary and Almshouse, in Poughkeepsie, New York, adapted to 85 residential units for the aged (2004), St. Luke's Hospital, in Chicago, adapted to 286 apartments for the aged (2004), and the Newberry Hospital, in Newberry, South Carolina, adapted to 36 residential units for the aged (2003). In the case of Newberry, the hospital, built in 1925, was to be abandoned in 2000. However, the local housing authority and the local Council on Aging wished to preserve this National Register building and convert it into much-needed affordable housing for seniors. The firm Landmark Group, of Winston-Salem, North Carolina, with Campbell Meeks and Associates, completed an adaptive use through an ingenious combination of low-income housing tax credits, historic property tax credits, a community development block grant, and a state-backed tenant-based rental assistance program. Precedent had been established: The Jersey City Medical Center adapted its 1930s art deco facility into upscale condominiums (1990), and built a replacement facility across the street. In New Orleans, a grass-roots effort was underway in 2009 to renovate the historic Charity Hospital (1935–1938), shuttered since being flooded by Hurricane Katrina in 2005 (see Chapter 5).[85]

In the U.S. alone, nearly a dozen pre-World War II twentieth-century hospitals have been destroyed since 2000, including the interpretive Nightingale high-rise Passavant Memorial Hospital (1927–1929) in Chicago, designed by the venerable firm Holabird & Root (demolished 2001).[86] As in the case of Charity Hospital, the administration dismissed its preservation and reuse amenity – in short, dismissing its continued sustainability. They took the position that Passavant would have been far too costly to renovate, was functionally obsolete and anachronistic with respect to current medical practices, and was in non-compliance with current building codes (Figure 2.38).[87]

A second historic hospital in Chicago was nearly lost recently, the National Register-listed Cook County Hospital (1912–1914). Portions of Cook County were demolished, leaving its ornate neoclassical front facade and colonnade, perched high above its surroundings, as the overall site awaits redevelopment. The facade appears to be held in mid-air suspension.[88] The historic St. Elizabeth's Hospital in Washington is threatened with destruction to make way for a new headquarters for the U.S. Department of Homeland Security. What would residents gain from the senseless loss of one of Washington's most historic places? Not much, according to a report from *The Brookings Institution*.[89]

Summary

In this chapter, various major developments in the history of sustainable architecture for health have been discussed. Fresh air, water, natural light, human scale, meaningful connections with the fabric of the adjoining community, natural, locally available building materials, and various construction technologies have been examined, premised on six provisos outlined at the beginning of this chapter. The ancient healing temples of Greece employed fresh air, water, and landscape in a unified therapeutic treatment regimen. The patient was cared for in the context of nature. Later, the mineral spring baths built by the Romans made use of water as a therapeutic and spiritual element. They constructed elaborate temples and bathhouses at these sites and towns soon grew around them. The hospitals of the Middle East, in Baghdad, Cairo, Damascus and elsewhere, were more advanced

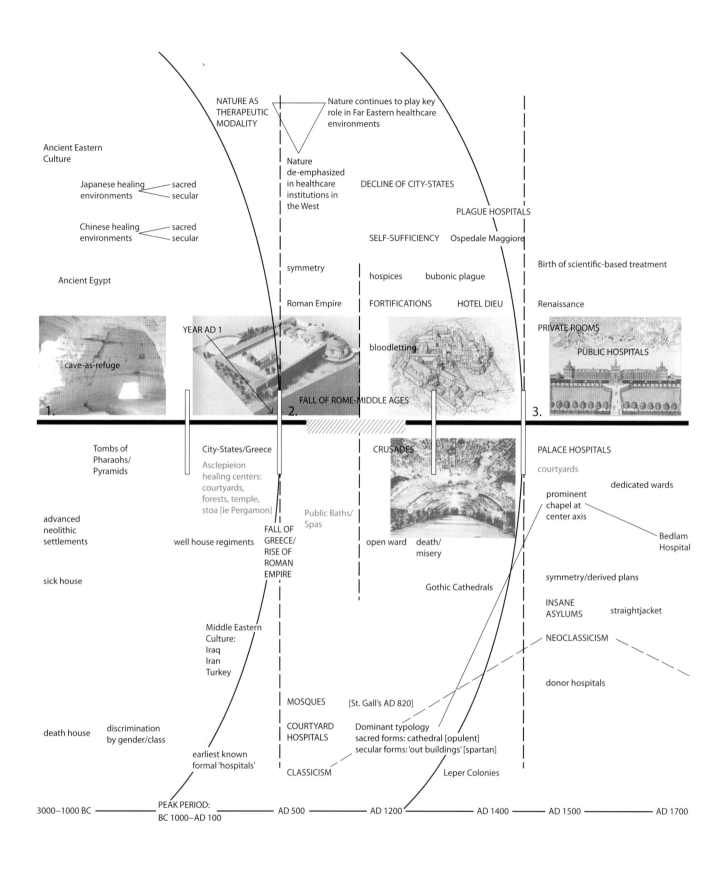

NATURE AS
THERAPEUTIC
MODALITY

Nature continues to play key
role in Far Eastern healthcare
environments

Ancient Eastern
Culture

Japanese healing ——— sacred
environments ——— secular

Nature
de-emphasized
in healthcare
institutions in
the West

DECLINE OF CITY-STATES

Chinese healing ——— sacred
environments ——— secular

PLAGUE HOSPITALS

SELF-SUFFICIENCY   Ospedale Maggiore

symmetry

hospices   bubonic plague

Birth of scientific-based treatment

Ancient Egypt

Roman Empire

FORTIFICATIONS   HOTEL DIEU

Renaissance

YEAR AD 1

PRIVATE ROOMS

PUBLIC HOSPITALS

cave-as-refuge

bloodletting

1.

2.   FALL OF ROME-MIDDLE AGES

3.

Tombs of
Pharaohs/
Pyramids

City-States/Greece

CRUSADES

PALACE HOSPITALS

Asclepieion
healing centers:
courtyards,
forests, temple,
stoa [ie Pergamon]

courtyards

dedicated wards

prominent
chapel at
center axis

advanced
neolithic
settlements

well house regiments

Public Baths/
Spas

Bedlam
Hospital

FALL OF
GREECE/
RISE OF
ROMAN
EMPIRE

open ward   death/
misery

symmetry/derived plans

sick house

INSANE
ASYLUMS

straightjacket

Gothic Cathedrals

Middle Eastern
Culture:
Iraq
Iran
Turkey

NEOCLASSICISM

donor hospitals

MOSQUES   [St. Gall's AD 820]

death house   discrimination
by gender/class

COURTYARD
HOSPITALS

Dominant typology
sacred forms: cathedral [opulent]
secular forms: 'out buildings' [spartan]

earliest known
formal 'hospitals'

CLASSICISM   Leper Colonies

3000–1000 BC ——— PEAK PERIOD: ——————— AD 500 ——————— AD 1200 ——————— AD 1400 ——— AD 1500 ——————— AD 1700
BC 1000–AD 100

2.37 Timeline of sustainable practices and building types in the history
of architecture and health

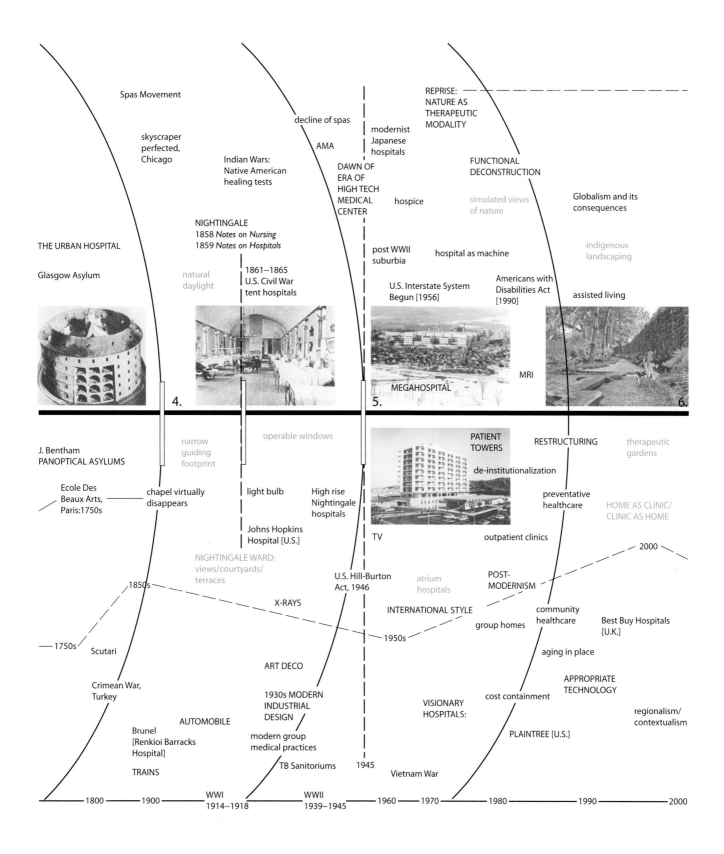

Spas Movement

skyscraper
perfected,
Chicago

decline of spas

AMA

modernist
Japanese
hospitals

REPRISE:
NATURE AS
THERAPEUTIC
MODALITY

Indian Wars:
Native American
healing tests

DAWN OF
ERA OF
HIGH TECH
MEDICAL
CENTER

FUNCTIONAL
DECONSTRUCTION

hospice

simulated views
of nature

Globalism and its
consequences

NIGHTINGALE
1858 *Notes on Nursing*
1859 *Notes on Hospitals*

indigenous
landscaping

THE URBAN HOSPITAL

natural
daylight

post WWII
suburbia

hospital as machine

Glasgow Asylum

1861–1865
U.S. Civil War
tent hospitals

U.S. Interstate System
Begun [1956]

Americans with
Disabilities Act
[1990]

assisted living

MRI

MEGAHOSPITAL

4.   **5.**   **6.**

J. Bentham
PANOPTICAL ASYLUMS

narrow
guiding
footprint

operable windows

PATIENT
TOWERS

RESTRUCTURING

therapeutic
gardens

de-institutionalization

Ecole Des
Beaux Arts,
Paris:1750s

chapel virtually
disappears

light bulb

High rise
Nightingale
hospitals

preventative
healthcare

HOME AS CLINIC/
CLINIC AS HOME

Johns Hopkins
Hospital [U.S.]

TV

outpatient clinics

NIGHTINGALE WARD:
views/courtyards/
terraces

2000

1850s

U.S. Hill-Burton
Act, 1946

atrium
hospitals

POST-
MODERNISM

X-RAYS

INTERNATIONAL STYLE

community
healthcare

Best Buy Hospitals
[U.K.]

1750s   Scutari

1950s

group homes

aging in place

Crimean War,
Turkey

ART DECO

APPROPRIATE
TECHNOLOGY

cost containment

AUTOMOBILE

1930s MODERN
INDUSTRIAL
DESIGN

VISIONARY
HOSPITALS:

regionalism/
contextualism

Brunel
[Renkioi Barracks
Hospital]

modern group
medical practices

PLAINTREE [U.S.]

TRAINS

TB Sanitoriums

1945

Vietnam War

1800 — 1900   WWI
1914–1918   WWII
1939–1945   1960 — 1970   1980 — 1990 — 2000

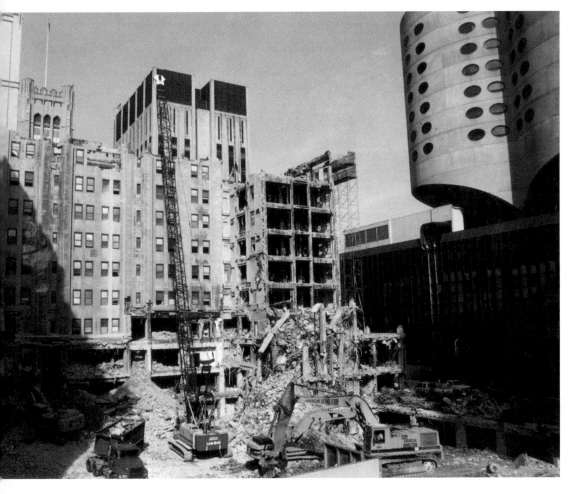

2.38 Demolition of Passavant Hospital, Chicago, 2001

2.39 Louise Coote Lupis Pavilion at Guy's Hospital, London,
2008. Note the operable windows

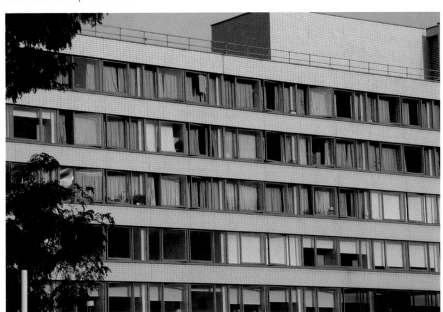

than their European counterparts during this period. They were designed with useful courtyards and wings for the transmission of fresh air and natural light into the patient wards.

The ecohumanist work of Florence Nightingale centered on the provision of clean, well-lit, and ventilated hospitals affording the patient a meaningful view of the outdoor natural landscape from within an open ward. Her passion and drive influenced generations of hospital administrators and their architects and her influence was international in scope. Nightingale hospitals were characterized by their low profile, relatively narrow open wards with interspersed landscaped courtyards, and the nursing station located at the inboard end of each ward, adjacent to a circulation artery.

In the late nineteenth century and early twentieth centuries, the mineral springs spa/retreat and sanitarium movements in the United States provided respite care and a means of escape from unhealthy urban conditions. Later, the pre-World War II modernist interpretation of these precursors was brilliantly expressed in Alvar Aalto's patient room and adjoining terrace at the Paimio Hospital in Finland (see Chapter 4). Meanwhile, as these retreats flourished and gradually fell into disfavor due to medical and public health advancements, a new generation of skyscraper Nightingale hospitals was built in the period 1910–1940. Nearly all of these hospitals are gone although those that remain afford unique opportunities for sustainable redevelopment and preservation. Now, 1950s-era hospitals are threatened, such as the Louise Coote Lupis Pavilion at Guy's Hospital in London, with its operative windows and narrow footprint (Figure 2.39). Many pre-1940 hospitals were demolished to make way for these International Style machine megahospitals. Today, the same is beginning to happen with hospitals built in the 1960–1980 period, as demonstrated in the battle fought by preservationists to save the modernist O'Toole Pavilion (1962–1964) on the campus of St. Vincent's Hospital, in Manhattan.[90]

The evolving role of site, landscape, and nature

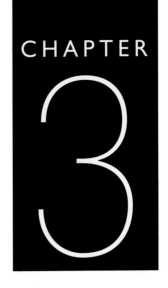

CHAPTER

3

Until recently, few hospitals relished taking on the role of environmental steward. Institutional policies frequently resulted in the dismissal of matters pertaining to ecological sustainability and conservation through the default posture of 'looking the other way'. A sustained commitment to the local community in this regard, however, takes time and effort. Paying attention to the local *community* can help to shape/reshape a hospital and a medical center's civic role in two ways. First, it can increase the community's social cohesiveness and its physical health. Second, it can increase the community's ecological well-being. Often, an attitude of respect for the local culture is a prerequisite to any serious broadening of an institution's stewardship mission. This is not always easy. Hospitals, in the face of daily operational pressures (not unlike virtually any other institution), tend to act inwardly and in their self-interest. This is complicated by the fact that an institution's public/civic identity and posture usually evolves gradually over time, sometimes centuries (see Chapter 5). Change often comes slow to this relationship.

With this said, a hospital's success in part hinges on its ability to contribute to a community's sense of place – its *genius loci*. An inability of a community to self-define its own unique identity makes it hard to define precisely those cohesive, indigenous cultural and vernacular qualities to critical value in defining a given hospital's *civic identity*. Hospitals that rapidly expand into new greenfield communities and put up generic buildings often have this problem because they find it difficult to achieve this (or any) degree of civic identity. The anywhere–anyplace appearance of the facility and the generic cookie-cutter image it projects may further exacerbate this. The hospital runs the risk of being equated generically with the nearest McDonald's.

Deeper qualities and sensibilities of *place* are rarely expressed in recent hospital architecture. The sad fact is that most recent hospitals often do not contribute anything of this sort to their community. They dilute the concept of civicness, environmental sustainability, and stewardship, therefore undermining the aforementioned qualities – resulting in *placelessness*. This symbolizes a dangerous weakening of the hospital's civic functions and potential. It is endemic to institutional rootlessness.[1] It is the reflective architect's task to assist the client to attain a civic, aesthetic, formal, and environmental presence that resonates. Striking a balance is prerequisite between local vernacular traditions, non-local technological imperatives, and ecological and human health promotion, which attainment of

3.1 Martini Hospital, Groningen, the Netherlands (2004–2007). The retention pond created on the site serves as an urban oasis for the hospital and for the community

a unique aesthetic expression. These factors are of high priority in this equation.

Genuine architectural expressions of local vernacular culture, human experience, and local ways of making buildings are becoming rare in this age of standardized franchise healthcare, global economic uncertainty, and monolithic top-down healthcare oligarchies. With economic survival sometimes hanging in the balance in a highly competitive healthcare industry, hospitals are pitted against one another in the open marketplace to lure and to retain the best staff and to garner the best reputation. *Genius loci* remains a powerful yet elusive vehicle to an organization reaching its fullest potential in this regard. An ephemeral, obsessively mobile, fast-food, of-the-moment culture runs the risk of perpetuating the mirror image of this in its hospital architecture. Three facets of genuine placemaking are discussed below – site planning, landscape design, and nature – each is viewed as a therapeutic intervention, from the scale of a community to that of a hospitalized inpatient's room.

Site – urban design

The Martini Hospital in Groningen (2004–2007), the Netherlands, was designed by Burger Grunstra Architects and Consultants. The three major design goals were to use industrialized prefabricated building components, to provide adaptable interior spaces, and to develop a demountable kit of parts to be used interchangeably as functional needs evolve over time. This system is called IFD (Industrialized, Flexible, Demountable). It received a demonstration grant from the Netherlands' Ministry for Housing, Regional Development and the Environment (Figure 3.1).

In plan, the hospital resembles two chromosomes that touch at 'junction points'. These nodes house vertical circulation (stairs, elevators, conference rooms, support). The two undulating bands are informally deployed on the site to allow for differing view orientations from within, and different perspectival vantage points when viewed from the exterior. In composition, eight 'blocks' each 16 meters in depth (as opposed to the typical depth of 25 meters) were created as a starting point in order to allow additional daylight into the building envelope. Each block's floor template is 1,000 square meters per floor. All mechanical and electrical support is provided to each block through a centrally located vertical core.

An important difference between Martini and prior Dutch hospitals is the use of this narrower 16-meter bay depth. This allows for significantly more daylight penetration and for the complete reconfiguration of the internal floor plans as needs change across an anticipated 40-year life span. The exterior facade is a layered demountable panel system. The outer skin of this double-layered membrane is made of low-e glass and possesses supplemental sound abatement properties. The inner skin of the vertical interstitial cladding system consists of demountable, moveable screens and panels. Window apertures of varying proportions are possible, and the interstitial space is 80 centimeters in width. Exterior windows are operable throughout the building envelope, in thin horizontal bands spanning the entire length.

The structural aperture and its exterior skin are standardized. Extensions or 'drawers' may be added to this frame allowing the floor area to grow outward – increased – by ten percent. For example, it is possible to add or subtract new functions, including up to 250 housing units, within the hospital's anatomical infrastructure and structural aperture. The aperture is designed to accommodate future non-hospital uses. All floors and walls are demountable for this reason. The hospital, at its opening, housed 570 beds, a 20-bed ICU (intensive care unit), and 17 operating suites. The Martini Business Centre houses a number of health-related commercial enterprises. Peter Stuycken, a well-known Dutch artist specializing in color abstraction, produced a matrix of 46 colors for 'random' non-place-specific application throughout the interior. Its random application ensures it is not associated with any particular unit, function, or room type.

The base level houses the majority of outpatient services, and levels two through five house inpatient housing, diagnostic, and treatment care units. The adjacent original hospital was retained for non-direct patient care functions including the central administration, and medical center general support. This expanded campus therefore makes maximum use of this amenity, ensuring it will have a continued life for years to come. It is a 'best of both worlds' scenario seldom pursued and seldom executed with such bravado, especially in recent American replacement hospitals.[2]

The Martini Hospital is also noteworthy because it is an infill replacement facility in a dense site context – the new hospital fits comfortably into its long-established urban neighborhood (Figure 3.2). The site was chosen because it was within the city center; it possessed excellent public transportation connections, and is easily reached via walking or bike by many of the 240,000 residents it serves.

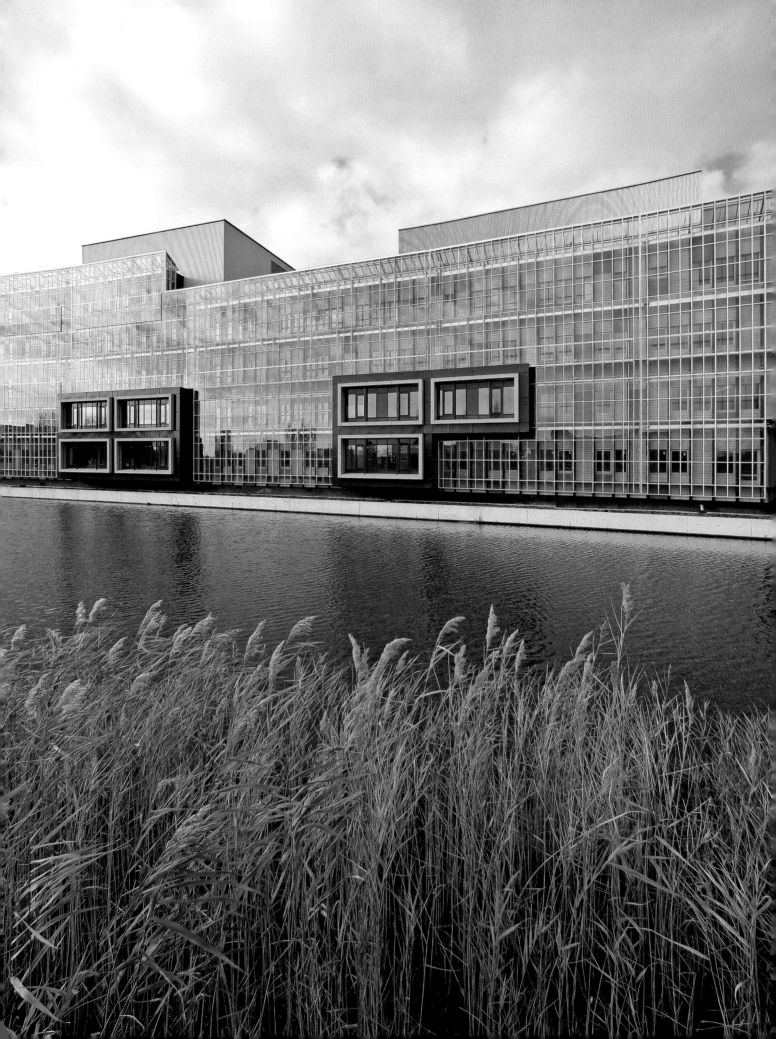

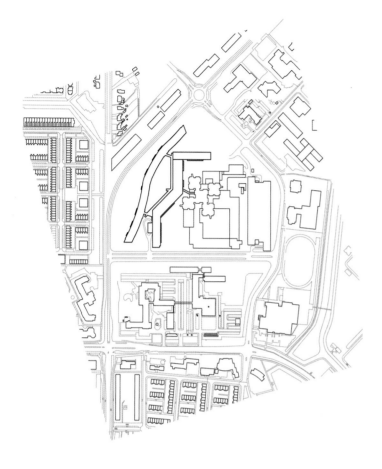

3.2 Site plan, Martini Hospital, Groningen, the Netherlands, indicating its relationship to its dense urban context

Landscape – anthropomorphism and biophiliaism

Buildings that symbiotically express the inner profundities of architecture, site, and landscape remain of enduring value and fascination. They are not about merely attempting to mimic a site's superficial attributes. They organically express a spirit and physicality of site and landscape. The strong affinity humans have for sustained engagement with the natural environment is at the core of the emerging field known as *biophilia*. Biophilic design is defined as the expression of the deep-rooted human preference for involvement with nature.[3] The fundamental dimension of biophilic design is an organic or naturalistic dimension. This affinity manifests in two ways. First, direct experience refers to relatively unstructured contact with self-sustaining attributes of the natural non-human built environment such as daylight, plants, natural habitats, and ecosystems. Humans' direct involvement with nature has been dominant, in an evolutionary context, in critical features such as light, sound, smells, wind, weather, water, vegetation, animal species, and the natural unbuilt landscape. Indirect engagement requires human involvement in the sustenance or management of nature, be it a fountain in a courtyard, caring for plants, trees, or a vegetable garden. Another type of indirect engagement involves symbolic, or surrogate contact, i.e. a wall mural, video, painting, or projected image of a natural setting (discussed below).

A second dimension of biophilic design is place-based and vernacular, defined as the interplay between landscape, its formal properties, built form, and formal geometries that symbolize the intrinsic human affinity for nature. Buildings and landscapes that express a local vernacular culture of a particular place or geographic region are at the heart of this interpretation of placemaking. Its advocates argue that landscapes and buildings expressive of these biophilic design principles become integral to their inhabitants' individual and collective social consciousness, and are capable, at their best, of being spiritual and transcendent.

Various architectural historians have described buildings that express the geometries of nature with the terms *biomorphic*, *organic*, and *anthropomorphic*. The art nouveau movement of the early twentieth century, best represented perhaps in the work of Hector Guimard, was laden with vegetational motifs, as evidenced in his Paris Metro Station gateways fabricated of cast iron (1899–1905).[4] Antonio Gaudi's Casa Batlló in Barcelona (1904–1906), perhaps his

The bikeable, walkable advantages of its location immediately set it apart from nearly every recent American replacement hospital. It is therefore of and about its place. Recent comparable campuses in the U.S. are constructed on greenfield suburban or exurban sites with little or no attention paid to the hospital's larger community footprint.

The Martini Hospital site includes a prominent man-made retention pond. An existing curved road defines one edge and the hospital, the other. Every citizen can appreciate this amenity. It further extends the civic footprint of the medical center little differently than if a new public park had been created on the site. On the other side, across from the main entrance, a pocket park features curving walkways, and landscaping. Both sides of the site provide places for socializing, private reflection, and health -promoting physical exercise. The presence of water and green space, it is hoped, will encourage staff and family members to take patients outdoors whenever feasible.

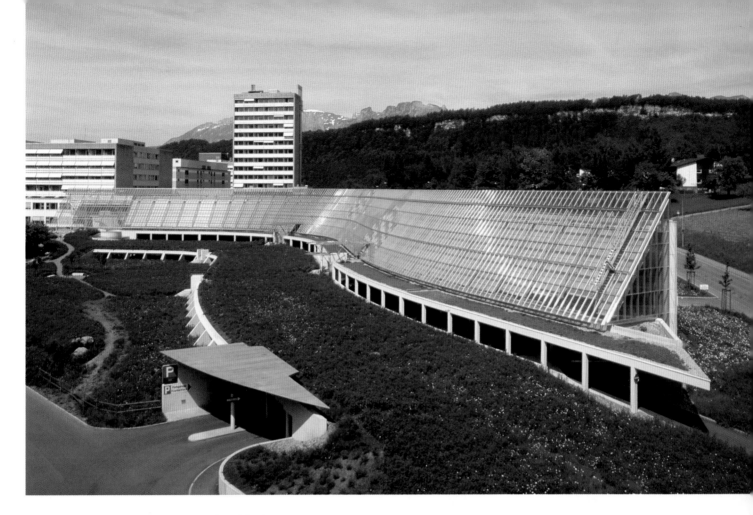

3.3 The serpentine public arrival spine at the Feldkirch
State Hospital (1992–1994), district of Vorarlberg, Germany

best-known building, featured swirling naturalistic geometries – both
compositional and ornamental – throughout the interior and exterior
surfaces.[5] In the case of Frank Lloyd Wright and the Prairie School, his
Robie House (1907–1909) in the Hyde Park section in Chicago was
organic in its composition, siting, materiality, and outward reach to
its context. His magnum opus in this regard was the Kaufman House,
known as Fallingwater (1934–1936), in Pennsylvania. The organic
tradition in modern architecture has consistently endeavored to resolve
the inherent contradictions and commonalities between nature and
vernacular culture, both in local and in cosmological terms.[6]

The recent work of Hungarian-born architect Imre Makovecz has
sought to resurrect modernist traditions from the early twentieth
century, then later dismissed. This work has sought to reconcile folk
architecture, green architecture of the 1970s, and anthropomorphic
metaphors. This work, notably his Spitalfields Park Shelter, in London
(1992–1994), with Jim Gomez and the Prince of Wales Institute,
made use of wood in a waveform, rolling composition punctuated
by folded planes. Makovecz values the organic tradition in both
ecological and cosmological terms. For him, according to Charles
Jencks, 'It [the work] includes not only the canonic figures – Frank
Lloyd Wright, Bruce Goff, Herb Greene, Lechner Odon, Kos Karoly,
Rudolf Steiner, Antonio Gaudi and William Morris – but [is] a response
to the environmental crisis'.[7]

The traditions of organic and anthropomorphic architecture have
always attempted to reconcile the inherent contradictions between
nature and vernacular culture, not their similarities, which is the
avowed goal of biophiliaism. Makovecz's cosmologic inspirations are
drawn from cultures of ten, twenty thousand years ago, are based
in the archetypes of Carl Jung and in the two great ancient cultures
of Central Europe, the Celts and the Scythians. This stream of work
is rooted in a basic, almost primitively embedded sense of place,
and a fundamental spirituality that relates to the earth and to the
animism of long-lost cultures.[8]

The additions to the Feldkirch State Hospital (1992–1994), in
the district of Vorarlberg, Germany, by Erich Gutmorgeth, express
the complex tensions between nature, organic architecture, and
key aspects of biophiliaism. But it goes beyond this: it is a high-
tech synthesis of all three influences. The existing hospital was
expanded, with buildings, laboratories, and administration space
plus an undulating glass atrium pedestrian 'street' that is 656 feet
in length (Figure 3.3). This element serves as the new main entrance
to the medical center and to a multipurpose building. The lobby,
flooded with natural daylight, houses a cafe and main waiting areas,
and provides ample space for social interaction between patients,
visitors, and staff.

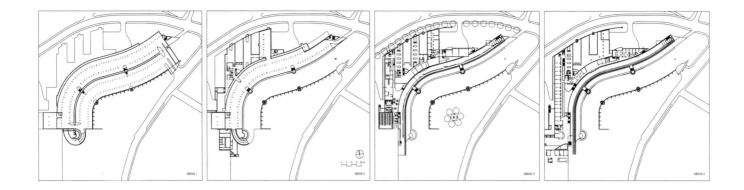

ERWEITERUNG LANDESKRANKENHAUS FELDKIRCH   1988 - 1993

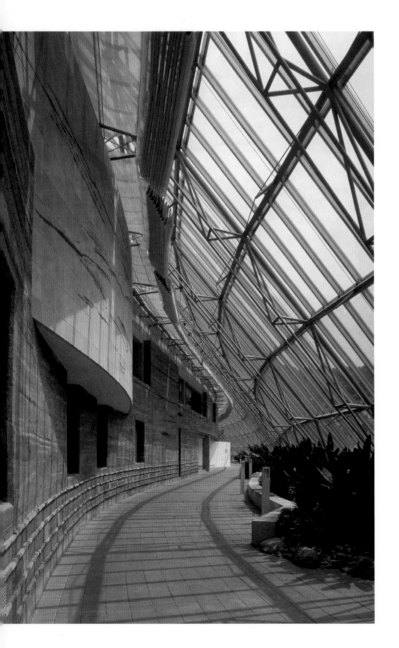

The curvilinear glass skin is 43 feet high, and spans the entire length of its civic promenade. This element references its topological parameters (whereby section and elevation provide interchangeable readings of the composition) and formally acts as a continuation of a segment of an undulating contour that continues 'infinitely' in both directions. The site plan describes the means by which the building at once absorbs and reflects its existing earthen contours (Figure 3.4). The interior space is ventilated by means of an elaborate system of louvered sunscreens to provide shade, and its earthen backwall is revealed at key intervals in a metaphorical reference to the self-restorative powers of Mother Earth (Figure 3.5). A water element and this episodically revealed earthen wall function in tandem to provide spatial delineation. Landscaping is used extensively to further express its biomorphic waveform parti'. A water-based passive cooling system cools the building in warm weather months; while the earthen retaining wall yields thermal mass properties during cold weather months.

The building is embedded *in* its site – not *on* it – and blends seamlessly by means of a judicious use of landscape elements at key intervals. A subterranean parking garage allows for additional green space on the campus. The intrusive visual effect of the automobile is avoided by means of the underground garage, with its car park entrance at the midpoint of the undulating waveform promenade. The staircase leading upwards from the garage is similarly expressed in an organic, or biomorphic, shape, and is fabricated in steel with a translucent glass canopy (Figure 3.6).[9]

Architects, and architectural historians, for that matter, have had an on-again off-again interest in the organic 'style' expressed in biomorphism and anthropomorphism. Wright himself was so committed to his version that in one lecture he offered 52 definitions of the term.[10] As mentioned, organic architecture had exponents in the industrial age in the late nineteenth century in the work of engineers and art nouveau architects, and 100 years later in the recent high-tech movement. Alvar Aalto's Paimio Hospital's organic metaphors at the scale of site remained limited although the buildings were themselves in sympathy with nature. Regardless, this work would appear to be of interest to proponents of the biophilia movement (see Chapter 2).[11]

3.4 Feldkirch State Hospital, Germany. Parking is provided below ground, with the building footprint expressing the site's undulating topography

3.5 Louvered sunscreens and natural daylight in public areas, Feldkirch State Hospital, Germany

3.6 Staircase with translucent glass canopy leading from the subterranean car park, Feldkirch State Hospital

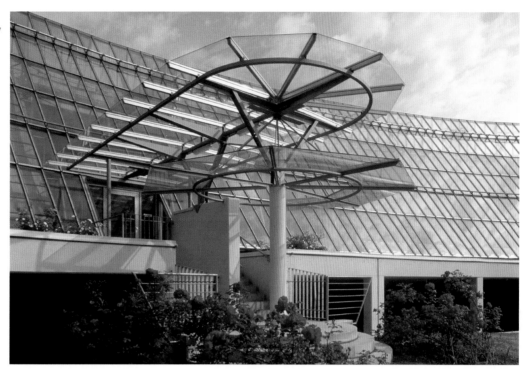

The recent high-tech movement in architecture, which emerged in the 1970s, was in part grounded in organic metaphors, though this influence would remain subservient to the machine aesthetic – which was not at all based in nature. However, now, it is almost the same cost to design bowed, curved roofs and wall systems, as it is to design these elements rectilinearly. The work of Archigram in the 1960s was visionary, and high-tech as an attitude flourished in the U.K. in the late-twentieth-century work of Sir Richard Rogers and Sir Norman Foster, Nicholas Grimshaw, Cedric Price, and in the rationality of Michael Hopkins (see Chapter 8). In Japan the work of the metabolists in the late twentieth century represented an alternate yet equally provocative interpretation of high-tech in architecture.[12]

The architecture of the Spanish engineer Santiago Calatrava is based in high-tech biomorphic and anthropomorphic formal vocabularies as opposed to expressly biophilic imagery or principles. It is therefore not about indigenous vernacular or about connecting a particular building to a particular or unique place. It is an international brand of biomorphism transposable in theory to any site and to any part of the world, as he has demonstrated as more and more of his buildings are completed. The bird-like form and silhouette of the Milwaukee Art Museum is stunning and universally appealing in its imagery. It is a bird poised to take off in flight, and yet a non-place-specific bird that can be found in many places on earth.[13] Would it have been considered a vernacular expression of biomorphism if this bird-like form were a species found only in the Upper Midwest? Calatrava's elliptical, swooping, animated, animal-like compositions are as a result generally not embedded in their sites, nor are they deeply sympathetic to local culture. They appear to be far more inspired by bridge forms than site contours, to any place versus a specific place. However, they do express a signature person–nature dialectic, and are iconographic. His buildings contribute on a certain level to an understanding of a global definition of placemaking. That is, at the very least they are curiosities – anomalies – thereby attracting tourists and wide attention.

Jencks writes:

Why give so much emphasis to an architecture of undulating forms? The partial answer is that wave motion, like nonlinearity, is so crucial and omnipresent in nature. At a basic level, in the microworld of quantum physics, the wave function of the atom is as fundamental as the particulate aspect. Every subatomic particle is both wave and particle. Every object and human being is composed of this bipolar unity, this double entity. The wave aspect is masked to us, however, because it is unobservable … an idea weighs nothing … is stretched out like a wave [in the brain], can travel at the speed of light, and is changeable like an ocean wave … [and] can contain many contradictory states within itself without collapsing.[14]

The extraordinary properties of quantum mechanics are embedded in nature and for this reason Jencks sees that they should be fundamental to the making of biomorphic architecture, whether about the *genius loci* of place or of a more universal architecture. In other words, vernacular, or folk, culture need not be the central concern. Biophiliaism, on the other hand, appears rather unconcerned with principles of quantum physics in favor of an indigenous vernacular architecture, its relationship to human experience, and the transactional person/building/earth relationship.

Nature – transparency and surrogates

Reinventing the relationship between site, landscape, and a building for healthcare requires the blurring of the often stark, abrupt line of demarcation between the interior and the exterior of a building. Such barriers are countertherapeutic and serve no purpose beyond a certain point. Five innovative strategies to break down the needless walls/barriers between a hospital and the natural environment are discussed below: water, roofscaping, surrogates, therapeutic (healing) gardens, and transparency, in a two-way continuum between the interior and exterior – giving rise to a new term, *theraserialization*. By peeling away, or dematerializing, the physical and symbolic barriers that cut the interior of a building off from the outside world, its true 'nature' can be revealed and the building can *breathe*.

Water

Water is essential to life. It is hygienic, aesthetic, spiritual, life sustaining, and symbolic. We are drawn to water edges, waterfalls, rivers, streams, and vistas overlooking water. Water has no shape itself; it is given shape by environmental forms and in turn water profoundly shapes the physical environment it touches. Still water is soothing. Its calming properties come from its movement, motion, force, directionality, and sound. A rushing waterfall or river, changes in current, turbulence, waveform rhythms, and the powerful force of a hurricane are awe inspiring and at once a source of fear and fascination in humans. Leonardo da Vinci was convinced that the motion of fluids was at the center of understanding the power of the universe.[15]

The sounds of water are analogical to music and this link has been attributed to our evolutionary past. Water is a source of visual, aesthetic, and recreational use. Human beings seek vital engagement with water for its intrinsic challenges, multisensory stimulation, and sustenance. It is both to be protected and to be challenged and provides opportunities for contemplation, respite, and spiritual restoration. Water has inspired countless works of art, literature, and music. In the medium of film, water is a consistent thematic element. Water holds a central pace in virtually every religion on earth. The Japanese Shinto place a water bowl in every shrine for purification. The writings of Muhammad discuss the inalienable water rights of Muslims, and the well of Zemzem at Mecca is considered sacred water.[16] In the urban environment, cities' identities are defined by their relationship to water (Venice, New Orleans, Amsterdam) or their lack of connection with it (Las Vegas, Phoenix, Santa Fe). In the past decade many hospitals have incorporated a water element either in their facility or somewhere on the campus. Water sculptures have been used with success at main entrances as a means to provide a soothing sound as one arrives. Fountains, ponds, and waterfalls are in more and more hospital lobbies and in outdoor courtyards for visual, auditory, and aesthetic reasons. They contribute in a positive, memorable way to the ambient environment. Water is therefore important in establishing a hospital's *genuis loci*.

The Bon Secours St. Francis Cancer Institute is the first major expansion on the recently constructed St. Francis Medical Center campus, in Midlothian, Virginia. A two-level addition (2003–2006) was designed by Odell Associates of Richmond, Virginia. The 55,000 square foot facility is prominently located as the gateway structure to the main entrance to the campus. The building features natural materials (principally wood), a stone base, cedar piers and soffit details, terracotta tile roofs, and copper gutters, and this element functions as the campus front door and 'living room'. Low, sloping roofs, masonry and timber pergolas, several water elements, including a central fountain in the main courtyard, and a heavy timber arrival canopy reinforce the imagery of a manor house or rural retreat. A three-level staircase-tower brackets the entrance to one side, at the main entrance. This element at once articulates the main entry portal and references the larger bell tower of the main hospital beyond (Figure 3.7). The interior features an indoor-outdoor continuum with extensive natural light and views to the courtyard, and the palette of colors, materials, forms and alcoves facilitate semi-private social interactions (Figure 3.8). The living room features a large stone fireplace (see Chapter 7).[17]

Extensive landscaping ingratiates the visitor to the scene and to its site context. Semi-sheltered seating nodes within this garden

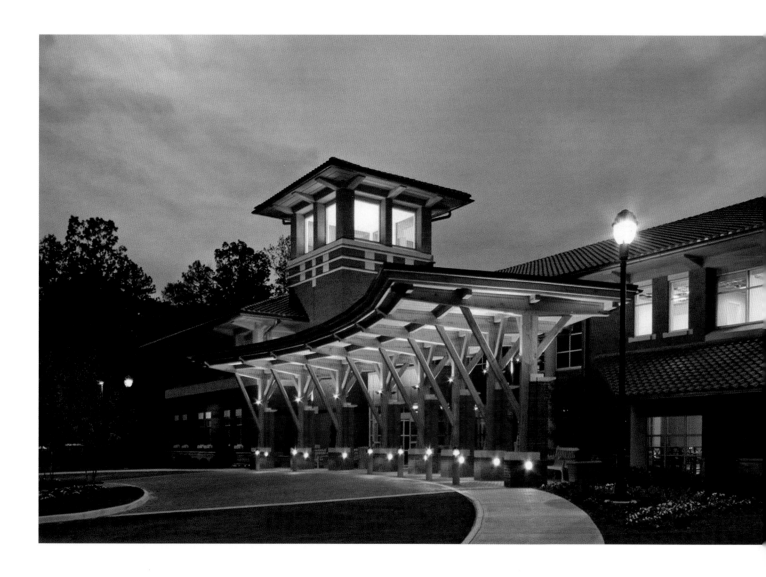

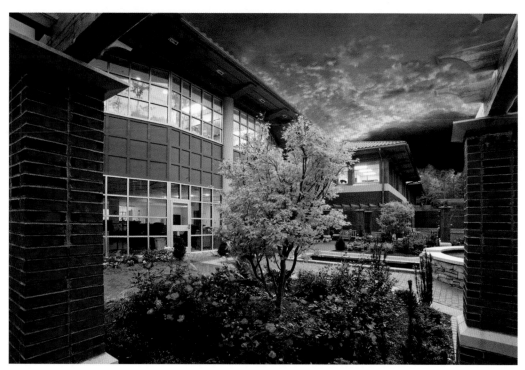

3.7 Main entrance, Bon Secours St. Francis Medical Center, Midlothian, Virginia (2003–2006)

3.8 Theraserialized courtyard, Bon Secours St. Francis Medical Center

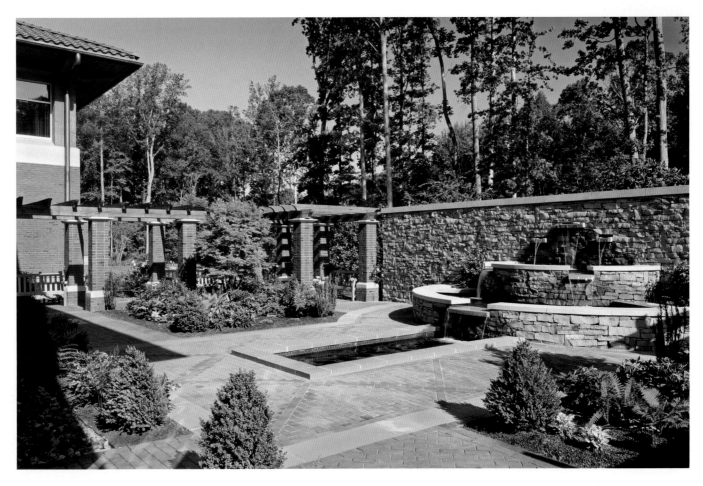

3.9 Theraserialized courtyard,
Bon Secours St. Francis Medical Center

and its water features invite year-round use by staff, visitors, and patients. Water flows from a stone wall into a two-tiered circular pond, from here into a rectangular pond at grade level. The lower tier also provides seating. A mature stand of trees on the campus was preserved and this contributes to the natural imagery and sense of enclosure within the courtyard (Figure 3.9). Water is used sparingly yet effectively. The courtyard provides respite and is transitional, as it leads to the main hospital immediately beyond.

By contrast, the desert is an extreme landscape context for a hospital. When one envisions a desert landscape, scorching temperatures come to mind, dryness, starkness, minimal vegetation, the absence of water, and general physical discomfort. The Banner Estrella Medical Center in Phoenix (2002–2005) designed by NBBJ Seattle, established a complementary yet high-tech counterpoint to this extreme site context. Banner Estrella embraces and expresses some of the surrounding desert landscape's most striking and extreme indigenous vernacular elements. Its architectural vocabulary fuses occupant needs, high technology, human comfort, energy conservation systems, and internal and external connections to its setting. It is a

human-scaled campus, aptly capturing elements of its vernacular context and local traditions in individual compositional elements, and yet its broader architectural vocabulary is high tech, even minimalist (Figure 3.10).

The campus' rock gardens and reflecting pools are serene and provide spiritual respite. Shades of copper, red clay, light brown, sienna, and earth tones in the hospital's public spaces mirror the hues of Arizona's nearby canyons and plateaus, further reinforcing its connection to its site-place. This 452,000 square foot hospital was masterplanned for expansion from an initial 63 beds to an additional 33 beds in the coming years (Figure 3.11). The central nervous system for the campus is housed along a linear internal spine from which the footprint can expand without disturbing other structures on the campus. Pathways and indigenous plant species surround the reflecting pool. It is a contemplative setting, affording respite to its users (Figure 3.12).[18]

A number of medical centers are converting conventional turf landscaping to native planting and xeriscapes. Innovative site landscaping embraces the use of indigenous native plantings. Their

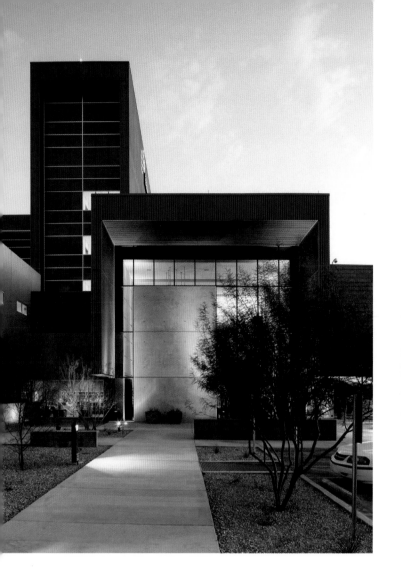

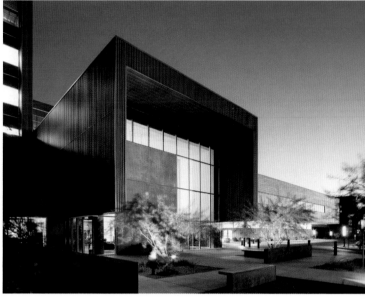

3.10 Main entrance, Banner Estrella Medical Center, Phoenix, Arizona (2002–2005)

3.11 A cantilevered roof brackets the main entrance and arrival plaza, Banner Estrella Medical Center

3.12 Reflecting pool and therapeutic landscape, Banner Estrella Medical Center

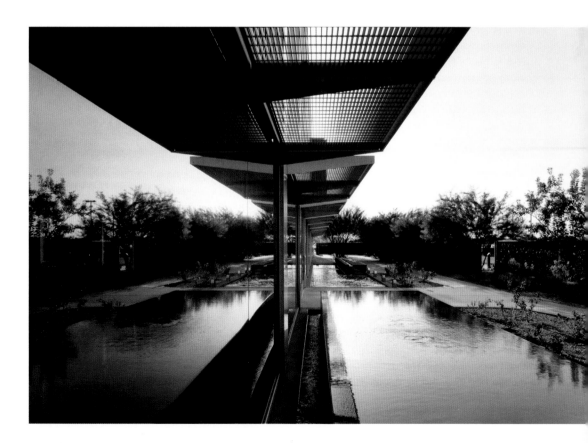

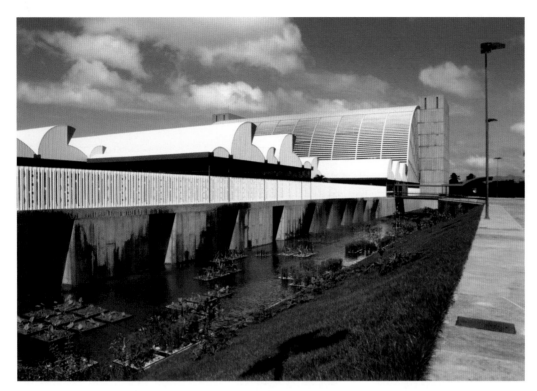

3.13 Reflecting pond adjacent to main entrance, Sarah-Fortaleza Rehabilitation Hospital, Brazil (1988–1991)

use conserves water, requires less maintenance, and greatly reduces the need to apply chemical fertilizers and herbicides. The Legacy Salmon Creek Medical Center (Chapter 8) created a healing garden with indigenous plant species in this manner.

The Sarah Network, named for Sarah Kubitscheck, wife of former president of Brazil Juscelino Kubitschek, was developed incrementally over a twenty-year period beginning in 1980. The first in this network was the 294-bed Sarah-Brasilia, which opened in 1980. The network provides rehabilitation inpatient and outpatient treatment for malformations, trauma care, locomotive systems diseases, and neurodevelopmental disorders. A total of 1,000 beds are distributed throughout eight hospitals built in six Brazilian cities. They are the work of the architect João de Gama Filueiras (known as Lelé). This network embodies sustainable design features, industrialized construction methods, and strong connections to the physical and indigenous vernacular landscape. Collectively, it is a powerful testament to the therapeutics of healing environments.

The Sarah Network hospitals are widely respected for the quality of care provided. Daylighting, natural ventilation, and passive cooling systems are attuned to users' preferences as much as to energy saving imperatives. Microclimate conditions are of high priority. The hospitals are visually striking, with playful color palettes, water elements, hydrotherapy pools and gymnasiums, and feature prefabricated structural systems and cladding systems manufactured in a factory built specifically for the Sarah Network construction program, located near the network hospital in Salvador, Brazil (since closed). Each new hospital has benefited from improvements made to various thematic elements, advancements in prefabrication and in standardization, without repetitiveness. The *camamaca*, literally 'bed stretcher', is a mobile bed invented by the architect, allowing patients to be easily taken outdoors to shaded courtyards next to their inpatient room (see Chapter 8). The Sarah-Fortaleza (1988–1991) is a 61-bed rehabilitation hospital. It includes an open-air physical therapy space in a landscaped covered courtyard setting, with a therapeutic pool at its center, for strengthening and conditioning programs. Filtered daylight is transmitted into patient rooms vis-à-vis sculpted rooftop vents. The hospital at Fortaleza also features a reflecting pool at the main entrance (Figure 3.13).[19] The retention pond at the Martini Hospital is more urban than its counterpart at the Sarah-Fortaleza and yet both speak to the therapeutics of water.

Roofscapes

The roof surface of a hospital is almost always dismissed. There have been few examples at any point in the past two thousand years where a hospital's roof was used by patients or for any other therapeutic purpose, for that matter. This is because they were usually steeply pitched and their sloping surfaces did not allow flat areas for walkways or overlooks. Their function was strictly perfunctory: to shed rainwater and snowfall, and to shade and protect the interior of the hospital from leakage or structural failure. Most modernist machine hospitals had flat roofs, by contrast. Often, the mechanical equipment for the elevator shafts and other infrastructure equipment were housed on the roof, even water reservoirs (as in the case of the pre-modernist Kirkbride asylums, see Chapter 2). The maintenance workers, and more recently 'facility management team', maintained sole jurisdiction over the hospital's roof. As medical centers expanded over the decades the addition of a wing here and a wing there

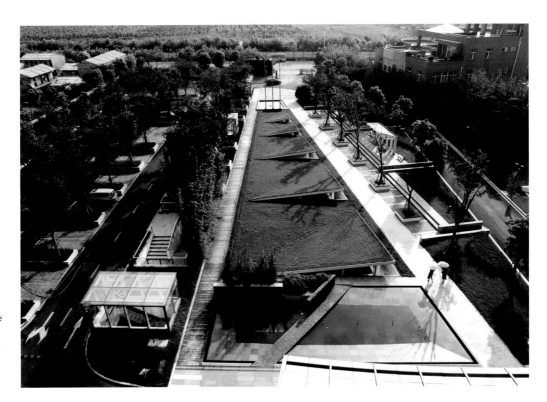

3.14 Angled roofplates atop the subterranean parking deck at the Pudong Huashan Hospital (2003–2006) in Shanghai, China, double as green spaces and transmit natural light to below

would often result in a series of cascading roofs. Too often, an unlucky patient's room would overlook one of these unfortunate appendages. The room may comply with basic code requirements, but the view outside is harsh. The brightness caused by a reflective roof surface causes undue glare and visual discomfort. In the worst cases the blinds have to always be kept drawn.

Many recent hospitals have been designed with cascading roof terraces. The spaces beneath the roof most often house diagnostic and treatment support functions, and general support. This platform base is generally wider and longer than the patient bed tower(s) that sit atop this base. But this is by no means a new strategy. In the 1960s this compositional approach was referred to as the 'matchbox on a muffin pan'. The support base could be expanded outward with additional patient towers added on top at a later date. The net result, then as now, remained the same – a dreadfully bland roof surface that screamed out for improvement.

In the past few years a number of older hospitals have attempted to ameliorate these negative outcomes by landscaping their roof surfaces. The term *green roofscaping* is apropos to describe this trend. New medical centers are featuring such roofs as integral to large-scale master planning and landscaping concepts and the results have been encouraging. Roofs are now incorporated either as part of a therapeutic (healing) garden, in rainwater harvesting, for cultivating vegetables, for solar collectors, and to shield the surface from solar heat gain. Municipalities in the U.S. are mandating that their public buildings be designed with green roofs to mitigate urban heat island effects and to capture storm water runoff for recycled use. The Meyer Children's Hospital in Florence, Italy, describes its green roof as an active skin membrane that mediates solar radiation (see Chapter 8).[20] The roofscape at Harrison Memorial Hospital in

Bremerton, Washington, features a winding path and rock garden. Their intersecting geometries create a third pattern at the center. A second path, radial in shape, of stone, bisects the garden, connecting to seating nodes. Indigenous plantings are featured.

The third floor roof terrace at the Bloorview Kids Rehab hospital in Toronto (2003–2006) provides patients and family with an opportunity to access the outdoors, and seating is provided overlooking views of a nearby ravine and pond. Wood is used as the decking material. Water is drawn through its openings and outward to the perimeter. It is a far cry from the barren roof surfaces of the recent past (see Chapter 8).[21] At the REHAB Basel Centre for Spinal Cord and Brain Injuries, in Switzerland, by Herzog and de Meuron (1999–2002) each room features, above the bed, a 6 foot diameter spherical skylight that bathes the patient room in daylight and the roof surface above is habitable, with its natural wood roof decking (see Chapter 8).[22]

Ground level surfaces can also be greened by placing certain hospital functions below ground and landscaping their roof surfaces. The Pudong Huashan Hospital (2003–2006), in Shanghai, designed by Wang Yan/Zhong Lu Architects, has 10 med/surgical PCUs and each unit houses 24–26 beds. In all there are 240–260 beds in the hospital. Huashan Hospital is located in a recent new town district on the edge of Shanghai. Comprehensive inpatient and outpatient services are provided on site. The density ratio called for an innovative solution to the need to park 300 cars on-site. In response, the parking deck was built beneath the hospital. The roof of the parking garage was landscaped and transformed into an aesthetic amenity (Figure 3.14). It is a park-like space for use by the general public. Patients and others can look out from the bed tower onto landscaped green space rather than a sea of unsightly autos and asphalt.

Therapeutic gardens

Hospitals can be extremely stressful places. The ability to draw upon the therapeutic qualities inherent in nature can extend one's capacities to cope with uncertainty and this in turn can potentially improve health outcomes. Since 1945 few hospitals had attempted to provide patients with any sort of meaningful contact with nature or with natural landscapes. This aspect of the hospital experience was dismissed outright, with the result that many medical centers built in the post-World War II period resembled stark factories and office parks. Air conditioning replaced natural ventilation; outdoor terraces and balconies vanished. Nature gave way to graceless, sterile parking lots and garages. Interior spaces were to be singularly about 'efficiency' and functionality; nature was often seen as an extraneous, costly distraction, at best. In many hospitals where landscaped open spaces once existed a parade of expansion projects would in time obliterate all of them.[23]

By the 1990s some hospital administrators began to awaken to the harsh reviews their facilities were receiving from patients, staff and others, from this standpoint. Soon, a trend was underway to transform otherwise dreary, concrete spaces through the use of softening elements drawn from landscape and nature. This first wave of site improvements were visible in the main lobbies and atrium of hospitals. These spaces, previously devoid of natural daylight and plantings, were suddenly being transformed into civic places once again with planters, faux waterfalls, flowers, and so on – a trend not seen since the grand urban hospitals of the late nineteenth century when statues and fountains adorned lobbies such as in the main lobby at Johns Hopkins.[24]

The term *healing garden* is most often used to describe an outdoor landscaped space on the grounds of a medical campus. These exterior spaces are designed specifically for human engagement and therapeutic use. This term, however, smacks too much of some slick unsubstantiated marketing pitch in a glossy public relations brochure so *therapeutic* is used here instead to describe these spaces. These provide instrumental therapeutic support – although they are not to be misconstrued as curative spaces in their own right (a garden itself cannot instrumentally engage in 'healing' anyone, neither is the term meant to imply that this type of garden is first and foremost about 'healing' itself). But they can *assist* in achieving the following benefits: help in stress reduction which helps the body attain a more balanced psychological state, help patients summon up their own inner healing resources, help patients come to grips with an incurable medical condition, help staff in administrating physical therapy, and horticultural therapy with patients. They can also provide caregivers with a place to obtain respite from daily stress, and provide a relaxed setting for patient–visitor interactions away from daily stresses.[25] The best of these therapeutic gardens are defined by the terms restorative, rehabilitative, and biophilic.

Activities occurring in a *therapeutic garden* can range from passive to active. These may include viewing the garden through a window, sitting outside, dozing, napping, or being engaged in meditation, prayer, exercise, walking to a preferred spot, eating, reading, working outside, viewing children playing in the garden, self-involvement in raised bed (platform) gardening, and light sports activities. They can help ameliorate stress and they are a source of positive distractions.[26] In addition, a well-designed therapeutic garden provides visibility, accessibility, familiarity, quiet, comfort, and unambiguously positive artwork. Precedents that designers have successfully drawn from in recent therapeutic garden design include precursive archetypal spaces (Institute for Child and Adolescent Development, Wellesley, Massachusetts), metaphor (Good Samaritan Hospital, Phoenix, Arizona), historical precedents (Hospice of the Texas Medical Center, Houston), regional vernacular (San Diego Children's Hospital, San Diego, California), works of art such as sculpture and fountains (West Dorset Hospital, Dorchester, U.K.), and as a stage for the reinterpretation and translation of medical diagnoses into built form (Good Samaritan Hospital, Portland, Oregon).[27] Successfully designed therapeutic gardens are having a positive ripple effect through the healthcare industry in the U.S. and elsewhere. Architects are encouraged to use the therapeutic garden as an opportunity for genuine placemaking. These *places* can express local and regional vernacular traditions, microclimate, geography, topography, plant species, and art traditions (see Chapters 7 and 8). It is expected (and hoped) that this biophilia-attuned amenity in hospitals will become a standard site amenity in inpatient care hospitals.

Theraserialization

Most healthcare facilities are freestanding, and therefore autonomous. Too often they are isolated, and, at worst, cut off from their surroundings. The outer walls of a hospital slam to the street like

3.15 Exterior, meditation space, Banner Estrella Medical Center, Phoenix

3.16 Interior, meditation space, Banner Estrella Medical Center. Transformable walls theraserialize connections with the outdoors

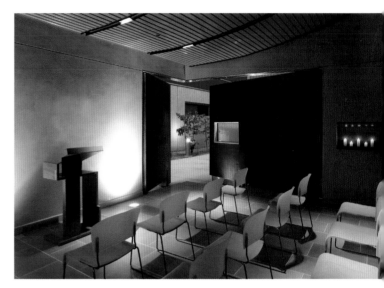

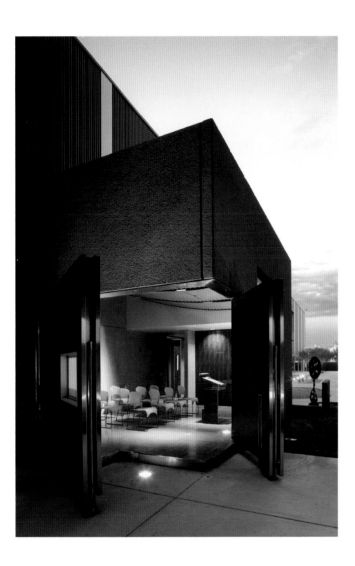

a giant guillotine. This unfortunate guillotine syndrome can occur either by design or by default, and some of the reasons for this sad reality are discussed later. Suffice to say, an entire book could be filled with images of only hospitals that relate very poorly to their sites. It is, by any measure, an unfortunate condition that precludes any genuine connection with the exterior world, and vice versa. The term *theraserialization* is a hybrid assemblage of the words 'therapeutic' and 'serialize'. It is a very promising alternative to the status quo. It is defined as a continuum of indoor to outdoor space consciously designed in support of biophilic environmental design principles. It entails the interpretation of space as being serialized, as layered, collaged, superimposed, transparent, and fluid. It is about the creation of serialized space from the public, to semi-public, to semi-private, to private. It is about the spaces in-between and about illusion. Theraserialization is applicable to a single continuum or multiple continua on the same site. It is horizontal and it is vertical, it can reach upward from subterranean spaces to the ground plane, ascending to the sky.

The meditation space at the Banner Estrella Medical Center, in Phoenix (2002–2005) comes close to illustrating this concept. It is transformable: at one moment it is enclosed and at the next instant can open directly onto the exterior realm (Figures 3.15 and 3.16). It is spatially interactive, and expresses transactive, biophilic, aesthetic, and indigenous vernacular influences. Visual and sensory connectedness is reinforced by a ground plane – or floor – a continuous, unbroken surface. By peeling away the walls (actually achieved through the use of a variation of a sliding/folding panel) the interior and exterior are joined. In so doing the space in between dissolves. The barrier posed by the walls dissolves, or dematerializes. The net effect is that the indoor and outdoor realms become transactive. This space can *breathe* in this manner after sunset on cool desert evenings, all year round. Dematerialization yields the architectural equivalent to a building's lungs expanding and contracting.

The work of Austrian-born architect Rudolph Schindler is a precedent for the theraserialization of architectural space in twenty-first-century healthcare architecture. After studying with Adolf Loos for one year, Schindler left Vienna in 1914 for the United States, including a stint in the office of Wright in Chicago (1917–1920). Work for Wright brought him to California in 1920, where he eventually set up his own office, although he continued to work with Wright until 1923. Schindler was influenced by the organic qualities in Wright's buildings, and his work came to emphasize topographical concerns and a keen interest in the fluid co-dependency between the indoors and outdoors. He sought to design from out to in – and vice versa. He used stepped sections to create gardens, terraces, and courtyards – elements found in Wright's best work. Schindler was influenced by Wright's introduction to the 1908 Wasmuth publication of his work in Europe, in which he advocated horizontal extension, sectional stepping, and the assimilation of the building into the 'prairie horizon'.[28] These concerns for a fluid translucency and transparency characterized all of Schindler's work from that point on. His deployment of these terms meant optical or visual serialization, the state of a given material being impervious to or in turn penetrable by light, or air, allowing one to see through layered, fluid, spaces either partially or completely. He became known for his private residences in the Los Angeles area in the 1920s through to the 1950s, beginning with his 'Translucent House' of 1927.[29]

Schindler's preoccupation with the relationship between a room and the world outside it centered on interconnectivity. This fascination between building and site was similar to Wright's emphasis on horizontality, but not identical. Wright argued for plasticity and organic synthesis and this was based on his severe criticism of boxed-in enclosures. Wright referred repeatedly to the prairie as an archetypal symbol of the American landscape, as if buildings were 'platforms' that were fitted in their totality into their terrain. Schindler, on the other hand, viewed this in somewhat more programmatic terms, insofar as individual functions of rooms within a dwelling needed to be connected to their larger site context, but each in its own way. He argued against compartmentalization and functional autonomy because they needed to 'flow' into their wider horizon line, as if a building were stretching its hands outward horizontally to embrace its neighbors. This view completely rejected neoclassicism and its obsession with formal facades, and base, body, cornice, and crown.[30]

The problem of being unable to break out of the hospital box begins with architects' obsession with perfecting the plan. The floor plan becomes the be-all/end-all medium. This shuts out the potential of the section as a medium to explore intrinsic *breathing properties* of the composition. This is unfortunate. Both plan and section deserve equal emphasis in healthcare planning and design in the creation of a sustainable architecture for health. Horizontal theraserialization can manifest in hospitals and in allied healthcare building types in other ways as well, including the use of large panel glass windows with sliding doors opening onto an adjacent terrace or healing garden, a water element that runs continuously from indoors to out, or vice versa, such as at the REHAB Basel, in Switzerland (see Chapter 8). In addition, the use of trees and various landscaping elements can help to establish screening in unbroken layered, fluid serialization,

perhaps further articulated by a retractable, transparent window-wall. Lighting and color can further enhance serialization, as can seating, and a pallet of natural materials consistently used across this spatial continuum. Vertical theraserialization is achievable, as mentioned, by connecting below grade to grade and the upper reaches of a building. Skylights, clearstories, and stepped or ramped grade modulations can achieve serialized modulation in this manner.

The therapeutic garden is by no means the centerpiece of theraserialization in architecture, although it must not be relegated to the margins either. Clare Cooper Marcus writes:

> Architects often 'think big' via computer drawn models, and outdoor spaces are sometimes seen as what separates buildings, or what's 'left over.' It is essential that a landscape architect be on the design team from the beginning to guide site planning so that outdoor spaces are in appropriate locations regarding access [and] microclimate … before the design of a garden reaches the schematic phase, it is essential that the design team consult with medical staff likely to use the garden for outdoor therapy, and with potential patient-users. Ideally, the team should annotate the final plan with presumed health benefits so that a later post-occupancy evaluation can be conducted to see if the garden functioned as expected. Research results should be [widely] disseminated … to encourage patients, caregivers, and families to make use of the garden.[31]

The major problem with most 'healing gardens' built to date is that they are treated as autonomous from their architectural context, that is, they are not *of* the architectural composition. In these cases they remain unrooted (pun intended) in the master planning and facility planning process from the outset. This allows for them to be easily dismissed later on. Or, too often they are created as afterthoughts: 'We have this extra space, why don't we put a healing garden there.' *That* is the wrong approach.

Virtual nature

Every hospital has one or more departments that are windowless or under-windowed. Some departments are not required to be windowed, such as materials management, central laundry, maintenance, or the central kitchen. Other departments may or may not be windowed, and may not be required as such by code, i.e. physical medicine and rehabilitation units, the exam rooms within an outpatient clinic, the nursing station within a med/surgical PCU, the medical records and admitting departments, or the chapel/meditation room. A third departmental type is often windowed, i.e. dining areas, dayrooms, art therapy rooms, wellness centers, central administration and conference spaces, and central atriums and lobbies. The fourth room type is always required to be windowed by code, i.e. the patient room.

Over the years many an institution expanded itself into a box-like, gridlocked configuration where windows, views, and daylight became scarce commodities. Departments that would ideally have been provided with these amenities became hamstrung through poorly executed master plans due to an administration that may have veered off course for whatever reasons. Ill-advised departures from an initial master plan for expansion often resulted in certain departments being shortchanged, such as the dialysis clinic, central laboratory, or other diagnostic and treatment areas that ended up confined to an internal zone somewhere deep within the bowels of the medical center, cut off from contact with the outside world and from nature.

The premise behind the nature surrogate – as an antidote to theraserialization – is to provide an 'artificial' or 'virtual' representation to ameliorate the sensory deprivation that can occur for the occupant through a disengagement from site, landscape, and nature. Since the 1980s it has been known that occupants of windowless and minimally windowed rooms in hospitals, from a psychological standpoint, have been found to equate these conditions as tantamount to being confined to an architecturally windowless room.[32]

Staff turnover is a chronic problem in many under-windowed (psychologically windowless) and architecturally windowless rooms and units within hospitals. Patient satisfaction may be adversely affected, and family members and direct caregivers may also experience sensory deprivation. A number of hospitals have recently taken steps to rectify this unfortunate situation by installing innovative surrogates. Many medical centers have transformed an otherwise blank wall or ceiling in their facility into a window aperture, a 'daylight activated' view of a natural scene – be it of a waterfall, forest, or windswept seashore – in MRI departments, outpatient surgery suites, waiting rooms, dining rooms, chapels, and other areas of the hospital where it would otherwise be impossible to provide the real thing because of budget, location, or site limitations.

Some see television as a surrogate that (at its best) reveals windows onto the world, so to speak. Yet television viewing is a distraction for many and remains a source of controversy in hospitals. In waiting rooms it has been found to be stressful and a negative distraction. A simulated view of nature, on the other hand, can be as effective as the real thing and a source of positive or restorative distraction, similar to the real thing. Interventions as benign as a wall calendar with nature scenes hung on a blood-draw cubicle in a lab can be effective. A more high-tech intervention is the use of nature programming on a closed-circuit television station. In the U.S., systems such as the Continuous Ambient Relaxation Environment (CARE) channel offer 72 hours of non-repetitive nature images accompanied by peaceful instrumental music. This has been found to be preferable to the often obnoxious, omnipresent mainstream programming on television monitors in patient rooms, in waiting areas and now even 'programmed' into the realm of the dining room and cafeteria.[33]

Jain Malkin writes:

It makes no sense to spend upward of $1 million on a piece of diagnostic imaging equipment without setting aside $10,000 to $20,000 for environmental amenities to distract patients and reduce their stress. The mere visual presence of such a large piece of equipment and the noises emitted during the procedure as the scanner gathers images can be frightening. Magnetic resonance imaging (MRI) can be particularly intimidating, especially after having to pass through a metal detector (a safety precaution in some hospitals) and having to answer numerous questions about implanted metal devices, orthopedic pins ... and so forth prior to the procedure. Having one's head inside a snug cylinder and having to lie perfectly still for a minimum of 45 minutes is pure torture for anyone who is claustrophobic ... certainly MRI suites should have soothing lighting and color palettes ... and images of nature to relax the patient ... headsets [can] enable patients to listen to their choice of music, which can help to block the noise of the machine.[34]

Progressive hospitals are responding to the biophilic predilections of patients and families by rejecting the sterile minimalism of internally windowless rooms and departments. Some are incorporating wall-based imagery with sounds and smells to recreate a multisensory surrogate experience, such as at a hospital MRI unit in Orlando,

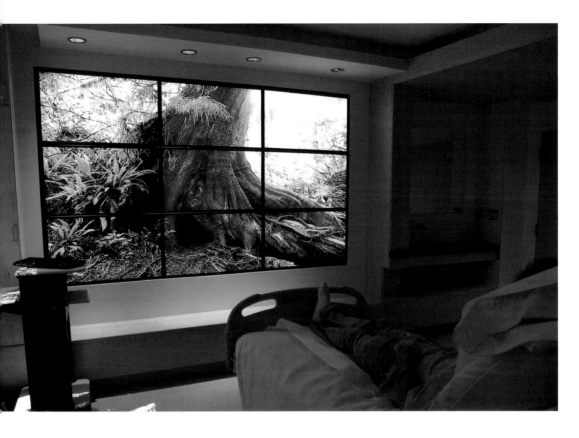

3.17 Self-selectable surrogate view representation, inpatient room of the future prototype, Clemson University (2008)

Florida, where patients hear, see and even smell a 'beach scene' while in the MRI unit. The use of evocative patterns on ceilings, and sculpture, can also create a positive distraction, combined with changing, evocative lighting that is orchestrated to provide the patient with dramatic reinterpretations of the subject matter while undergoing a diagnostic testing procedure, such as at the Scripps Center for Integrative Medicine, in La Jolla California.[35]

At Clemson University, the patient room of the future project has tested the use of a built-in inset wide screen digital e-wall that is controlled by the patient or family member. Various scenes are programmed and can be changed at any time in any combination of nine wall monitors that together appear as a large multi-panel window through which a single scene can be projected and viewed, or as many as nine different scenes at once. This provides the patient with personal choice to self-select his or her degree of engagement with the 'un/natural' environment (Figure 3.17). In the future, surrogate therapeutics will digitally portray a world where natural habitats such as rainforests, snow-covered mountain peaks, and remote undeveloped coastlines once existed. In addition, the patient and family member can use one or more such *e-apertures* on their e-wall for Internet-based video communications with friends, family, and caregivers. In hospitals, the architectural possibilities for digitally based person-nature transactions are wide open (see Chapters 6 and 7).

Alternatives to placelessness

The modernist megahospital was not about site, landscape, nature, ecology, or environmental stewardship. Because it was self-referential it, by default, rejected the value and meaning of locality, the particulars of site, local vernacular, and the intrinsic therapeutic amenity to be found in nature. Its alternative, residentialism, as a stream of postmodernism, valued elements of home, manor, neighborhood, natural materials, and human scale.[36] At first these experiments were executed in small-scale projects such as clinics and specialty hospitals: a gabled roof pitch, a stone walkway, an expanded color palette, carpeting in heretofore all-tiled zones, an arrival canopy at the main entrance, a balcony off a patient room, or a dayroom opening onto a terrace.[37] Early postmodern hospitals in the U.S. included the Martha's Vineyard Hospital (1973–1975), in Massachusetts, Arbour Hospital (1980–1983) in Jamaica Plain, Massachusetts, the Renfrew Center (1983–1985) in Philadelphia, and the Shenandoah Regional Rehabilitation Campus (1989–1991) in Manassas, Virginia.[38] In the U.K. the rejection of brutalism began earlier, with the opening of the Slough District General Hospital (1962–1965). Its low profile and wards reprised the classic Nightingale wards of nearly a century earlier.[39]

When postmodernism finally reached the hospital, it took on a second expression, functional deconstruction. It fractured the hospital into *parts* that were then redistributed elsewhere (or sometimes elsewhere on the same campus) – in the community. The former puzzle pieces of the hospital – not unlike an iceberg breaking apart – were recast as freestanding outpatient diagnostic and treatment centers. As fragments of a former whole, they became dialysis centers, primary care clinics, ophthalmology centers, heart institutes, emergicare centers, oncology centers, dental clinics, pediatric care clinics, sports medicine clinics, wellness centers, hospices, and so on.[40] Functional deconstruction and (new) residentialism occurred due to a similar yet different set of circumstances. The best of these places expressed a critical regionalism and local vernacular while simultaneously keying-in to broader national and global trends in healthcare.

Sadly, tens of thousands of poorly designed freestanding clinics and wellness centers have been built in the U.S. during the past twenty-five years. Most of these missed opportunities were built in suburban roadside strip malls and in 'medical malls'.[41] Most, unfortunately, were constructed as a direct result of functional deconstruction, but they had little to do with any sort of genuine sense of place. These buildings made a lot of money for some hospital organization, but they contributed little if anything to the quality of the built environment or to deeper, more resonant aspects of local culture. They were a far cry from a place where anyone would want to hang out, compared to if the clinic, say, had been built on a pedestrian-scaled town square next to an outdoor performance stage or as an integral part of a shopping arcade in the city center.

Tens of thousands of these healthcare non-places contributed mightily to sprawl, cultural rootlessness, and the ever-outward reaching tentacles of senseless development. Why does a hospital or clinic have to be built way out at the suburban fringe? Why not at the center of the town? What about the sustainable design precedent set by Wright, Schindler, and others? What about the merits of place, of civic life, of a critical regionalism in architecture?[42] A paradigmatic shift toward the rejection of sprawl and an embrace of place is now underway across the healthcare landscape, but it is still in its infancy. These three dimensions in healthcare architecture will aid in this search:

- *Site* – buildings for healthcare that are carefully composed and in harmony with one another and with high priority accorded to environmental stewardship. Their *civic footprint* extends far beyond the physical parameters of the building or campus site.
- *Landscape* – buildings for healthcare that reject suburban sprawl. High priority is given to locating hospitals and allied healthcare facilities in urban and town centers and in so dong contributing to a broader *sense of place* in harmony with the community's indigenous cultural fabric.
- *Nature* – buildings for healthcare that express and celebrate the *therapeutic amenity* inherent in the natural environment. This can occur at all levels of inquiry from the scale of the site to that of an individual room.

These three tenets are about the search for authenticity. The over-homogenization and widespread inauthentic debasement of the everyday built environment must be rejected. Placemaking calls for far more than a simplistic mischaracterization of cute, poorly fabricated vernacular motifs, construction methods, and materials, i.e. synthetic stucco in New Mexico, or fake slate roof tiles in Maine as if the clinic were a Taco Bell outlet. This theme is reprised later (see Chapters 6, 7, and 8). In sum, innovative healthcare environments – from the scale of site, landscape, to that of a room – deserve thoughtful care and consideration to people, history, local precedent, nature, *genius loci*, vernacular cultural traditions, and above all, authenticity.

The evolving patient room and PCU

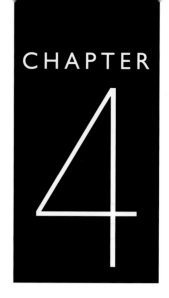

Human beings prefer environments and spatial conditions that provide safety, intrinsic meaning, and value. These timeless predilections manifest, at the most fundamental level of daily existence, in our species' survival instincts – as we attend to matters of life and death. This need for survivability is at the core of human experience. When one becomes ill and is hospitalized, uncertainty reigns. This uncertainty makes it difficult to predict what will happen next, and can result in isolation, alienation, and depression on the part of the patient.[1] The hospital environment can have a bearing on these outcomes in terms of the patient's level of acceptance of, and satisfaction with, its physical appearance and design. One facet, the role of the private room during hospitalization, continues to be a source of much attention with respect to the patient and the degree of control he or she experiences.[2] Privacy and safety have grown in importance to be considered precious commodies – entitlements – and their absence has been associated with patient deficits in emotional outlook, attitude, and health status.

The debate over the role of privacy and safety in patient well-being, and particularly in the context of the architecture of the patient room, has a long history within the history of the hospital.[3] The debate over their influence as healing agents has been at the center, and of that of its spacial context, the patient care unit (PCU), since the nineteenth century. Recently, the merits of the private room and the privacy and safety it affords have been pitted directly against other options. But this topic has challenged architects and their clients for 150 years. Johns Hopkins, founder of the hospital and medical school that bears his name, left funds in 1873 for the construction of a medical center that would rival the best in the world.[4] He consulted closely with his architects on the matter of patient privacy and safety but at the time the need for patient privacy, especially in a private room, was considered secondary to the need for proper indoor air quality and adequate ventilation as a means to control the spread of infection.[5]

Florence Nightingale believed that single-bed patient rooms were unsanitary, i.e. unsafe, and caused the spread of infection because they were so small and confining (Figure 4.1).[6] She considered fresh air, cleanliness, and openness as far more important than privacy and whether or not *it* was a source of patients' stress, outlook, or satisfaction. In a large open-plan ward proper air circulation within could be monitored better, she reasoned, and noise could more easily be kept to a minimum, reducing the role of these two variables as a source of stress.[7] This was considered a strict

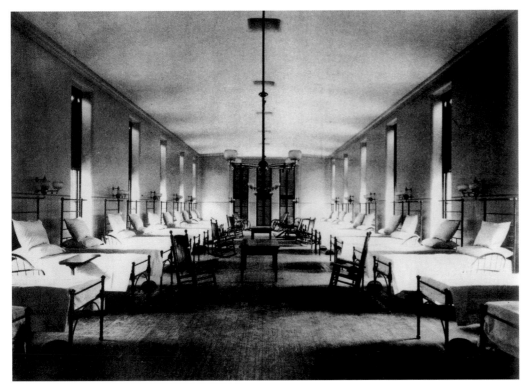

4.1 Inpatient Nightingale ward, Johns Hopkins Hospital, Baltimore, circa 1890

requirement for a state-of-the-art acute care facility.[8] At Johns Hopkins, the campus plan selected by Dr. John Shaw Billings featured five pavilions built in a row, the foremost priority being that well-ventilated air could freely circulate and recirculate within the open wards.[9] The attached main corridor functioned as a commons, or public area.[10] Hopkins' hospital boasted several different types of wards (including some private rooms), each with a technically advanced ventilation system, and safety issues took precedence over whether the vast majority of patients may or may not have experienced stress or related deficits over the less critical matter of personal privacy.[11]

From 1860 on, Nightingale was a firm non-believer in patient safety and privacy if it meant having to be confined in a small room, alone. Hospitals built in subsequent years for the most part provided some single-bed rooms, primarily for the purpose of isolation and as VIP suites, but the vast majority of configurations were open wards ranging from 4 to 24 patients.[12] The single-bed room in the pre-World War II hospital was championed by those who saw it as the ideal means to achieve isolation for victims of plague, leprosy, violent outbreaks, tuberculosis, and those who championed it for socio-cultural purposes – and of course for those who could afford to pay for a single-bed room and the privacy that came with it. To its advocates the private room was and remains the ideal to strive for, the gold standard.[13]

Nightingale considered a single-bed patient room as an unnecessary appendage that drew staffing resources away from the vast majority of other patients. As for the upper classes, who could pay for privacy because it signified a certain social stature, Nightingale chided hospitals that furnished their VIP rooms with fine

carpets, drapes, ornamented recliner lounges, and artwork. In 1878, *Harper's* published a view of a room in New York Hospital that aptly fitted this description. By comparison, a single-bed inpatient room in the pay ward at Johns Hopkins was somewhat more functional in its amenities (Figure 4.2):

> Thirteen rooms on each of the two pay floors are singles, and one is a two-bed room. The pay wards were in a building of their own, as were the single rooms of the isolating ward, a very different form bristling with ventilation. The isolating ward was based on Folsom's plan. Each isolating room … has its own fireplace and chimney, and the bed stood on a floor with 5,000 quarter-inch holes in it, the object being to have a large amount of air pass constantly upwards … Johns Hopkins' forward-looking plans were initiated in other hospitals even before its buildings were finished. In this one institution were combined the plush housing of private pay hospitals with the stripped, utilitarian common wards of the voluntary charity hospital – but not in the same building.[14]

As early as 1908 an all-private-room hospital was in operation at the King's Daughters Hospital in Temple, Texas, for paying and non-paying patients alike.[15] Other experiments at the time resulted in the first hospitals with a row of semi-private rooms with the bath/shower room on the inboard (corridor) side of the rooms.[16] By the 1960s the racetrack nursing unit configuration dominated the hospital industry in the U.S. although the ward remained the dominant form in most other places.[17] Hospitals by then were being built in both the public and private sectors with a higher percentage of private

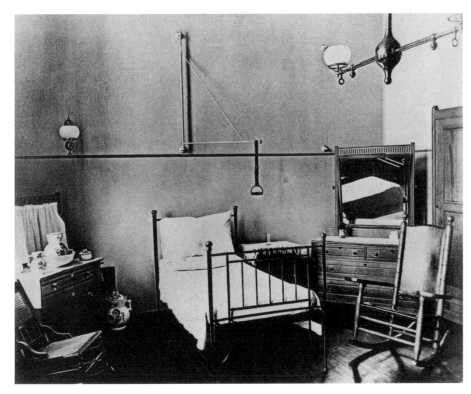

4.2 Private inpatient room, Johns Hopkins Hospital, circa 1890. Freestanding furnishings (in addition to the bed) included chairs, dresser, and side table

rooms.[18] Currently, well-being in the PCU and the patient room is predicated on a combination of influences including:

1 *Environmental control* – temperature, air quality, ambient humidity levels and the presence of non-toxic furnishings, building materials, and finishes.
2 *Aesthetics and appearance* – the visual setting, its formal attributes and ambiance.
3 *Patterns of occupancy* – the spatial and temporal movement of people and supplies and the ability to maintain spatial and cognitive control.
4 *Maintenance and upkeep* – ability to maintain a clean, sterile care setting devoid of contamination, and the resources required to sustain this outcome.
5 *Scale and configuration* – volume, size and massing from the overall building to the nursing unit and inpatient room.
6 *Daylighting, nature, and view* – transmission of natural light to the interior, contact with nature, landscape, and view amenity.
7 *Site context and orientation* – hospital setting, whether in a dense urban to suburban to rural location, and the orientation of interior spaces to exterior environs.
8 *Socio-cultural influences* – the function of culture, race, ethnicity, social class, and family influence in the patient experience.

These eight contextual factors define key physical features and the overall quality of the PCU and the inpatient care experience. Taken together, and when considered in direct relation to privacy and safety, a more complete picture is revealed of the role of the built environment on occupant well-being during hospitalization. *Privacy*

is an umbrella condition, or state, consisting of the sum total of five interrelated dimensions: auditory privacy (sound), visual privacy (sight), tactile privacy (touch), spatial privacy (personal space), and olfactory privacy (smell). In the patient room, this translates into whether the room is sufficiently quiet (sound), whether it affords a sufficient amount of visual privacy from outside the room either from the outdoors or from the adjacent interior corridor (sight), whether there is a sufficient amount of territorial control over space so that personal possessions are not disturbed (touch), whether there is a sufficient amount of physical space in the room (personal space), and whether the patient is sufficiently buffered from unwanted aromas and scents (smell).

These variables play out in numerous scenarios. These scenarios are the net outcome of various combinations of the five dimensions of privacy combined with various permutations of the eight contextual factors that define the form and function of the setting. Therefore, this matrix expresses eight form/function factors (8) x five (5) privacy type factors. These forty scenarios form the basis of person–environment transactions that play out with great fluidity on a daily basis in the patient care setting in a hospital.

Critical discourse on the inpatient room and the patient care unit has come a long way in the past decade. At present the patient housing realm is the subject of considerable systemic analysis especially with regards to its *digital tectonics*. Since 2000, experiments have been undertaken on nearly every surface and feature – wall surfaces, floors, windows, ceilings, color, windows, screens, lighting, built-ins – with every major interior element examined (except for the tectonics of the patient bed, which somehow still unfortunately remain outside the design purview of architects). For example, with respect to the

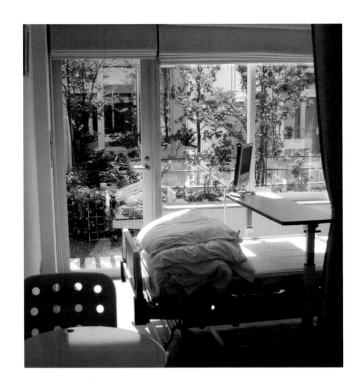

4.3 Inpatient room and adjacent landscaped courtyard, Katta Public General Hospital, Japan, 2007

4.4 Courtyard and exterior mounted sunscreens, Robert Koch Clinical Center, Leipzig, Germany, 2004

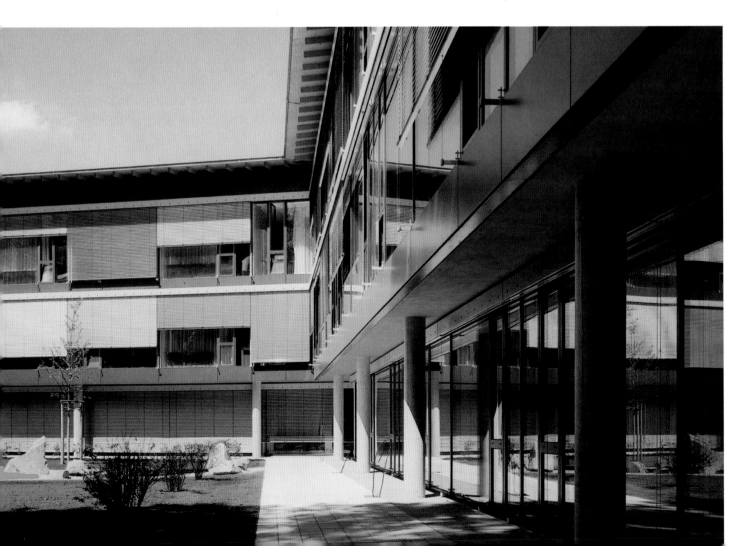

4.5 Sliding doors, Southwest Washington Medical Center, Vancouver, Washington, 2007

4.6 Inpatient room, Southwest Washington Medical Center

4.7 Built-in desk, inpatient room, Southwest Washington Medical Center

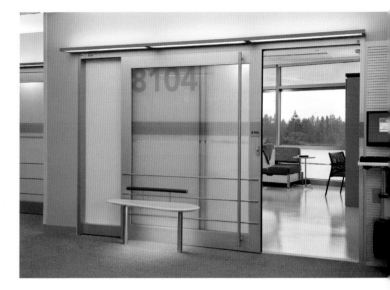

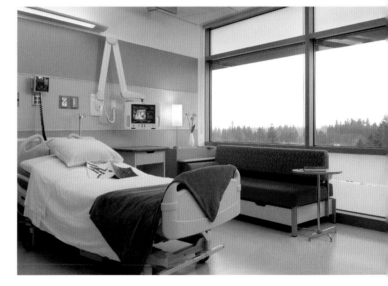

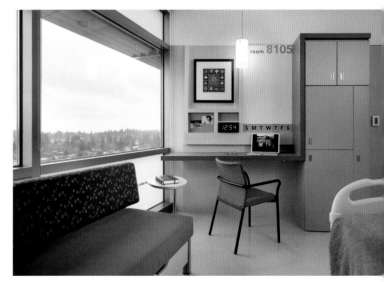

provision of visual privacy, the window aperture and screen has been receiving critical reappraisal in a number of countries. In the 2-bed room at the Katta General Hospital in Japan (see Chapter 8), a door with full height glass provides natural daylight and access to a landscaped roof terrace (Figure 4.3). The interior window screen is operated manually. Window screen tectonics are advancing as well. The Robert Koch Clinical Center in Leipzig, Germany (2001–2004) designed by HPP Laage & Partners, features electronically controlled exterior sunscreen devices. The patient rooms overlook a landscaped courtyard in this 144-bed addition to an existing acute care hospital. The second and third floors house the nursing units. The windows are recessed beneath extended overhangs, and full height apertures are provided in every patient room, and which include an operable window. Transparency is achieved by means of full height glass window walls (Figure 4.4).[19]

Exterior screening devices such as at the Koch Center are being integrated with other design elements. The Southwest Washington Medical Center, in Vancouver, Washington, open since 1858, was the first permanent hospital in the Pacific Northwest. The eight-level E.W. and Mary Firstenburg Tower (2004–2007), designed by NBBJ-Seattle, houses a heart and vascular center, 15 surgical suites, and 144 all-private patient rooms. Sawtooth walls in the hallways help to contain corridor noise and are sheathed with sound attenuating materials. Bathrooms are pivot-free, with wide openings.[20] All patient rooms are *same-handed*, meaning the headwall is on the same wall in every room (see Chapters 5 and 7). Two central nursing stations are linked with decentralized bedside and individual monitoring stations in the corridor, next to the rooms (Figure 4.5). A sliding door with full height glass opens to the left side, behind a fixed seating element. The staff workstation is to the right of the door. Sliding doors, so common in contemporary Japanese hospitals, remain rare in the West. Within the room at Southwest Washington, a bed for family members is positioned along the exterior window wall parallel to the patient's bed (Figure 4.6). The footwall houses a built-in desk and laptop workstation for patient and visitor use. A wood cabinet houses the television and drawers (Figure 4.7). Each bath/shower room was rotated at a 20-degree angle, creating the sawtooth pattern, in plan (Figure 4.8).[21]

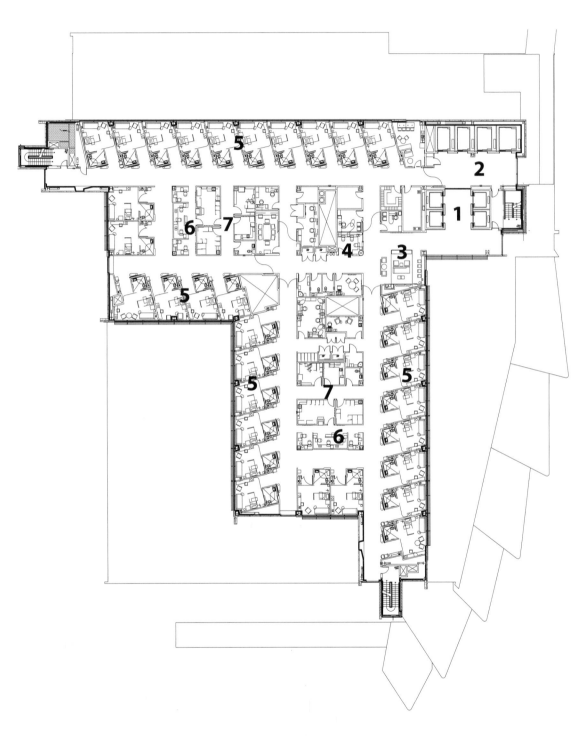

LEVEL 7 - LEGEND

1.	VISITOR ELEVATOR	4.	RECEPTION
2.	PATIENT/ SUPPORT	5.	PATIENT ROOM
	ELEVATORS	6.	NURSE STATION
3.	FAMILY WAITING	7.	STAFF SUPPORT

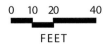

0 10 20   40

FEET

N

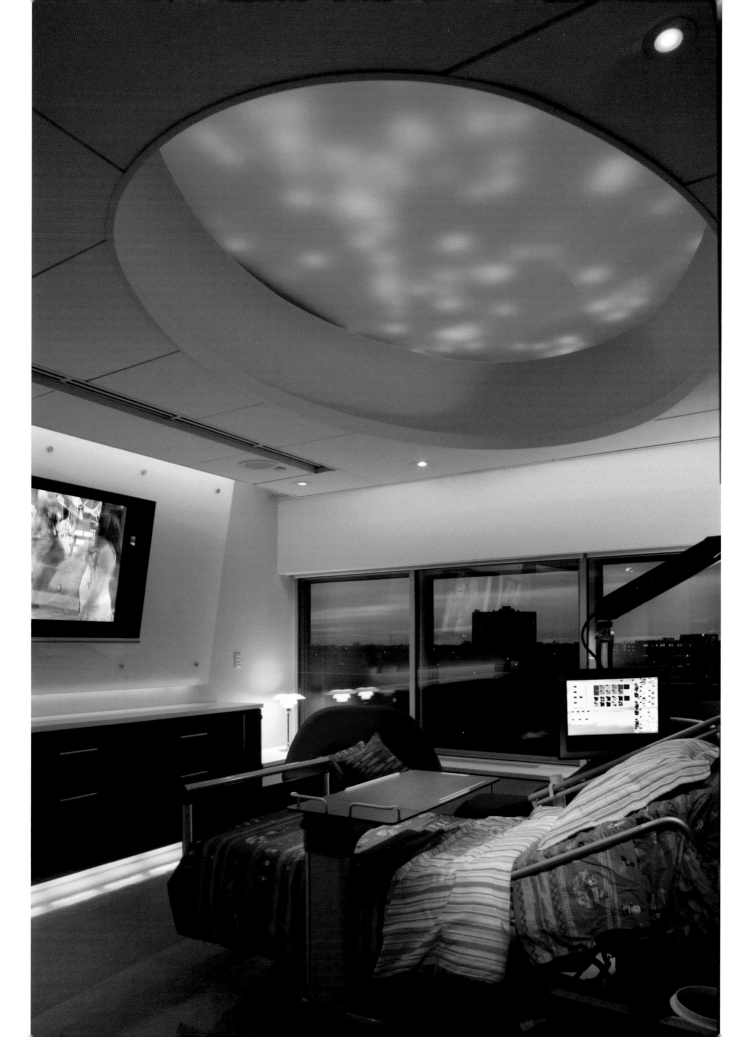

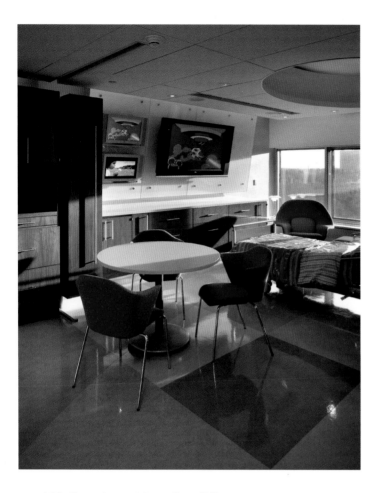

4.10   Parental zone, Adopt-a-Room (AR) prototype

4.11   Food prep amenities, AR prototype

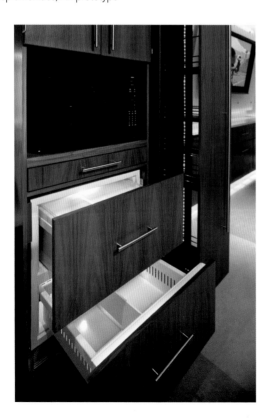

The Adopt-a-Room prototype

In 2006, Perkins+Will, Minneapolis, introduced an innovative patient room prototype for young patients who experience extended hospital stays. Two demonstration installations were built at the University of Minnesota Children's Hospital – Fairview, based on research and design work conducted over a two-year period.[22] The project focused on four aspects of the inpatient experience: sense of control, comfort, connectedness with life beyond the hospital, and family involvement. Multiple rounds of interviews, on site observations, drawings, and scale models were used to elicit users' feedback. The models allowed for furnishings and built-in room elements to be manipulated by the 'users'. Conventional room configurations were eschewed. Instead, the family zone was located on the inboard side of the room adjacent to the caregiver zone. This allowed for the direct sharing of information between parent and caregiver, and parents can come and go without disturbing the child by having to cross directly in front of him or her.

A foyer provides visual and acoustical privacy. Extra-absorptive walls mask unwanted noises from the hallway and bathroom, similar to what is found in a home theater. The patient bed area is beneath a recessed circular ceiling; its multiple lighting scenarios are controllable from the bed (Figure 4.9). As for its tectonics, the ceiling houses twenty LED lights to vary the entire room's color, with the recess able to simulate a blue afternoon sky, dusk, or a night sky, complete with stars. Fifteen theatrical 'scenes' (visual representations) are possible in this ceiling. A large flat screen television/monitor with two side-wall-mount monitors is for DVD and Internet use. The patient bed is located near to the door to the bathroom. The headwall is curved and sheathed in wood panels in order to provide the patient with semi-enclosure and to mask medical equipment and monitors. The nerve center for the room is located in a computer closet on the corridor wall outside the room. However, parents can control remotely the room's tectonics, and can modify ambient room conditions while their child is asleep or away from the room. For parents, additional autonomy is provided in the form of a computer workstation with a glass sliding door. Since parent overnight stays are common, the parent/visitor bed can be moved to be parallel with and set at the same height as the child's bed. This was requested by children during the pre-design process.

A computer workstation for parents plus a table and chairs is provided in the parental zone (Figure 4.10). This is a 'den' or

4.12   Headwall amenities, AR prototype

4.13   Transitional zone in corridor, AR prototype

4.14   Bath/shower room amenities, AR prototype

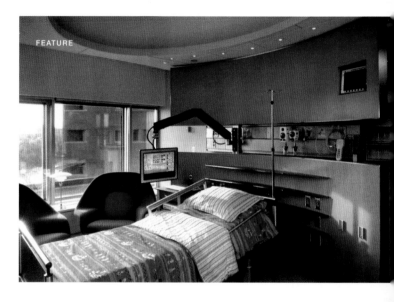

retreat space within the room, allowing for relaxation. It contains comfortable seating, a refrigerator, microwave, and coffeemaker because the research indicated that engagement with food and beverages contributes to a residentialist atmosphere, not unlike that at home (Figure 4.11). A HEPA filter controls odors that may otherwise emanate from the food prep area. Parents preferred this as it precluded the need for them to make frequent trips away from the room. An unusual amount of storage space is provided thereby making it possible for a parent to 'move in' with clothing and personal artifacts during their child's hospitalization. This also functions to further replicate the home environment. This amount of storage space does not exist in the typical inpatient room at this time.

In terms of digitization, the room supports an usually high degree of occupant control, particularly of the room's aesthetic/prosthetic

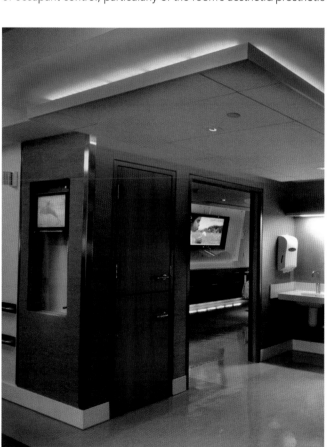

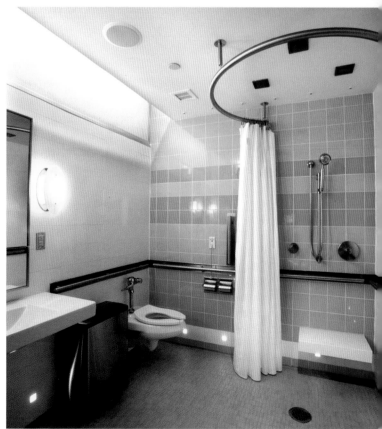

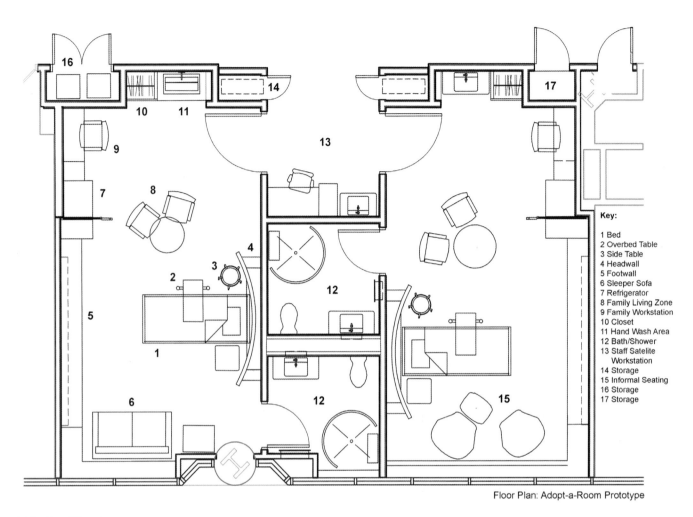

Floor Plan: Adopt-a-Room Prototype

Key:
1 Bed
2 Overbed Table
3 Side Table
4 Headwall
5 Footwall
6 Sleeper Sofa
7 Refrigerator
8 Family Living Zone
9 Family Workstation
10 Closet
11 Hand Wash Area
12 Bath/Shower
13 Staff Satelite
   Workstation
14 Storage
15 Informal Seating
16 Storage
17 Storage

4.15 Plan, AR prototype

personality options. At the bedside, a universal LCD screen with touchpad empowers the patient, and others. The patient can control the lighting, light-block window shades, temperature, and media technology options (Figure 4.12). The footwall is an oversized plasma screen and one screen can show images of exterior public areas of the hospital. At the front door to the room, a LCD panel allows for the display of photos, artwork, and messages. This screen allows staff to convey messages to family and visitors, affords additional privacy, and controls the occurrence of nosocomial infection (Figure 4.13). All furniture is freestanding and able to be relocated based on family and patient preferences. Tables are also height adjustable for ease of use. The bath/shower room features an ergonomically designed sink, shower, lighting fixture, materials and colors, and continuous grab bars (Figure 4.14). The complexity of this high-tech patient room is such that each family and patient is actually provided with a 'user's manual' (see Chapter 7) that demonstrates, in the form of an instructional video, how to 'operate' the room (Figure 4.15).

The Clemson experiments

Healthcare providers through the years have taken the extra step to fund the construction of full-scale mock-ups of various diagnostic, treatment, and patient rooms to test their functionality and performance. This has been done as part of new construction and in renovation projects in many countries. Staff, patients, and visitors are able to evaluate a mock-up and the feedback provided can be incorporated in the design process. This technique has been proven to be cost effective and a source of valuable information. Successive iterations are possible whereby a mock-up can be altered iteratively in order to achieve the best fit between the designed space and its functionality. An evidence-based research and design team at Clemson University in 2006 launched an innovative research project sponsored by the Spartanburg Regional Health Care System, in South Carolina, to fundamentally rethink the role and function of the digital inpatient room. The prototype that emerged was the product of an iterative evaluative process with staff and patients. The

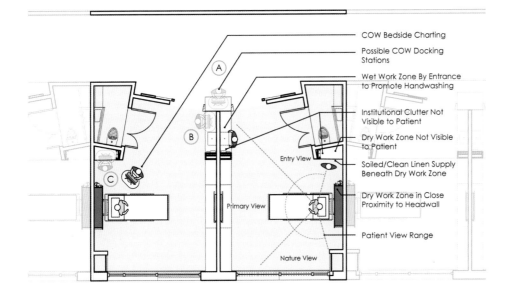

COW Bedside Charting

Possible COW Docking Stations

Wet Work Zone By Entrance to Promote Handwashing

Institutional Clutter Not Visible to Patient

Dry Work Zone Not Visible to Patient

Soiled/Clean Linen Supply Beneath Dry Work Zone

Dry Work Zone in Close Proximity to Headwall

Patient View Range

4.16 Annotated plan, inpatient room prototype, Clemson University evidence-based design initiative, 2006

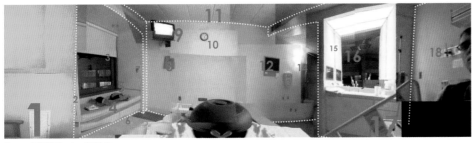

Current SRHS Footwall Clutter

1	Uncomfortable bedside chair	10	Time difficult to read
2	Peeling, yellowish wallpaper	11	Ceiling tiles stained, institutional
3	No patient control of shading	12	Noise of chalkboard painful
4	Poor insulation makes 'bed' cold	13	Sharps container in plain view
5	Window view angled, poor	14	Glove boxes tacked on wall
6	Storage too small, not secure	15	Mammoth paper towel dispenser
7	Yellow light hard on patient's eyes	16	Light off mirror intense
8	Guestbook covered with dust	17	Bed uncomfortable, stiff
9	TV small and hard to see	18	Headwall gases exposed, cluttered

4.17 Examples of institutional clutter that function as sources of stress for patients, visitors, family members, and staff

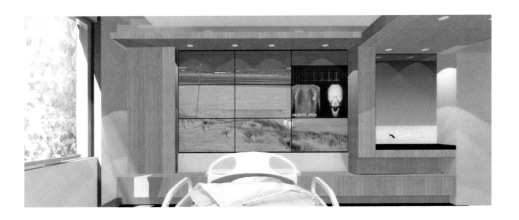

4.18 Footwall amenities, inpatient room prototype (IRP), Clemson evidence-based design initiative

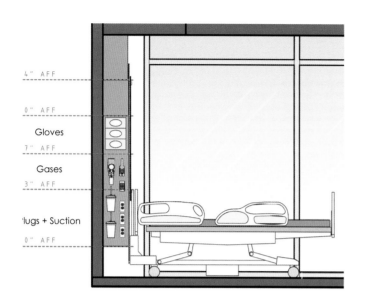

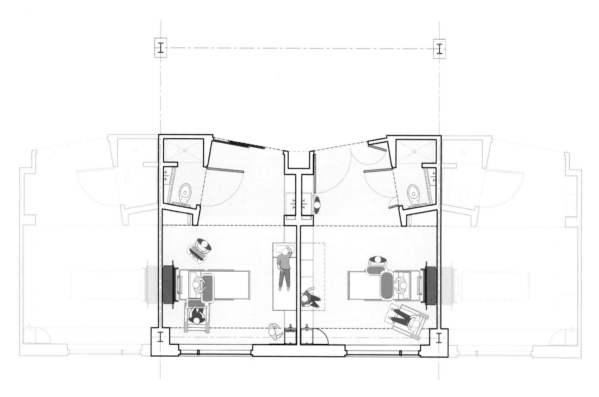

4.19   Section, Clemson IRP

4.20   Plan, Clemson IRP

4.21   Bedside/overbed smart table, Clemson IRP

4.22   Translucent headwall panel, Clemson IRP

findings were translated into the design of the patient rooms in the 48-bed Village Hospital at Pelham, in South Carolina (2005–2008), designed by Karlsberger, of Columbus, Ohio.[23]

Among its noteworthy features are visitor amenities, natural light, patients' interaction with various room components, and an innovative solution for the bath/shower room. This hospital is planned for a maximum number of 150 beds. The prototype chassis is intended to be adaptable for all acute care and telemetry beds. A 3,000 square foot facility was built in on the campus at Pelham specifically for the full-scale testing of various prototype room configurations and their attendant components and furnishings. The four goals were to provide a restorative care setting, to rethink the relationship between caregiver, patient, and family, to provide a functional and efficient care space, and to design for adaptability. The entry and sliding glass doors are designed to optimize sight lines and access, and a staff handwash sink is located near to the door. The ceiling is lower to create a threshold transition from the corridor to the patient bed and family zones within the room.

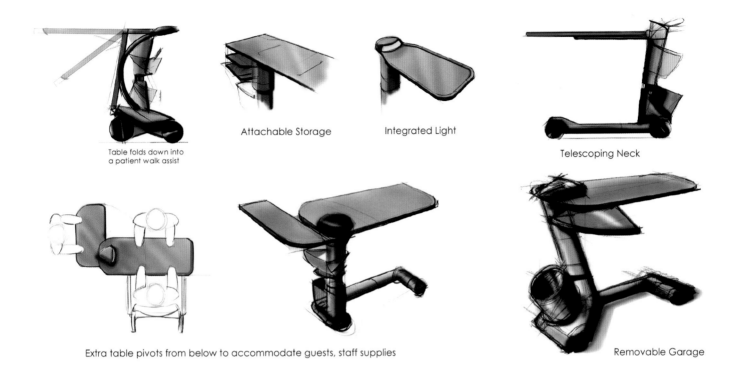

Table folds down into
a patient walk assist

Attachable Storage

Integrated Light

Telescoping Neck

Extra table pivots from below to accommodate guests, staff supplies

Removable Garage

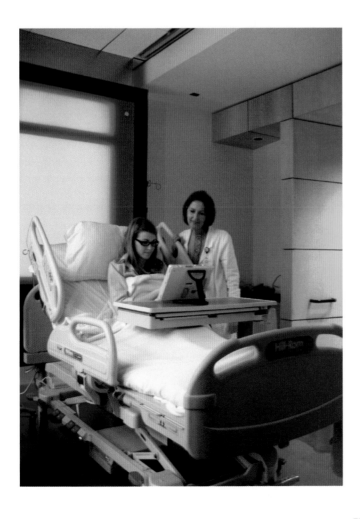

The bath/shower room is located on the headwall to allow for direct access, whether by the patient or staff-assisted. The standard commode chair was eliminated, allowing closer proximity to the bed. This distance is further reduced because the bed pivots towards the commode. Three staff work zones were identified: a mobile staff zone accommodates a computer on wheels (COW) for staff use and medication dispensing while allowing for eye contact with the patient (see Chapter 7), a wet work zone and the aforementioned sink at the entry to the room to promote hand washing upon entering and exiting the room, and a staff storage and dry zone housed at the headwall and out of the sight line of the patient, when in the bed (Figure 4.16). A primary objective was the elimination of visual distractions, or *institutional clutter*. A post-occupancy assessment illustrates this condition (Figure 4.17). The footwall was conceived as the 'hearth' of the room. It is the visual focal point for the patient, is free from visual clutter, and provides seating, storage, and a forward opening bed for family use during overnight stays (Figure 4.18).[24]

The headwall is the most equipment-intensive fixed feature part of an inpatient room. For this reason, considerable staff and patient input was elicited. The placement of the headwall equipment was determined through extensive nurse testing of numerous preliminary mock-ups (Figure 4.19). Panels conceal some apparatus while other items are revealed not unlike on the dashboard of a high-end sports car. Objects are positioned to minimize bending and reaching by staff, and the headwall can be reconfigured as staff needs evolve over time.

The overbed table is a critical element in patient care. It is typically the closest bedside element to the patient, houses myriad personal care artifacts (MP3 player, food, laptop, tissues, eyeglasses, and so on), and is used on a 24/7 basis by the patient and others (Figure 4.20). A proposal currently in testing is multifunctional. It is at once a table that can transform into a walking assistance device, it has an onboard light, a telescoping neck, an extra table that pivots outward at an orthogonal angle for use by family, visitors, and staff, and also an onboard, removable trash receptacle (Figure 4.21). Every effort has been made to incorporate recycled materials and furnishings in this prototype room, including cork flooring, recycled fiber carpet, maple panels, low-e glass, and a biodegradable *EcoResin* headwall panel. All temperature and lighting controls, including the recessed ceiling above the bed, can be controlled by the patient, including the backlit headwall panel. This translucent panel can be activated by the patient in any one of twelve colors (Figure 4.22).[25]

Planetree and beyond

With the nursing station so pivotal in the life of the PCU environment, it became the first target for reinvention. The long, drab, sterile-looking *infinity corridors* of most hospitals together with the nursing station were in need of complete reconsideration through the lens of postmodernism.[26] Previously, harsh, fluorescent light fixtures were seemingly everywhere, with drab color schemes (white, white, and more white) and the most perfunctory accommodations for equipment, supplies, and people. Many seminal innovations in PCU design stemmed from the pioneering *Planetree* program launched in 1985 at the Pacific Presbyterian Medical Center in San Francisco. The basic premise of the first Planetree case study, a prototype 13-bed unit, had been to radically alter the design of the nursing station, the nursing service core, and the semi-public realm. This was achieved by adding room-to-room windows, removing walls, providing lounges for family members and visitors, and through the creation of a deinstitutional, residential aesthetic. This work is discussed in detail in the book *Putting Patients First*.[27] The Planetree demonstration projects in hospitals across the U.S. and beyond were highly influential to what is widely known today as *patient-centered care*.[28]

The nine elements of Planetree patient-centered care are: the importance of human interaction, informing and empowering diverse populations including the creation of consumer health libraries and patient education, healing partnerships centered around the family and friends, nutrition and the nurturing aspects of food, spirituality and drawing upon inner resources in healing, human touch as an essential medium for interpersonal communication, the therapeutic value of the healing arts, the integration of complementary and alternative medicine into conventional care theory and practice, and the restorative role of architecture and interior environments in the healing process.[29]

Privacy, safety and the incomplete case for the all-private-room hospital

Planetree had a major impact in the reinvention of the nursing station within the PCU but somewhat less of an impact regarding the reinvention of the inpatient room. Planetree hospitals placed the family in a more prominent role compared to the past. Family members used to be considered as visitors, as opposed to partners, in the healing experience. Often, access to the patient was therefore limited. Patient and family centered care is grounded in mutually beneficial partnerships among the patient, family, and healthcare professional. It centers on the positive dimensions this brings to the healing process. It involves educating the family about the patient's injury or disease, and how the pre- and post-hospitalization phase can be more fully understood by this knowledge.[30] Hospitals in the U.S. have gradually become more receptive and far more now allow family members to stay overnight. Children's hospitals had been at the forefront of this trend, i.e. the Planetree demonstration hospitals, and the Adopt-a-Room prototype.[31]

The Center for Health Design's *Pebble Project*, begun in 2000, extended the innovative philosophy and precedent established by the Planetree projects.[32] The Pebble Projects were directly inspired by Planetree and sought to push the envelope in this regard.[33] Fifty active Pebble Project case studies have been completed to date (plus twelve 'alumni' institutions) and the settings where these have occurred include many large healthcare systems in the U.S. Nearly 40 percent of these case studies are now open, with another 40 percent currently under construction (2009). Within the mainstream evidence-based design research community in the U.S., including the Pebble Project case studies, it has been all but concluded that the all-private-room hospital is the superior option and this recommendation is based on these five points:

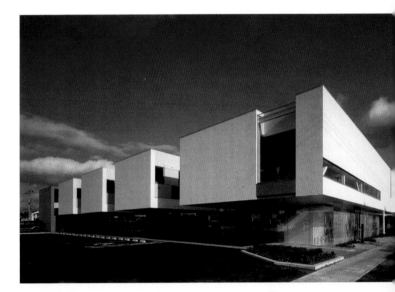

4.23 Sekii Maternity Hospital (2000–2001), Sekii, Japan. Inpatient suites appear as if floating above a semi-transparent support base

4.24 Inpatient semi-private rooms, Sekii Maternity Hospital

- *Nosocomial infection control* – infections spread between patients and the longer the patient remains in the hospital the incidence of hospital-acquired nosocomial infection rate increases.
- *Control of personal space* – cognitive and spatial control is highest when the patient and family are in a space of their own, undisturbed by outsiders, and where persons unfamiliar to the patient and family do not share the same zone of personal space.
- *Provisions for family and visitors* – ample space is available for overnight stays by family and friends not dissimilar from what would occur at home. Multiple zones of personal space exist for occupants' use.
- *Minimization of disruptions* – the abatement of unwanted noise, excessive, spontaneous events, and the maximization of privacy for the patient, family, and visitors. Staff monitoring occurs at the nursing station, bedside, or in an alcove adjacent to the inpatients' room.
- *Acuity adaptability* – the inpatient room and its tectonics can be reconfigured for varying levels of patient acuity levels and technology support requirements. This requires a private room that can be modified to step up or step down in its level of acuity-support.[34]

Japan is a mountainous island nation, and 90 percent of the nation's population live on little more than 10 percent of the land. For this reason, through the centuries, Japanese cultural traditions have emphasized making the most of tight quarters. This remains equally the case in the domestic milieu as in the hospital milieu. At the Sekii Maternity Hospital, in Sekii, Japan (2000–2001), designed by Atelier Hitoshi Abe, patient suites are housed above a transparent base, housing all administrative, diagnostic, and treatment services (Figure 4.23). The pateint suites are cantilevered outward, projecting as a series of bandwidths from within the building, appearing as if afloat on water. The upper level houses thirteen 4-bed suites, fourteen 1-bed rooms, and four 2-bed rooms. In the 4-bed open suites the bath/shower room is situated as a buffer zone. The fenestration pattern on the outer wall is highly orchestrated, with small-framed views accessible from both a supine viewing angle and also from an upright standing position. Privacy curtains are provided between beds, and the room conveys an inviting communal ambience despite the fact that four patients occupy the same room (Figure 4.24).

At the Martini Hospital (2004–2007) in the Netherlands (see Chapter 3) a typical, 32-bed PCU is comprised of a complement

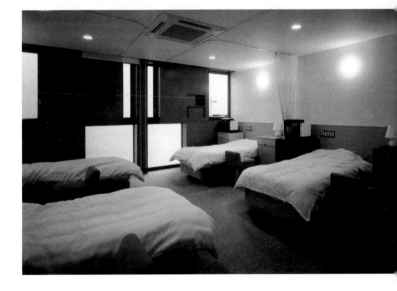

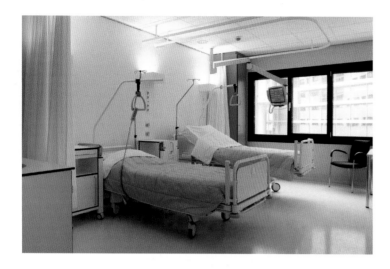

4.25 Semi-private inpatient room, Martini Hospital, Groningen, the Netherlands

4.26 PCU, Martini Hospital

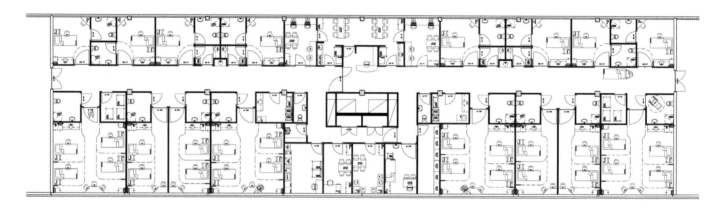

of 4-bed patient rooms and eight single-bed rooms. The 4-bed room has a minimalist headwall design in a white room, with built-in cabinets that provide a modicum of color. Minimal accommodations are provided for the family. This room would be considered sparse and dysfunctional by American standards due to its non-homelike ambiance and the fact that more than one patient is in the same room (Figure 4.25). The nursing station is located at the center of the unit (Figure 4.26). These two examples of the Sekii Maternity and Martini hospitals underscore, in many ways, the vast difference between current American, European and Asian thinking.

Infection control is a core American justification for the all-private-room hospital.[35] Despite this, relatively little direct empirical evidence directly correlates patient room design (whether private or semi-private rooms) to increased rates of nosocomial infection.[36] In actuality, other factors can have far more of an impact, principally the frequency of handwashing by caregivers prior to engaging in patient care activities, and this has been proven to influence more significantly the spread of infection within hospitals than whether one or more patients share the same room.[37] In fact, it was recently reported that the empirical evidence remains inconclusive on this point.[38] Given this, the provision of a well-located handwashing sink in the room can achieve the same outcome, rather than isolating every patient in his or her own separate room.[39]

In reality, a growing number of U.S. hospitals need more than ever to maximize the number of paying patients admitted every day in order to maintain overall financial solvency. Similarly, the NHS in the U.K. now fosters between-hospital competition. Understandably, nosocomial infections can delay patient recovery and discharge, thereby resulting in fewer available beds.[40] Moreover, in the U.S. beginning in 2009, Medicare (the federal government health insurer provided for the elderly and disabled) no longer reimbursed the costs of preventable conditions, including nosocomial infections and medical errors resulting from a hospital stay. A highly publicized report from the *Institute of Medicine* in Washington D.C. cited medical errors as a leading cause of death and injury in the United States, claiming approximately 98,000 lives in any given year.[41] In fact, deaths in hospitals due to preventable adverse events of hospitalization in 2008 exceeded the number attributable to motor vehicle accidents (43,458), breast cancer (42,297), or AIDS (16,516). The rationale supporting single occupancy rooms also stems from the notion that they are safer because they eliminate the possibility of errors and omissions associated with the mishandling of charts, medications, and dietary regimens.

People – not architecture – are responsible for such errors. Indeed, medical errors still occur in private patient rooms despite the absence of a roommate to potentially distract or confuse the caregiver. Human factors, particularly fatigue and stress, are documented contributors to medical mistakes. *The New York Times* recently reported the negative influence disruptive doctors often create and the mistakes that may occur as a result:

> A survey of health care workers at 102 nonprofit hospitals from 2004 to 2007 found that 67 percent of respondents said they thought there was a link between disruptive behavior and medical mistakes, and 18 percent said they knew of a mistake that occurred because of an obnoxious doctor … another survey by the Institute for Safe Medication Practices, a nonprofit organization, found that 40 percent of hospital staff members reported having been so intimidated by a doctor that they did not share their concerns about orders for medications that appeared to be incorrect. As a result, 7 percent said they contributed to a medication error.[42]

A hundred and fifty years ago Nightingale prescribed light-filled open wards to facilitate patient surveillance access, and patient safety. The private room, in her view, represented its antithesis, separating each patient into their own compartmentalized experience – world – and thereby closing down informal social interactions among patients. In the contemporary sense, a private patient room is seen as delimiting patient transfers due to infections and personality conflicts, and this thereby lowers the risk of the patient acquiring an infection during transfer. Also, associated demands on staff may be less, with fewer misdirections and miscues, and less overall confusion caused by transfers. These scenarios, repeated in thousands of hospitals, exist independently of the debate over the private versus the semi-private room. To this extent, even the most strident proponents for all-private-room hospitals concede that further studies and demonstration projects are needed to fully ascertain the safety advantages of private rooms.[43]

Core determinants of semi-pivatisation include the following:

- *Expense* – from a capital expenditure perspective, the all-private-room hospital may dramatically expand the overall building's size and cost, i.e. its height and/or its footprint, in contradiction with sustainable site planning and design principles. This can place further strain on already stretched capital and staff resources. Second, all-private-room nursing units result in greater staff walking distances, an average of fifteen feet or more per bed compared to semi-private-room PCUs which average only eight feet of corridor

per bed.[44] Therefore, all-private PCUs require nurses to travel greater distances to monitor fewer patients whilst semi-private units by comparison reduce nurse travel distances for patient surveillance and access, thereby streamlining care and response times.[45]

- *Privacy and personal control* – lighting levels, spatial props, furnishings, noise, temperature, daylight, view, and so on are believed to influence patient outcomes.[46] The inability to adjust one's immediate personal space is asserted to impact adversely the healing process and to manifest in adverse behavioral outcomes including sleep disorders and noncompliance with medication regimens.[47] The overriding consensus at present in the U.S. is that patient control is greater in private rooms, as patients can adjust lighting and sound levels according to their needs, without having to be concerned about the needs of others.[48] However, in the digital age patients sharing a room can in fact control their immediate surroundings – air quality, lighting, view, screens, television, for example – relatively simply and probably more easily than ever before in history. Beyond this, anyway, is it not logical to assume that every patient upon admittance to a hospital inherently accepts that they will have to relinquish *some* degree of privacy and personal control?
- *The family* – since 2000, the family has assumed an increasingly higher profile in the healing process, in many countries. The social support provided by family members and friends is believed to have a positive impact on patient outcomes. Contemporary patient room designs provide for more space and furniture to accommodate the family and others than did their semi-private-room predecessors. However, the support and insight patients and others are able to share in a semi-private room can help one another. From this standpoint this experience of sharing cannot be underestimated or easily dismissed. A recent study found that 'a positive aspect of sharing a room was highlighted by comments that ranged from a sense of support proffered after discussion with the health professional to companionship in an otherwise lonely environment'.[49] Therefore, the family and friends of patients who share a room can serve as an important support network for one another during hospitalization.
- *Socio-cultural factors* – it appears that the *ideal* of privacy underlies the argument for the all-private patient room. Although difficult to define, and therefore difficult to measure scientifically, nearly every advocate for the all-private-room hospital returns to this fundamental issue.[50] However, privacy depends on individuals'

different understanding of the concept within the values and normative behaviors that govern their lives. These vary dramatically between individuals and, more importantly, between different cultures.[51] From a cultural perspective, it is well known that Americans in particular tend to have higher needs for privacy than do members of other cultures.[52] The private patient room therefore is a logical extension of the built landscape within the United States whereas in other parts of the world the multiple-patient ward remains an accepted reality, by and large, as an equivalent expression of those built landscapes. In a recent study in the U.K. it was found that most patients preferred a communal space to an individual one, usually citing anxiety about the fear of isolation as the main reason.[53]

- *Confidentiality and the role of government* – the U.S. federal government enacted legislation in 1998 to protect patient heath information and this law has had significant architectural ramifications. Considerable cost has been incurred as a direct result of the renovations and amenities required to provide adequate provisions for patient confidentiality in healthcare facilities. The *Health Insurance Portability and Accountability Act* (HIPAA) elevated the importance of reasonable safeguards to protect the confidentiality of staff conversations, with and about patients.[54] This legislation further fueled the drive towards the all-private-room hospital. For example, patients who fail to answer questions related to sensitive matters in their medical history completely, or honestly, risk misdiagnosis. Also, a limited exchange with one's physician may result in incomplete or inaccurate information regarding one's condition or options for treatment. Is it believed that being in a private room can alleviate this?

- *The physician* – physician bedside manners further obfuscate patient confidentiality when the caregiver fails to sensitively and fully communicate with the patient. While drawing a cubicle curtain track closed may protect a patient's visual privacy, caregivers must realize that this fails to attenuate sound and accordingly that any and all information shared in confidence ought not to be broadcast in a manner whereby others in the same room can overhear what is said. Patients and their doctors could stand closer instead of from the end of the bed, and proceed to quietly discuss a matter rather than speak in a loud voice for all to hear in the room or beyond.[55] Instead, U.S. hospitals are closing in on legislating the all-private-room hospital as the sole means to ensure patient confidentiality and privacy.

Hospital as hospitality

For better or worse, the debate over privacy remains amorphous and difficult to define with incontrovertible precision. The empirical literature remains inconclusive. Too many studies either rely principally on anecdotal evidence or opinion to frame their core arguments, or utilize research population samples too miniscule to generalize to the broader contexts to which their authors seek to generalize them. Consequently, the architectural profession has anchored itself to a spurious position in the midst of a construction boom, the effects of which will be felt a half century into the future. The consequences of decisions made today extend far beyond the immediate horizon line. The matter of the increasing fiscal and environmental unsustainability of the all-private-room hospital is worth careful re-analysis. Issues of sustainability have come to the forefront of global attention as scientists uncover the consequences so-called human 'progress' has reaped on the environment. The built environment has been exposed as one of the main culprits, responsible for 72 percent of the electricity and 13.6 percent of the potable water consumed annually as well as 39 percent of the carbon dioxide emitted into the atmosphere each year, contributing more than either transportation or industry.[56] In response, the building industry has endeavored to take steps to ameliorate its adverse practices in order to reduce the carbon footprint of the constructed landscape. Despite this, hospitals lag far behind other market sectors.

Meanwhile, the 'directive' for the all-private-room hospital in many ways directly contradicts sustainability – principles that can greatly reduce a hospital's carbon footprint. An all-private-room scenario can increase a hospital's carbon footprint, inevitably resulting in a demand for more resources, both financial and material-wise, to finish and furnish. Energy costs can rise by as much as one-third compared to the alternatives that are available. The uncomfortable truth remains that the demands hospitals place on the environment are necessarily more pronounced than other building types due to their highly specialized and intensive use. However, an all-private-patient-room hospital tends to exacerbate its negative impact on the environment.

The trend of *hospital as hospitality* further exacerbates this dilemma for the healthcare industry, as semi-private rooms and appropriately scaled waiting rooms give way to overscaled private suites, in places featuring materials and furnishings more indicative of a hotel or resort than a hospital. These not only inherently expand the hospital's carbon footprint but also add significantly to costs. Private patient rooms, often more expensive than semi-private rooms, result in higher first-time costs per patient. An analysis of ten nursing units with varying configurations, some featuring exclusively private patient rooms and others a combination of both types, and based on an equivalent unit (per square foot) construction cost, averaged $182,400 per patient, relative to only $122,550 per patient in comparable hospitals' mixed private and semi-private room arrangements.[57]

To compensate for this hospitality bias, many hospitals find it necessary to augment their billings, off-loading their capital investments and quotidian expenses to their patients and their insurance companies. This is also happening in other aspects of hospital operations in the U.S., whereby a patient with insurance currently pays for the patient without insurance. The irrationality of the present situation is apparent as ever larger, more lavish rooms result in ever-higher costs, in turn requiring more beds to offset the initial capital investment. Yet this dictate for all-private-room nursing care unit intrinsically *doubles* the number of rooms necessary for a hospital to defray its costs. This is especially paradoxical relative to the lower costs associated with the semi-private room. An unsustainable, costly cycle of hospital expansionism is being perpetuated and the end of this trend is in clear sight unless something changes.

And what about the nurses who staff the PCU? By 2004, the average age of a nurse in the U.S. had climbed to 43 years of age.[58] Strains on nursing staff stem from high turnover rates (20 percent per year as of 2002) resulting in an overall nursing shortage that directly relates to the quality of patient care and safety. *The Joint Commission on the Accreditation of Healthcare Organizations* (JCAHO) examined 1,609 hospital reports of patient deaths and injuries since 1996 and found that low nursing staff levels were a contributing factor in 24 percent of cases, indicating the troubling implications of this shortage and its future consequences.[59] Ironically, the authors of these reports did not cite the architectural design of the PCU as having a direct bearing on any of this.[60] It would appear that expansive hospital designs with exclusively private rooms would overextend an already overextended nursing profession.

The case for reconsidering the virtues of the semi-private room and open suites of up to six beds may be summarized in these four points:

- *Reduces sensory deprivation* – the patient in a room with one or more other patients can interact with them and their families

and visitors, therefore reducing the loneliness and isolation that may otherwise occur. This is a particular problem among patients who are new to an area and may not have many family or friends nearby. Infection control remains a legitimate concern although no empirical evidence to date has definitively concluded that nursing unit design per se is the cause.

- *Relieves otherwise unsustainable staffing patterns* – with the current shortage of trained R.N.s it is becoming increasingly difficult to fully staff the hospital inpatient care nursing units in the U.S. This is also a growing concern in a number of other countries. Semi-private and mini wards and suites offer a more sustainable and elastic staffing model in the face of growing nursing shortages in the coming decade. The alternative is to have fewer staff personnel stretched more thinly, or to mothball the furthermost rooms when feasible.

- *Reduces otherwise unsustainable construction costs* – it can cost up to 40 percent more to construct an all-private-room hospital unless its total number of rooms is greatly reduced. Difficult trade offs will have to be made between a given hospital's size versus the overall number of rooms. By contrast, a hospital planned and designed for either a majority of semi-private inpatient rooms or a balance between private and semi-private inpatient rooms may offer a more sustainable strategy from a fiduciary perspective. Excessive up-front costs played a similar role in the demise of the interstitial hospital of the late twentieth century.

- *Supports acuity adaptability* – a semi-private (2 bed) inpatient room or suite (3–6 beds) can be reconfigured as patient needs change and as nursing staffing models change. Transprogrammation is one means to achieve this (see Chapter 7). Interior non-structural partitions can be removed and/or relocated as functional requirements evolve in response to new treatment regimens, shifts in acuity levels, types of patients, evolving organizational systems, and financial models. It has not been empirically proven that flexible partitioning strategies reduce personal control, privacy, safety, or increase infection rates.[61]

A call for a balanced typology

Since 2000, many countries have experienced tremendous growth in their healthcare sectors.[62] Yet this period of growth has been a

4.27 Semi-private room with
expansive views, Kempten-Oberallgau
Clinic, Germany, 2006

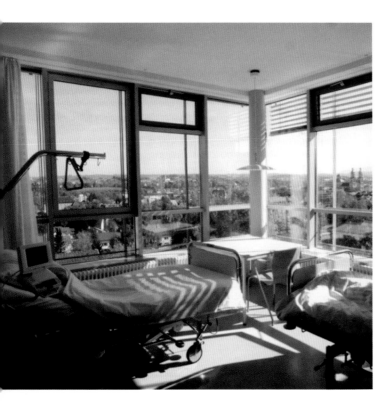

repeating pattern throughout the past 150 years, as periods of expansion have been followed by periods of economic stagnation and drought from the standpoint of capital improvements and design innovation. International trends are in flux at the present time with respect to the private versus semi-private inpatient room. Despite this, the mainstream evidence-based research and design community clearly supports the all-private-room hospital above all other options. Nevertheless, the design considerations (see Chapter 7) and case studies (see Chapter 8) presented later in this book emphasize the accruable benefits of a hospital's ability to provide a reasonable balance between at least two types of rooms: single-bed rooms, and suites housing either 2 beds, and from 3-beds up to 6-beds. The ratio of one room type to the other room type(s) will vary of course in response to local circumstances and there are many ways to achieve a balanced mix in response to institutional, direct caregiver, patient requirements, and family concerns. The either/or arguments – for or against the all-private-room hospital – as simplistic as they are, and with the all-private contingent lacking conclusive empirical evidence, are by no means over. Meanwhile, from reading the most recent evidence-based research and design literature it can be concluded that the semi-private room and open ward are on the verge of being sent to their deathbed once and for all:

> The years 2006 and 2007 will be remembered as seminal years for research and analysis of patient room planning options. In a fairly brief period, enough research was gathered on the subject of single versus semiprivate rooms to culminate in the American Institute of Architects (AIA) *Guidelines for Design and Construction of Health Care Facilities* (2006) standard of one bed per room unless the functional program demonstrates the necessity of a two-bed arrangement. This is a victory for patients and families on all fronts ... a survey of more than two million patients in 1,500 hospitals by Press Ganey Associates in 2004 revealed that patients in single-bed rooms were much more satisfied. Findings from several studies indicated that the presence of a roommate is usually a source of stress, not social support ... in fact, patients often ask to be moved due to lack of compatibility with a roommate.[63]

This raises two concerns. First, is the term 'necessity' in the above passage an escape clause in the face of global climate change, a global financial crisis, resource depletion, carbon neutrality, or excessive population growth? Second, would these factors not have the cumulative effect of trumping in priority, real, but by comparison somewhat less critical concerns such as roommate compatibility? Moreover, when considered from a broader socio-political context, a strong case can still be made for the virtues of the multi-bed room, as at the Kempten-Oberallgau Clinic, in Germany (2003–2006), designed by RRP Architects/Engineers. This room allows opportunities for social interaction, or privacy, and direct connections with nature in the form of its large corner windows and the ability to open the window for fresh air (Figure 4.27).[64] What would Nightingale say today about all this? The 150-year debate continues.

The evolving role of memory, place, and sustainability

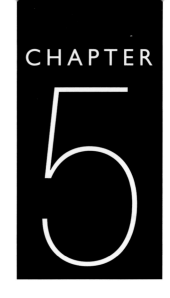

A worrisome trend is undermining the continued evolution of the international movement towards carbon neutral healthcare environments. This threat is due to actions at times paradoxical and which run counter to the core principles of sustainable urban development and the tenets of the *Smart Growth Movement*.[1] Often, a decision is made by elected officials and the leadership of healthcare organizations to construct a new replacement hospital on suburban and in distant 'fringe site' contexts. Many of these replacement medical centers are being built in outlying areas at the far edge of their communities. On the surface such a strategy for relocation to a new site may make sense. And in past decades no one would have raised an eyebrow. It would have appeared to make good common sense that high land costs in urban centers, the difficulty involved in the assemblage of the large developable tracts, and an enhanced ability to attract and retain top staff at the new location would be powerful justifications.[2] Additional ammunition for relocation could easily be justified on the basis of on-site parking requirements, space needed for the mechanical plant, open space requirements, and having enough space for future expansion.

With these justifications in hand, thousands of hospital administrators had been successful in relocating their institution to new sites, often many miles from the original legacy neighborhoods. For those institutions that opted to remain in their legacy neighborhood the options usually consisted of:

1 Expansion though land expropriation and the use of eminent domain powers with the backing of the local, state, and federal government.
2 Reinvention on-site by employing a strategy of expansion combined with the construction of new satellite facilities elsewhere.
3 The purchase (or takeover) of, or the forging of partnerships with, allied care providers in order to create a coordinated network of care providers within a large metropolitan or regional market.
4 Various combinations of strategies 1, 2 and 3 implemented over a multi-year period.

During the past quarter of a century, hundreds of historic hospitals have been destroyed in the name of progress (see Chapter 2). This inventory of hospitals is vast. The corresponding cultural currency, heritage, and traditions they represented to their communities is lost. Nearly every city has experienced the loss of a landmark hospital. At the present time many more are threatened with destruction.

Nearly all of these threatened hospitals and portions thereof were built in the period 1935–1970. The 1930s hospitals that remain in the U.S. were usually built in the art deco style and stand as exemplars of that period. The more recent (post-1945) hospitals were nearly always designed in the International Style. These hospitals and parts thereof are also being lost by the thousands. Most of these facilities had been added on to haphazardly over the years with the result being – from an aesthetic, functional, and operational standpoint – a case of the sum total not performing to the level of any of its constituent parts.[3]

The megahospitals of the late twentieth century represented the apotheosis of an unyielding belief in the power of medical science in the post-1945 era. By the 1960s the International Style dominated the hospital as a building type in nations around the globe. The movement to incorporate advanced building technologies resulted in a quest to develop a hospital template that 'would never become obsolete' in the words of Eberhard Zeidler (see Chapter 2).[4] Healthcare facility planning, systems engineering, and interior design emerged as specialized fields apart from architecture. Health-centered political bureaucracies grew in their size and complexity. The regional teaching hospital evolved in recognition of the need to allow for internal flexibility and external extension in a highly complex, dynamic organism and in so doing became almost completely self-referential. Worse, this obsession with size, bed capacity, and technological prowess pushed aside any possibilities to create a sustainable hospital – resulting in a tightly bundled machine hospital extremely costly to run from an energy standpoint.[5]

Beginning in 1946 in the United States, with the advent of the federal urban renewal programs sponsored by the Department of Housing and Urban Development (HUD), the race was on to construct ever larger and more complex hospitals and medical research centers. This often happened at the expense of long-established adjoining ethnic neighborhoods. Neighborhoods were disfigured, and at worst completely eradicated in the name of progress. Medical centers were transformed into behemoths – energy-hungry 'medievalist' enclaves. Institutional out-migration was made possible by the interstate highway system, launched in 1955. This network of high-speed arteries cut through and flowed outward from city centers. By the 1960s, critics began to assail the new machine-driven megahospital because renovations were always required to keep apace with new diagnostic methods, equipment, and departments.[6] The modern hospital was chastised for its premature obsolescence. This gave rise to a new wave of thought with the result even more costly to operate from an energy standpoint.[7] The interstitial medical center was a direct response to the rejection of the 'obsolete' art deco hospital.[8]

It is now only a matter of time before the modernist behemoths of the late twentieth century will be themselves threatened with extinction in the name of progress, that is, more sustainable alternatives. In the meantime, evidence-based case studies are needed to demonstrate the viability of retaining the older landmark hospitals and in resuscitating them for new lives. It is highly probable that the total carbon footprint of a new replacement hospital is significantly greater than that of a historic hospital reborn, when all the variables are looked at together in a single equation. Yet in the absence of any broad-based statistics on this point it remains an uphill battle to try to argue for their preservation and/or adaptive use versus their demolition. As is shown below, it is far harder to argue effectively for the preservation of an historic hospital in the aftermath of a major catastrophe, as is the case in the aftermath of Hurricane Katrina in New Orleans.

The battle to save Charity Hospital and a historic neighborhood

New Orleans continues to struggle to rebuild from the massive devastation caused by Hurricane Katrina in 2005. Nearly 1,800 deaths were directly attributable to the catastrophe and at $13 billion in federal mitigation costs Katrina ranks as the costliest disaster in American history. Eighty percent of the city flooded, inundating 122,000 residences, businesses, and civic institutions with toxic floodwater for up to three weeks.[9] The city's healthcare infrastructure was put on life support: official data indicate that there are now (2010) 25 percent fewer hospital beds in New Orleans than before Katrina hit and there are at the time of writing less than two beds per 1,000 residents as compared to over three beds before the disaster. Major healthcare institutions were damaged and many never will reopen, including three hospitals and nearly a dozen neighborhood-based primary care clinics, in addition to dozens of private physicians' offices, dental clinics, and counseling centers. Only one general hospital is functioning at pre-Katrina capacity and

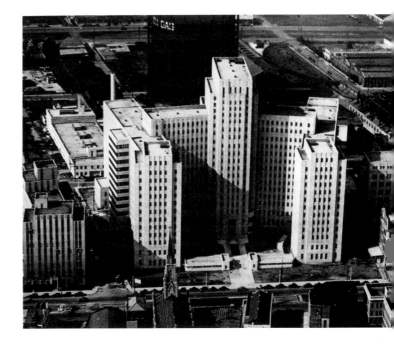

5.1 Medical Center of Louisiana at New Orleans (Charity Hospital), New Orleans, 1948 aerial photo. Charity Hospital is an iconic landmark in the city

16,800 fewer healthcare sector jobs exist (down 27 percent) in the post-Katrina urban landscape.[10]

The basement and part of the first floor of Charity Hospital, located in the Central Business District (CBD), flooded in Katrina's aftermath and it was forced to shut down. It remains closed at the time of writing. Next door to Charity sits the Department of Veterans Affairs New Orleans Medical Center, known locally as simply the VA Hospital. The main hospital opened in 1949. Its basement also flooded in Katrina's aftermath and remains shuttered. This current iteration of Charity Hospital (1935–1938) was designed by the firm Weiss, Dreyfous and Seiferth and is the fourth Charity Hospital (whose official pre-Katrina name was the Medical Center of Louisiana at New Orleans) on the site (the first Charity Hospital opened in 1728). This firm also designed at about the same time the 35-floor skyscraper art deco State Capital in Baton Rouge (1933–1936). Charity, affectionately known as 'Big Charity', features a 20-level main tower with two 14-level hyphens and two 12-level side wings (Figure 5.1). The adjacent 15-storey VA Hospital campus now includes a 12-level parking ramp with a two-level nursing home on its top (1987–1989), plus a medical research building (1981–1983). For generations, both Charity and VA hospitals served as training centers for physician residents and nurses from the adjacent Tulane University, and Louisiana State University (LSU) medical schools.

The owner-operator of Charity Hospital is the Louisiana State University Health Sciences Center (LSUHSC). Charity, prior to Katrina, was in a deteriorated condition due to years of deferred maintenance, lack of renovations to keep apace with medical advancements, and political bickering over its future. This had resulted in periodic accreditation compliance problems that were frequently solved in a makeshift ad hoc manner on a case-by-case basis. Prior to Katrina, the LSUHSC had been lobbying state politicians for more than a decade for construction of a completely new replacement hospital on a new site. Meanwhile, the 1938 facility was now eligible for placement on the U.S. National Register of Historic Places (henceforth referred to as the National Register). Big Charity served the poor for over 250 years and was the oldest continually operating hospital in the U.S. until being inundated by Katrina's floodwaters.[11]

In the days immediately following Katrina the LSUHSC announced it was permanently closing Charity Hospital and would seek federal mitigation funds from the Federal Emergency Management Agency (FEMA) to build a replacement facility in a nearby neighborhood, across the Interstate 10 from the current VA/Charity campus. The

DVA (Department of Veterans Affairs) similarly announced at about this time that it too was also seeking funds from the U.S. Congress to permanently close its facility. The DVA was appropriated more than $600 million to build a replacement medical center on 37 acres of a 71-acre site targeted in the Lower Mid-City neighborhood. The two organizations signed a formal Memorandum of Understanding (MOU) in October 2006 to jointly construct two freestanding yet interconnected hospitals that would share certain support functions, i.e. parking, dietary, central mechanical plant, and public spaces.[12] The site is adjacent to the Central Business District and across the aforementioned interstate highway from the two shuttered hospitals.[13] The New Orleans Redevelopment Authority (NORA) was put in charge of assembling the land, through the use of Federal Community Development Block Grant (CDBG) funds given to the city after Katrina. The DVA site alone contained 188 separate properties. It promised to be an arduous task.

Everyone in New Orleans knows Big Charity. This art deco landmark skyscraper hospital commands a lofty position in the city's urban landscape and even more so in its collective psyche.

It is a cultural touchstone, a place widely celebrated in song and verse. Many important jazz musicians were born there, including the immortal Louis Armstrong (born in 1900 in the 1938 building's predecessor facility). In the case of a 300-year-old city such as New Orleans, the continued vibrancy of such places is key to retaining a community's history and its cultural identity.[14] Charity was a place where generations worked, worshipped, socialized, grieved, commiserated, and celebrated life. Places such as this in the United State are rare, as they are at once ordinary, transcendent, and inimitable.[15] This art deco skyscraper Nightingale hospital was the nation's largest urban hospital when it was dedicated by President Franklin D. Roosevelt in 1938.[16]

The joint LSUHSC/DVA proposal immediately stirred controversy and resentment in the community. The National Trust, and the Foundation for Historical Louisiana (FHL), based in Baton Rouge, the state capital, argued that while the return of healthcare and a teaching hospital was a critical issue supported by all in Louisiana, the site for the two replacement hospitals was the most costly, most time consuming, and most destructive of all options explored by decision makers representing LSU and the DVA. The LSU/DVA strategy called for the use of eminent domain, forcing the dislocation or destruction of 263 nineteenth- and early-twentieth-century homes and businesses in an historic neighborhood to build a project costing $1.2 billion. Nearly 100 percent of the buildings in the 71-acre tract would be bulldozed, the old Dixie brewery, a school, and a 124-year-old German heritage community center, the Deutches Haus, would also be destroyed. Furthermore, a collection of reusable buildings totaling over two million square feet in the downtown medical district would be abandoned, with no plan proposed for their reuse by the LSUHSC or the DVA.[17] The National Trust named Charity Hospital and this threatened neighborhood on its 2008 list of the eleven most endangered historic places in the nation, to focus national attention on the controversy:

> On November 25, the U.S. Department of Veterans Affairs and Louisiana State University announced the selection of the Mid-City neighborhood as the site of their replacement hospitals and this action will destroy the historic neighborhood around Charity Hospital where residents have been rebuilding their homes in the aftermath of Hurricane Katrina. Once a prestigious center of medical training and a beacon for public health care, Charity Hospital now faces an uncertain future.

Surrounded by floodwaters when Hurricane Katrina shattered the levees around New Orleans, the art deco icon has been shuttered and vacant for more than three years. Despite its legendary role in serving hundreds of thousands of uninsured patients and the critical need for medical facilities in New Orleans, this historic building continues to languish and remains vulnerable to demolition. In the wake of Hurricane Katrina, the basement of Charity Hospital suffered water damage and some of the electrical and mechanical systems were damaged or destroyed. After the water receded, the medical community, the military, and a number of volunteers pumped out the flooded basement, cleaned out the debris and restored electrical power to make the building useable again, but the doors to the hospital were permanently locked when the building was deemed unsafe and unusable by the Louisiana State University (LSU) leadership.[18]

The National Trust for Historic Preservation called this decision a serious error and in a press release urged the VA and LSU to reconsider. *The New York Times*, in its typical, often-glib post-Katrina role as devil's advocate with regards to any grass-roots historic preservation effort in the hurricane-battered city, wrote:

> Local and federal officials on Tuesday announced plans for a 71 acre medical campus in the heart of New Orleans to replace two hospitals damaged during Hurricane Katrina, a $2 billion investment that supporters say will create thousands of jobs and begin to rebuild the city's shattered health care system … One of the hospitals … would replace the city's landmark Charity Hospital, a lifeline for generations of the city's poor … the other would replace the vacant Department of Veterans Affairs hospital, also severely damaged by the flooding. The old hospitals and adjacent buildings will be abandoned under the plan, which officials described as the foundation for a new economy for New Orleans, and the largest investment in the area since Katrina. But the plan, brewing for months, has drawn strong criticism from preservationists and neighborhood activists … officials said steps would be taken to mitigate the loss, including moving some houses in the way of the proposed development. But they suggested the city's higher priority was to begin rebuilding the economy with a high-impact project. 'Today we are not thinking small, we are thinking right …

we're talking about something spectacular,' said Mayor C. Ray Nagin. James P. McNamara, who heads the Greater New Orleans Biosciences Economic Development District, said the campus was the most important project in the city. 'For us, that is enormous,' he said. That some will lose their homes as a result, he added, is 'just the reality of life.'[19]

The article went on to note that critics claim this strategy will be the most costly, time-consuming, and complex to implement, and will needlessly destroy a historic neighborhood where residents are struggling to rebuild while its proponents claimed it would create thousands of jobs.

Nossiter continued:

The long shadow of this city's recent natural disaster has redrawn the odds on even the most unassuming districts, promising obliteration for some, like this composite of ghostly wrecks and painted shotgun house gems a single room wide, adjacent to downtown … [yet] many residents are mystified by this logic [of leveling the neighborhood and abandoning Charity], in a city with vast stretches of underused, unused and downright derelict property … 'It's a terrible idea,' said Wallace Thurman, who lives on Palmyra Street in the heart of the [targeted] new campus, in a handsome Arts and Crafts style house that went partly underwater after the storm. 'I was born in my house, and I'm going to lose it to put up a hospital?' He spent $50,000 to get his house back in shape after Katrina, he said, 'and they're going to tell me I can't live here?' So why get rid of a neighborhood that is functioning, in its teetering New Orleans way, when so much of the city lies empty and unused? Many residents have urged the state to renovate Charity Hospital rather than build a new one, and said the veterans hospital could go on the site of the ruined Lindy Bogs Medical Center, a dozen blocks away … 'We're talking about a total redefinition of the future,' said Edward J. Blakely, executive director of the city's Office of Recovery and Development Administration. He added, 'I'm the last one that wants to destroy a neighborhood'.[20]

The LSU replacement hospital proposal remained severely underfunded, however. The University was in the midst of a pitched battle over the assessed mitigation cost to be paid out by FEMA, under the provisions of a convoluted law called the Stafford Act. LSU wanted $480 million and the most recent federal reimbursement figure was a mere $150 million (mid-2009). It was estimated that the full cost of the new facility would reach $900 million, including land acquisition and demolition. The replacement was first planned for 424 beds, later downsized to 300 beds, and its opening date had not been set, although architects had been hired. The firm of NJBBJ, its Portland and Columbus offices, was hired, in a joint venture with Eskew/Dumez/Ripple Architects of New Orleans.

At this time, local community grass-roots groups began to turn up the heat on the LSU/DVA Memorandum of Understanding that had been signed some months earlier. That agreement was reached prior to the FEMA Section 106 Review (see below) and any public meetings. Its legality was immediately questioned by attorneys representing the to-be-displaced residents of the targeted Lower Mid-City project site. The New Orleans-based Internet site *Squandered Heritage* posted many video interviews with affected residents in the neighborhood.[21] *Squandered Heritage*, founded by Karen Gadbois and Karen Lentz in the aftermath of the storm, had by then garnered national attention for its tireless efforts to call public attention to the urban demolition crisis occurring in Katrina's aftermath. Each resident interviewed told his or her personal story and how they had struggled to return to the city to live and to rebuild their life. Every building in the neighborhood was photographed and posted to the *Squandered Heritage* home page or on other Internet blog sites based in New Orleans. The National Trust continued to post updates on its Internet site *Preservation Nation*.[22]

In June 2008, the FHL commissioned the Philadelphia office of the U.K. firm RMJM Hillier to assess the feasibility of preserving and redeveloping Big Charity into a state-of-the-art medical facility. Their report, released in September 2008, concluded that the facility could be rebuilt from within with a new atrium lobby in three years at a cost of $484 million. Building a new replacement would take five years and cost at least $620 million. No property owners would be displaced. The hospital's building envelope, exterior walls, windows, and roof were fully restorable. The structural system was sound and this fact alone would shave two years off the construction timeline. The building's footprint, with its H-shape, fully complied with 'modern hospital design goals of enhancing daylighting and providing views from all rooms' (Figure 5.2). Up to 446 inpatient all-private rooms would be provided (see Chapter 4). The existing floor plates were workable for a first-class health facility, except for the third floor,

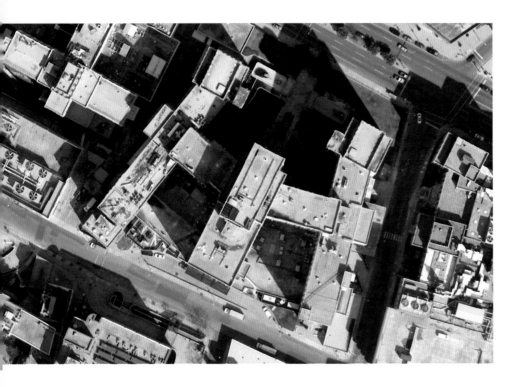

5.2 Charity Hospital, New Orleans, aerial photo. The hospital's footprint personifies vanguard pre-1940 hospital architecture in North America and Europe

5.3 Annotated site plan for the renovation of Charity Hospital and its campus, RMJM Hillier, 2008

5.4 Historic shotgun house in neighborhood slated for demolition for the LSUHSC/DVA replacement medical center, New Orleans, 2009 photo

which the A/E team proposed enlarging (Figure 5.3). The report recommended the new DVA hospital should be built on a smaller site that did not require the destruction of the historic homes and businesses in the nearby Lower Mid-City neighborhood (Figure 5.4). The report also cited the value of retaining an historic neighborhood that provided ample affordable housing for thousands of healthcare workers and others within close walking distance of a revived medical district. These positive outcomes were cited as being in keeping with sustainable and ecologically sound architectural and urban design principles.[23]

The RMJM Hillier report stated, in part:

Before Katrina, all floors of Charity Hospital were in use. Newly renovated facilities sat next to outdated, noncompliant departments. Hazardous materials such as asbestos, lead and mold, as well as outdated mechanical systems were a major concern. The fact that the facility had to remain up and running made needed renovations almost impossible … without massive temporary relocations of departments and the disruption that such an approach would cause. Now that the

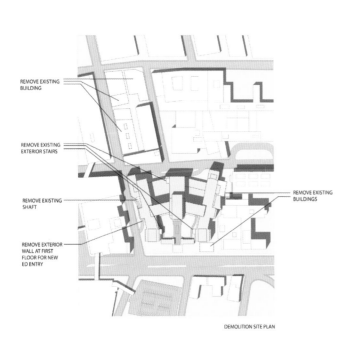

REMOVE EXISTING BUILDING

REMOVE EXISTING EXTERIOR STAIRS

REMOVE EXISTING SHAFT

REMOVE EXTERIOR WALL AT FIRST FLOOR FOR NEW ED ENTRY

REMOVE EXISTING BUILDINGS

DEMOLITION SITE PLAN

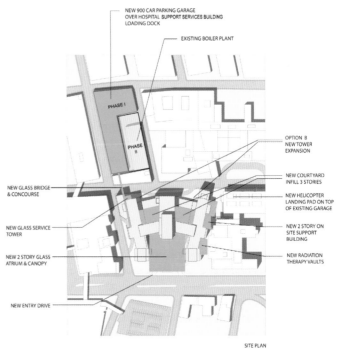

NEW 900 CAR PARKING GARAGE OVER HOSPITAL SUPPORT SERVICES BUILDING LOADING DOCK

EXISTING BOILER PLANT

PHASE I

PHASE II

OPTION B NEW TOWER EXPANSION

NEW GLASS BRIDGE & CONCOURSE

NEW COURTYARD INFILL 3 STORIES

NEW HELICOPTER LANDING PAD ON TOP OF EXISTING GARAGE

NEW GLASS SERVICE TOWER

NEW 2 STORY ON SITE SUPPORT BUILDING

NEW 2 STORY GLASS ATRIUM & CANOPY

NEW RADIATION THERAPY VAULTS

NEW ENTRY DRIVE

SITE PLAN

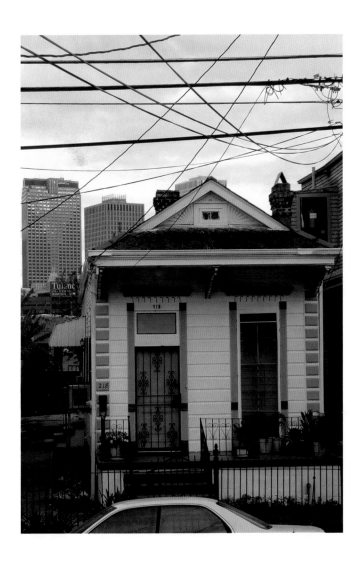

trauma facility, and respect and enhance significant historic features. This comprehensive renovation work would use available funds promptly and effectively, and be completed within three and a half years – quicker than it would take to build a new structure, and at lower cost. This approach also takes advantage of existing associated structures on adjacent sites in order to house necessary support systems.

It continued:

Using the existing infrastructure of tunnels, utilities and bridges that connect these sites, support facilities would be upgraded to meet current code requirements … its revitalization will be an important step in the redevelopment of New Orleans, reinforcing the value of sustainability – not demolition and social displacement – as a key component … it also underscores how sound preservation principles can be creatively integrated with modern design parameters, including the most stringent healthcare requirements. The rich history of the architecture in the city is a fundamental part of the city's success, and there can be no better example of leadership and commitment to sustainability, redevelopment and growth in areas ravaged by Katrina, than the re-use of a nationally significant and iconic historic landmark, such as Old Charity.[24]

The reinvented Big Charity would have a new glass-enclosed atrium front court facing Tulane Avenue, with a curb cut and drive at the main gateway (Figure 5.5). A pair of well-composed and ornamented one-level sentry structures flank the entry in the courtyard leading to the main entrance. These were originally used for outpatient services and a dispensary. They would now become a bookstore and a pharmacy (Figure 5.6). The atrium would allow for dramatic views of the front facade (Figure 5.7) and all renovation and restoration work would be in conformance with the U.S. Secretary of the Interior's Standards for the Treatment of Historic Structures (1995). The 150-page RMJM Hillier report to the FHL contained schematic floor plans of all levels, elevations, and building sections, as well as a detailed floor-by-floor narrative.[25]

The Main Level plan indicates all vertical circulation systems would be reorganized to allow for distinct separation between staff and support services and direct patient care services. Visitor elevators would be reoriented towards the main entrance. All infrastructure

building has been vacated, a new opportunity presents itself … the condition assessment findings demonstrate that many issues requiring remediation affect the building as a whole … The design team concludes that the best approach is to address the entire Charity structure, with a comprehensive, innovative design that would allow a permanent re-use of the core and shell of the building, provide state-of-the-art facilities and amenities for a modern hospital and Level 1

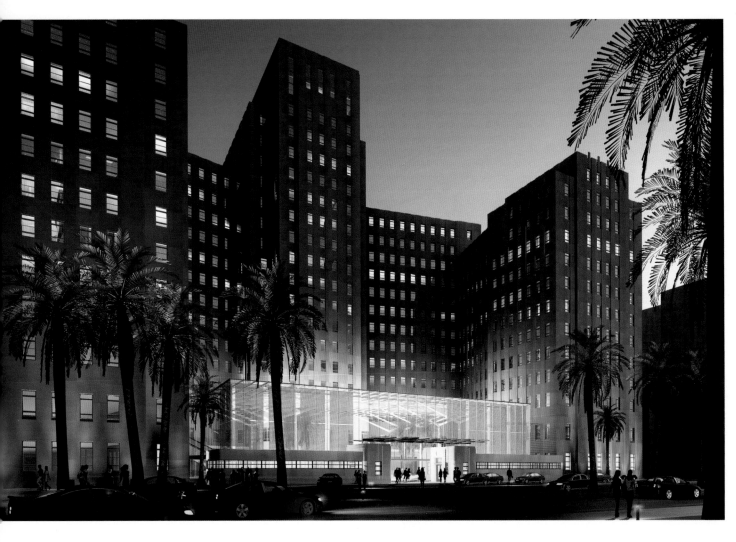

5.5 Rendering, front facade of Charity Hospital, RMJM Hillier, 2008

5.6 Main arrival court, Charity Hospital, RMJM Hillier, 2008

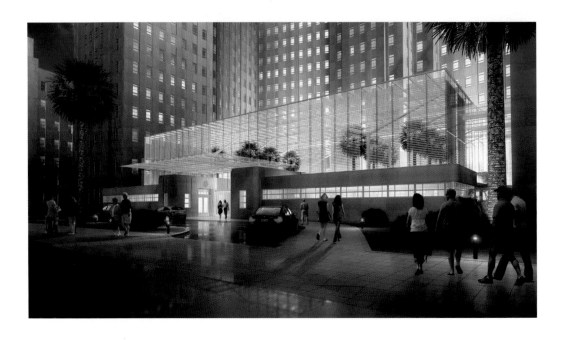

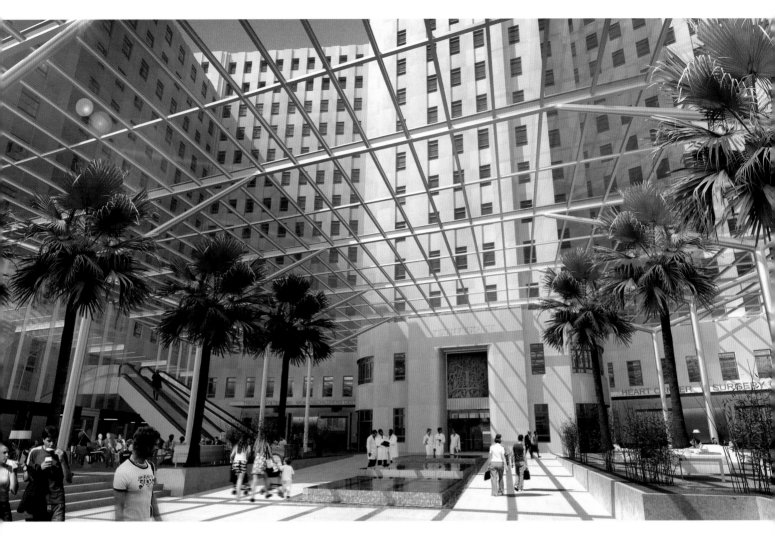

5.7 Enclosed courtyard atrium,
Charity Hospital, RMJM Hillier, 2008

support would be housed on the first level and above in order for the hospital to remain functional in a catastrophic event. The Basement Level would provide the option for below grade parking. The Main Level would house the Level 1 Trauma Center and related support functions.

The Second Level would house the center for interventional procedures, surgical pre- and post-op, and diagnostic imaging, including radiation therapy. The Third Level would house an 8-bed labor and delivery (LDR) unit, and a 22-bed postpartum unit and related support. The Fourth Level would be strictly devoted to mechanical support, functioning as an *interstitial* floor. Levels 5 to 12 would be reconfigured to single bed inpatient care units (PCU) and associated support functions. The Fifth Level would house a 24-bed women's services unit, endoscopy, and a 24-bed clinical research center IP unit. Levels 6 to 8 would house PCUs – each floor with two 24-bed units – 16-bed ICUs, and related support. Levels 9 and 10 would house additional PCUs, dialysis and rehabilitation serves, and the CIU services. Level 11 would house an on-call suite, pulmonary services, patient escort unit, environmental services, staff

lounge, biomedical engineering, and the central pharmacy. Level 12 would house two 30-bed behavioral health units and related support. Level 13 would house an 18-bed acute behavioral health unit. Levels 14 to 20 would house the administration and support, including an auditorium on the top floor.[26]

The patient rooms within the various PCUs would all be same-handed, identical rooms in terms of their layout. As discussed in Chapter 4, this strategy was preferable and in keeping with current national best practices in nursing care compared to mirror-image A/B A/B inpatient rooms (with back-to-back patient headwalls). The patient room would be fully standardized in all respects. The architects acknowledged, however, that this method at this time was yet to be definitively proven as 'safer' for the patient. However, the RMJM Hillier team asserted that as more hospitals were built in this manner in the next few years, nursing-based medical errors in the PCU setting were likely to decrease significantly (Figure 5.8). Moreover, the slight shift, or angling, in plan, of the all-private inpatient rooms would yield a sawtooth pattern along the corridors, yielding additional privacy for patients and family (Figure 5.9).[27]

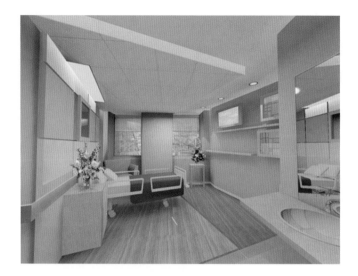

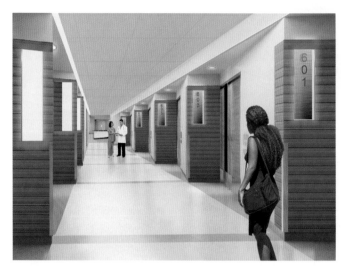

5.8 Inpatient room, Charity Hospital, RMJM Hillier, 2008

5.9 PCU corridor, Charity Hospital, RMJM Hillier, 2008

The Section 106 Review

The mission of FEMA is to function as a first responder agency to provide emergency disaster relief for victims of national disasters and related emergencies. FEMA is quick to point out that it is not in the hospital construction business. In the context of historic preservation, however, FEMA is empowered by the U.S. Congress to ensure that any disaster mitigation funds it disperses to organizations and municipalities locally do not occur in a manner that violates federal policies and mandates. In Katrina's aftermath FEMA opened a large New Orleans field office. FEMA is mandated by the U.S. Congress to comply with the provisions of the Section 106 Review process. This legislation is administered by the Advisory Council on Historic Preservation, an independent federal agency that promotes preservation nationally by providing a forum for influencing federal actions, programs, and policies that impact on historic properties. As part of the National Historic Preservation Act (NHPA) of 1966, Section 106 of NHPA is a critical component.[28] This is because it requires:

> The consideration of historic preservation in the multitude of federal actions that occur nationwide … the Section 106 Review encourages, but does not mandate, preservation … [it] ensures that preservation factors are factored into federal agency planning and decisions. Because of Section 106, federal agencies must assume responsibility for the consequences of their actions on historic properties and be publicly accountable for their decisions.[29]

At the state level of government, the State of Louisiana operates the State Historic Preservation Office (SHPO). This agency is under the auspices of the governor and is housed within and staffed by the Lieutenant Governor's office. In each of the fifty states, the SHPO coordinates the state's historic preservation program and consults with federal and local agencies during the Section 106 Review process. It issues independent reports and recommendations that are a key component in the Section 106 Review. The Louisiana Office of Community Development (OCD) is an organization within the State of Louisiana Division of Administration. The primary goal of the OCD is to improve the quality of life of the state's residents through its three programs: the Community Development Section, the Disaster Recovery Unit, and the Local Government Assistance Program. Grants are administrated to local organizations by these entities.[30]

The Section 106 Review centered on more than 150 National Register-listed historic homes situated within the 71-acre neighborhood slated for destruction. The neighborhood includes, specifically, the aforementioned historic Dixie Brewery (1922–1926) on Tulane Avenue, and the modernist landmark former Pan American Life Building (1961–1963) on Canal Street. The aforementioned Memorandum of Understanding (MOU) signed a year earlier between the DVA, the city, and LSU committed the city and state to spend up to $79 million to acquire and completely 'cleanslate' the site of all structures. A series of 'information gathering' meetings were held with affected residents. This 'consultative phase', as FEMA calls it, appeared, at least on the surface to casual onlookers, to be above board and properly conducted, but opponents suspected that something was amiss from the outset.[31]

Opponents contended that while it appeared on the surface and from a public relations standpoint that FEMA and the SHPO had properly conducted the Section 106 Review, in actuality these two entities were put under intense political pressure to support 100 percent the MOU signed by LSU, the DVA, and the City of New Orleans. Second, opponents contended that the impacted neighborhood's residents had been dismissed in the Section 106

Review. Grass-roots preservationists and the National Trust argued that it would be entirely feasible to relocate intact dwellings to vacant tracts in adjoining residential areas presently offering a multitude of available existing vacant lots at a relatively low cost or, better yet, to simply chose the alternate site that was offered and remained available nearby – a site that did not require the demolition of a single historic building or forcibly relocate a single citizen.[32]

The Section 106 Review concluded that the LSU and the DVA had properly gone through the motions and were therefore on solid legal ground to pursue their vision. Opponents, however, contested this conclusion. Also, this ruling now qualified LSU to receive the disaster mitigation funds they were counting on to build their hospital. In a letter to the State of Louisiana Legislative Appropriations Committee on Health and Human Services, dated 4 December 2008, Sandra Stokes, of the Foundation for Historical Louisiana, wrote:

I would like to thank you for your graciousness in the aftermath of the Charity Hospital incident on Tuesday 2 December 2008 when the Foundation for Historical Louisiana (FHL) and the principal architect from RMJM Hillier, along with a physician, were excluded from attending the inspection of the Charity Hospital building in New Orleans by the House Committee on Appropriations, Subcommittee on Health and Human Services. We were obviously surprised and disappointed that we were unable to observe or participate in the committee's tour of the building. We have accumulated a great deal of information about the building, its condition and its future viability as a re-built medical center. We thank you for your interest and concern regarding this important issue and we await the opportunity to present the findings of the Charity Hospital feasibility study in a public hearing before your committee.

We do wish to state what we observed regarding the events which transpired at Charity Hospital. The FHL and the architects responsible for the independent study for re-use and adaptation of Charity Hospital were invited by state representatives to explain parts of the study on site. We were stopped at the door by Charles Zewe, spokesperson for LSU, saying 'I strongly object to you being here.' When asked exactly who was blocking our entry, Mr. Zewe replied 'I'm stopping you, on behalf of LSU.' He also said the tour was only for representatives, even though we observed other

non-representatives had been allowed entry. We observed that Mr. Jim McNamara, who is not a state representative and is an active advocate for building a new LSU hospital, was allowed through the doors after this encounter. When we asked Mr. Zewe about this discrepancy, Mr. Zewe said Mr. McNamara was an invited guest of LSU. It was very clear to us that LSU was acting as the gatekeeper on who would be permitted into the building.

It is our understanding that the issue regarding state funding of LSU's plan to abandon the Charity building as a medical center and build a brand new hospital is very much an open question at this point in time. We are aware (however) of LSU's public position that the issue is 'closed' and that LSU is planning on proceeding with construction. If this is true why would the committee have gone to Charity Hospital to seek information on 2 December?

It is our understanding that, despite these statements, the financial issues underlying this project are still very much unresolved. We are especially concerned that the actual cost of this LSU-proposed project greatly exceeds what has been publicly stated ($1.2 billion). Further, LSU's refusal to seriously consider the less costly and more expedient alternative of restoring the existing Charity Hospital building has serious consequences both financially and with regard to timely restoration of accessible health care in New Orleans. We look forward to a full and open discussion on this important issue. We are also available to revisit the Charity Hospital site with the committee should that be helpful in this process.

Of most urgent concern is that the U.S. Department of Veteran Affairs has announced selection of a site co-located to the proposed new LSU hospital site in New Orleans. We believe the selection of this site by the VA was heavily influenced by LSU's public statement of their intention to build the new LSU hospital. If the VA builds on the site selected, and the state does not proceed with LSU's new hospital, the VA will be left isolated from the Medical District.

The issue has been quite controversial since the location of these two hospitals will require the demolition of hundreds of historic buildings, including private homes and businesses, covering 71 acres in Lower Mid-City. The State has agreed to carry out the expropriations of these homes and businesses on behalf of the City of New Orleans. Based on the representation that the new LSU hospital is a 'done deal' demolitions of homes will begin soon in the densest part of this historic neighborhood. The citizens who are facing the loss of their homes and businesses are the same people who were encouraged to come back and rebuild after Katrina. They struggled to reestablish their community, only to now face losing their homes again – this time to bulldozers. Many of these taxpaying citizens have stated their intention to leave the state altogether if these expropriations go forward.

If, in fact, the best solution is to restore and reuse Charity Hospital as the site for the LSU hospital, the location of the VA hospital needs to be reconsidered and reconfigured. There is urgency to this matter, as the VA has announced their intention to proceed. The VA has assured all parties in the Federal Section 106 Historic Preservation Review process that they are committed to building in New Orleans. There are other alternatives that could be a win–win for all.

The vacant Charity Hospital building presents an opportunity the State has never had before: the complete transformation of a historically significant icon into a world-class medical facility. The building is currently unoccupied. This is a new, extremely rare opportunity that allows the entire building to be gutted. The one million square foot, structurally sound shell could be fitted out into a modern, sustainable medical marvel. Such a restoration would send an important message about the progressive stance of the State of Louisiana in creatively integrating new facilities into the fabric of our historic communities and buildings. We would become a nationally recognized leader and model for other communities.

Such an outcome would also allow medical care to be made available more quickly and at significantly less cost than the current LSU plan to build an entirely new facility by destroying an historic neighborhood and abandoning the existing Charity building. LSU could rehabilitate Charity into a 21st century hospital, the VA could build on a much less densely populated site near Claiborne Avenue, thereby creating a medical corridor consistent with proper urban design, and synergy with other medical facilities in the district. Downtown New Orleans would be revitalized instead of abandoned, and the residential neighborhood would be saved. We would have the same jobs, the same economic opportunities, and the same medical corridor – sooner, at less cost, and with

less destruction. We have approached this question from a perspective of common sense and careful analysis and are deeply concerned that the proposal now on the table is the most expensive, time-consuming and destructive option.[33]

Meanwhile, as this controversy grew in intensity, the DVA, authorized to build a 200-bed facility, was, behind the scenes, quietly being courted by another healthcare provider organization in the metro area (Ochsner Medical Foundation Hospital) and beyond (the community of Gulfport, Mississippi). Ochsner offered the VA a parcel of land directly across the street from its main campus on Jefferson Highway just across the Orleans Parish (County) line in Jefferson Parish. Jefferson Parish has had a long history although the vast majoring of its growth occurred in the post-World War II period and it is now a suburban community. Its population totals more than 600,000 at present. As politicians in the region became aware of the fracas they also sought to woo the VA to their turf. The U.S. congressional delegation from the Mississippi Gulf Coast region made a pitch for the new VA medical center to be built in their district. This would place it as far as 75 miles from downtown New Orleans. This strategy would be counterintuitive to the avowed goal of then-President George W. Bush to do 'whatever it takes' to rebuild New Orleans, as he proclaimed two weeks after Katrina in front of an emergency power-generated floodlit speech in front of St. Louis Cathedral, while the entirety of the city remained desolate and without electrical power.[34]

On 29 January 2008 a pro-new hospital letter was published in the local daily newspaper, The Times-Picayune, authored by John Lombardi, the president of the LSU System. His editorial reiterated the same argument that had been made for months – in fact from the days immediately following Katrina in the fall of 2005. It was a propaganda war at this point that was being waged by LSU. The newspaper (and the public) lapped it up like a cat goes for fresh spilt milk.[35]

Louisiana State University proceeded to launch a public relations campaign to discredit the countervailing arguments of the local grass-roots preservationists, the Mid-City Neighborhood Organization, the National Trust, the FHL for its sponsorship of the RMJM Hillier report, and the soon-to-be-displaced residents of the targeted historic neighborhood:

After months of relatively quiet planning for a new medical complex in New Orleans, the temperature is rising between

LSU system officials and opponents of the school's proposed site in lower Mid-City. LSU leaders say they are reacting to what they characterized as misinformation and cheap shots by preservationists and other opponents of the proposed complex. 'It's going to be tough to get this project built; it's always been tough,' LSU spokesman Charles Zewe said, 'And we are frankly sick and tired of people trying to define us as secretive, mean-spirited and focused only on the aggrandizement of the institution … We're simply not going to stand for it anymore.' Walter Gallas, the New Orleans field director for the National Trust for Historic Preservation, said LSU officials have earned the criticism, and he said the University is to blame for any rhetorical escalation. 'Their attitude has been, "If we get any opposition, we'll just attack the opposition," Gallas said. LSU (and the VA) are proposing a $1.2 billion academic medical complex that would be built … on a 71-acre footprint bounded by Claiborne Avenue, Tulane Avenue, Rocheblave Street and Canal Street. Local preservation groups are pushing the VA to build in the lower nine blocks of the larger footprint, with LSU rebuilding a new hospital from within the shell of Charity Hospital … the plan calls for LSU also to assume control of the old VA campus, which sits across Gravier Street from Charity.[36]

The newspaper account continued:

Behind the back-and-forth are reams of competing architectural and building analyses, federal environmental reviews, transcripts of review sessions convened under federal historic preservation law and letters from both sides making their cases to state and federal lawmakers … [state officials] also refute the idea that Charity could be gutted and rebuilt in less time and for less money than a new hospital, insisting that architects and builders who say so are underestimating the ease of rehabilitating a 70-year-old building. Zewe said the idea of a refurbished Charity is 'fanciful nonsense.' When preservationists invited LSU and VA officials to speak alongside them at a series of neighborhood meetings to discuss the project, LSU and the VA declined … 'These [preservationist] groups have gone from historical to hysterical … It's time to move on with this.' Zewe said.[37]

Sadly, and paradoxically, in the aftermath of Katrina, New Orleans experienced the destruction of its twentieth-century architectural landmarks at an accelerated and alarming rate, at a time when every extra effort should have been made to preserve landmark buildings from the city's long legacy of world-renowned architecture. Many important buildings worthy of placement on the National Register have already fallen to the wrecking ball, post-Katrina, including the modernist masterpiece St. Frances Xavier Cabrini Church, designed by the firm of Curtis & Davis (1960–1963).[38] If a city's urban landscape is the manifestation of its citizens' shared sense of purpose and identity, its historic hospitals notwithstanding, then the conservation of this heritage should be first and foremost on the civic agenda.[39] At the time of writing the outcome of this controversy was yet to be determined although there were some signs that a growing number of local and state officials were beginning to listen to the arguments made by the by-then 30 or more various preservation, and healthcare advocacy, organizations in the battle to save Charity Hospital. Above all, ironically, more than 50 percent of the funding needed for the LSU/HSC replacement hospital proposal remained unsecured.[40]

Historic hospitals and the need for confluence

The case of Big Charity demonstrates that urban redevelopment and on-the-ground realities sometimes do not share the same universe. Let us first examine the role of urban redevelopment from the standpoint of cultural cleansing and how this may relate to carbon neutrality. Voltaire once said that it was dangerous to be right in matters on which the established authorities are wrong. Unbridled power is an intoxicant. The leadership of LSU engaged in questionable decision-making and it is arguable that the seeds of their motivation to abandon Charity had been planted in the public consciousness years before Katrina. Charity had for years prior to Katrina been underfunded and had, by default, become a model of hospital obsolescence. The institution muddled along with as little public operational funding as absolutely required to maintain its accreditation. Accreditation agencies, notably the JCAHO, regularly cited the administration for being in non-compliance with building codes.

Urban myth had it that the facility had fallen into obsolescence, especially in the view of local citizens who had private medical insurance. At least ten years prior to Katrina (1995) the administration publicly stated its interest to build a replacement facility.[41] However, no money was forthcoming from the state legislature. In addition, the public had come to regard Charity as at best a second-tier hospital, because it cared for mostly poor African-Americans. Unfortunately issues of race and class inequities constituted the heart of this myth, two factors historically at the root of everything in New Orleans throughout its 300-year history. The effects of this policy were clearly visible even to the casual observer. The interior was dated. It was drab in appearance. Charity Hospital looked tired, as if just hanging on by a thread. Because of this, the middle and upper classes in the metro area developed a very negative overall image of the hospital.

To critics, Katrina was seen as a godsend for the LSU administration. It was their once-in-a-lifetime chance to get out of Big Charity. More importantly, the possibility that FEMA might actually foot the bill for a new hospital was simply too irresistible to pass on. The LSU public relations spin put on the flood damage was instantaneous and consistent from the first week after the catastrophe (exactly the same strategy as that taken by the Archdiocese of New Orleans in the case of Cabrini Church). Their PR machine proclaimed the hospital was *destroyed* and unsalvageable. With this justification LSU felt justified in its decision to padlock the hospital and declare it a total loss. There would be one small complication to their logic: the FEMA/Stafford Act's 51 percent rule.[42]

The FEMA 51 percent rule reads that any structure that is damaged in a federal declared disaster zone is eligible for total replacement costs if it is declared to be 51 percent or more destroyed.[43] Of course, LSU's public relations people declared the hospital totaled, so they, from that point on, had banked on getting the full replacement cost to build the new hospital they had envisioned for a decade or more, only now completely paid for by the American taxpayer, thanks to Katrina. It was a dream come true. Based on this, LSU had to adopt a hard line on this point – that their hospital was far beyond 51 percent destroyed. The problem with this strategy was that in reality Charity Hospital was nowhere near 51 percent destroyed by Katrina. The first FEMA estimates were only in the 20 percent range. This news was not received well by the LSU leadership team. The first amount agreed to by FEMA was $20 million; later this was increased to $150 million. But this was still far short of the nearly half a billion that LSU was expecting from Washington.

In *The Power of Place: Urban Landscapes as Public History*, Dolores Hayden argues that places such as Charity Hospital have proven to be at once ordinary, transcendent, and inimitable.[44] To critics, the dismissal of Charity post-Katrina was tantamount to an act of cultural cleansing and urban myth perpetuation. It was a strategy justified through a combination of expediency and opportunism. It symbolized the dismissal of the power of place, the premeditated dismissal of civic memory, and that of an African-American community so fundamentally woven into the tapestry of the city's long cultural history. Where LSU saw this as a win–win, others did not. It was a lose–lose proposition for those about to be forcibly displaced from their neighborhood, a lose–lose for the immediate neighborhood in the CBD where Charity now sits, and a lose–lose for a civic building that is among the most significant in the entre city.[45] As mentioned, to critics public officials' antipathy towards Charity Hospital was deeply rooted in long-standing race- and class-based divisions. Most of the to-be-displaced residents of the targeted construction zone were African-American, as were nearly all of the patients (and many staff) who received care at Charity.

The strategy developed by LSU to abandon Charity has been used with regularity in post-Katrina New Orleans. It seemed that anyone who had wanted to tear down a building that they didn't like for whatever reason before Katrina now was able to use Katrina as the perfect excuse to do so. Thousands of old buildings were eradicated from the urban landscape in the months and years after the disaster, and this number included many nationally significant buildings. It was not unlike the aftermath of a war.[46] In addition to the art deco period landmarks, it seemed now that post-World War II modernism was also under attack. The city's modernist landmarks became easy prey.[47] Modernist landmarks destroyed as a result of this demonstration of post-Katrina irrational exuberance included the aforementioned St. Frances Cabrini Church, the Longshoremen's Building on South Claiborne Avenue, the State Supreme Court Building and adjacent State of Louisiana Office Building (both 1955–1957), a number of minimalist public elementary schools, and public libraries.[48]

Esther Charlesworth argues that architects miserably failed to provide effective reconstruction strategies for cities polarized by ethic and economic conflict after World War II.[49] She proposes architects should work as part of interdisciplinary teams (as in the battle to save Charity Hospital). She also argues that any planning process should be incremental and not governed by abstract, top-down bureaucratic machines, such as LSU, or the DVA. Those who are fighting at the grass-roots level to save this neighborhood and this landmark hospital were being drowned out by a large chorus of ill-informed naysayers and anti-preservationists uninterested in hearing anything about compromise, uninterested in hearing anything about any both-and possibilities. As for Charlesworth's second point, the hyperacelerated race to abandon one (hospital), destroy another part of the city (the nearby neighborhood), the reckless FEMA-driven Section 106 Review, the LSU (and to a lesser extent VA) PR machine, and local and state elected officials' desperation to build the new Charity 'yesterday' in an act urban renewal through removal made meaningful discourse next to impossible.[50]

Now enter the role of carbon neutrality in this controversy. All of these lost buildings would be extremely expensive to build today from scratch.[51] It would have been a far more sustainable strategy to simply renovate them and bring them back to life. It is interesting that in the chaotic, haphazard atmosphere of clean-up after Katrina virtually no flood or wind-damaged debris was recycled. Moreover, Charity Hospital and the targeted neighborhood deserved to be sustained and enhanced, not obliterated. It was a viable building in a viable community and this community had demonstrated it was resuscitating itself back to life, building-by-building, street-by-street. It did not help that the public's 'built environment literacy' level was very low in general prior to Katrina and especially on the matter of saving Big Charity. But curiously, few in the general public attacked Charity as being 'ugly'. Most of the public's ire was directed towards its poor condition prior to Katrina. However, to critics, this was the strategic intention after Katrina.

Next, let us examine the role of evidence-based research and design for health in relation to the saga of Charity Hospital, and particularly from the standpoint of the goal of carbon neutral healthcare architecture in the twenty-first century. In the 1960s and 1970s the interstitialists and assorted proponents of the high-tech megahospital convinced themselves their innovative building chassis would remain functionally viable 100 years or more into the future. No evidence-based research was conducted at that time to prove their claims. As mentioned, their vision of the never-to-be-obsolete hospital was a radical reaction to the accelerating rate of facility obsolescence occurring in hospitals at the time. Their construction proved to be the costliest experiment in the entire history of hospital architecture. Their then-radical arguments were directly and intentionally framed against the generation of 'obsolete' high-rise Nightingale hospitals such as Charity. It was only learned later it would cost so much to sustain these facilities because they consumed 30 to 40 percent more in annual energy consumption

costs compared to their predecessors. To critics at the time, the megahospitals were viewed as gluttonous behemoths for their energy consumption (after the 1973 Arab Oil Embargo), and for their wayfinding challenges, overwhelming scale, and threatening appearance. Natural daylight and ventilation was limited due to the unprecedented widths of the floor templates.

By contrast, as proven in the case of Charity Hospital, some surviving high-rise Nightingale hospitals remain beloved. Charity had attained urban mythical status. It was an icon. It is highly doubtful if this will ever be the case for the late-twentieth-century high-tech megahospital. Compared to the narrow footprint of the earlier skyscraper hospitals, the exaggerated massiveness of the building floor templates in interstitial and similar megahospitals is dysfunctional from a carbon neutrality standpoint. With so many departments now so far away from a window and a view to the outside, or any chance for fresh air or natural light, even staff morale began to be adversely affected.[52] More recently, attention has been redirected in the U.K. as to how these places can be operated with fewer toxic discharges, and modified based on safer construction practices. At the community scale parallel efforts are underway to reduce the number and length of automobile journeys to and from British hospitals and to locate health facilities in more walkable communities.[53]

It is too late to bring back the inventory of pre-World War II historic hospitals lost in countless cities (see Chapter 2).[54] Historic hospitals such as Charity were demolished long ago in other parts of the U.S. to clear land for their replacements – all in the name of *progress*. As discussed above, myth perpetuation on the part of elected officials remains a political and cultural impediment to the challenges of an already mammoth rebuilding progress in post-Katrina New Orleans. These same myths also affected the inability to resuscitate many neighborhood primary care clinics.[55]

A city's urban landscape is the manifestation of its citizens' shared sense of purpose, place, and identity.[56] Charity Hospital – symbolizing the intersection of health inequalities, race, class, and urban myth – merits a second look. This and other surviving historic hospitals can have new lives (see Chapter 2). It is within this framework that historic preservation and sustainable healthcare design must be viewed as seamless, as one rather than two disparate or parallel endeavors. Without this, synchronicity will be unattainable. An older hospital located in an established neighborhood near to public transportation can lessen that institution's carbon footprint, compared to it being located somewhere/nowhere out on the suburban fringe far from public transportation. In the face of global climate change, when so many new buildings are built on what was previously farmland, historic hospitals are worth reconsidering because they symbolize a place's collective memory and its cultural heritage. Many staff and patients rode the bus to and from Charity. It was a three-minute walk from the Tulane Medical School to Charity. In other words, a hospital's carbon footprint is more than its own campus and buildings. Its footprint extends broadly throughout its local community.

Doug Farr, in his book *Sustainable Urbanism: Urban Design with Nature* (2008) singled out two significant drawbacks to the current LEED system in the U.S. The first is the relatively low total number of buildings that have received LEED certification in comparison to those that have applied or are somewhere in the review process. This creates a bottleneck because LEED and the USGBC (United States Green Building Council) wish to greatly increase the number of recognized projects. But at the same time it wishes to elevate its criteria for carbon reduction. Hospitals old and new were being caught in a conundrum because they are so big and complex.

The second drawback was, in his words, 'LEED's building-centric focus and the low value it places on a project's location and context, particularly concerning auto dependency'.[57] The prerequisites and criteria weightings in the LEED system remained heavily weighted toward the building itself – and not much to its ripple effects in the community – and this had remained unchanged from the start of the program in 2000. There were no specific criteria for this aspect of a project and no more than 6 percent of all credits addressed these issues, greatly limiting the consideration of urban context or their immediate surroundings. Efforts are underway to launch a LEED program for urban neighborhood redevelopment in collaboration with the Congress for New Urbanism. This broadened view of sustainable urbanism and historic preservation would greatly aid the grass-roots local effort to save Charity Hospital and the 71-acre neighborhood slated for demolition.

Beyond the LEED system, specialists in preservation, conservation, and sustainable architecture and urbanism need to work together to broaden the definition of 'evidence' gathered and presented in support of carbon neutrality. Preservationists typically use due diligence, cultural inventory, recognizance, archival research, and fieldwork in their research and the Section 106 Review protocols include seven litmus test questions to assess if a given building or place is culturally and/or architecturally significant. Specialists in healthcare, for their part, typically use interviews, satisfaction surveys, patient medical records, staff records, behavioral observation, and workflow analyses in their research.[58]

The health needs of medically underserved populations remain acute in post-Katrina New Orleans. Nationally, as stated earlier in this book, nearly 48 million Americans lack medical insurance. However, the southern region of the U.S. has the highest percentage of uninsured – 19 percent (compared to 15 percent nationwide). With a statewide population of 4.2 million, the percentage of medically uninsured and underrepresented persons in Louisiana reached 750,000 in 2007 and this exceeded the national average.[59] It is well known that medically underserved populations have less access to care options in their communities and as a consequence, diagnosis and treatment often occurs too late. When this happens, the emergency departments of acute care hospitals, i.e. places such as Charity Hospital, become overwhelmed with patients with no way to pay for their care. This is a crisis in both the public and private sectors.[60]

Let this be a cautionary tale to others trying to save an historic hospital or any other type of historic healthcare facility. Even in normal times it is an uphill battle. Those responsible for this innovative alternative to the abandonment of Charity are to be commended for their strategy of hiring (at their own personal private expense) an experienced team to provide a feasible counterpoint – specialists with a strong record in historic preservation and current best practices in new hospital construction. Regardless, the jury remains out on whether the politicians, hospital officials, and community representatives will reach a consensus in Louisiana (as well as anyplace where such controversies exist) on the growing problem of how to address the critical intersection between sustainable urban design, architecture, and historic preservation in the arena of environments for healthcare. However, and sadly, in New Orleans it appeared that the local business community had cast its lot in full support of building the two new hospitals on the 71-acre site of an historic neighborhood.[61] Meanwhile, a local coalition of citizen-led community groups filed a lawsuit in Federal Court to block the permanent closure of Charity Hospital.[62] The architectural profession is just now beginning to sponsor workshops to aid architects seeking to recycle their clients' older healthcare facilities in the U.S.[63] These themes are reprised in the chapters that follow.

Prognostications

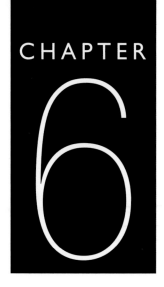

6

From the epochal events of 11 September 2001, to the inability of a mother in Ethiopia to obtain life-saving immunizations for her infant, a confluence of geopolitical and population growth challenges is resulting in highly pressing global health conditions. The world's 6.1 billion population increases by nearly 9,000 persons each hour. Several worldwide population institutes estimate that, by 2050, between 9 and 9.5 billion people will be living on the planet.[1] Populations in need of global architectural intervention include communities ravaged by HIV/AIDs, malaria, tuberculosis, plagues such as the virulent Ebola virus in Africa, and new strains of yellow fever. Add to this the profound pain caused by new settlements built in places where they should not be, such as in low-lying coastal zones, earthquake-prone regions, and in the midst of notorious hurricane 'alleys'. Ecologically sustainable buildings and typologies for health are needed in support of diverse occupants, their aspirations, and functional requirements. In a world of high construction costs and diminishing natural resources, we are being forced to relearn useful lessons from practices known for hundreds of years.

The field of architecture for health is at a turning point. In the coming years uncomfortable trade-offs will be made, although critical discourse on the challenges that lie ahead remains fragmented. The hospital, both as an idea and a building type, warrants reconsideration. It is teetering between an unsustainable status quo and an uncertain future. As a force that strives to promote human *and* ecological health, either/or trade-offs will no longer suffice. An environmentally compassionate future is the future of the hospital. The two principal aims of the following discussion are first, to delineate a road map of sorts for architecture for health within the broader discipline of architecture, and second, to prognosticate likely challenges to the discipline and practice of architecture for health between now and the year 2050. These are discussed from a dual present/futurist perspective. Nine prognostications are presented below and these are keyed to a diagram to portray visually how events may shape the healthcare landscape against a backdrop of geopolitical and technological events likely to unfold by then (Figure 6.1).[2]

The final chapter in my 2000 book consisted of six 'megatrends' likely to guide developments in the coming decade. These were:

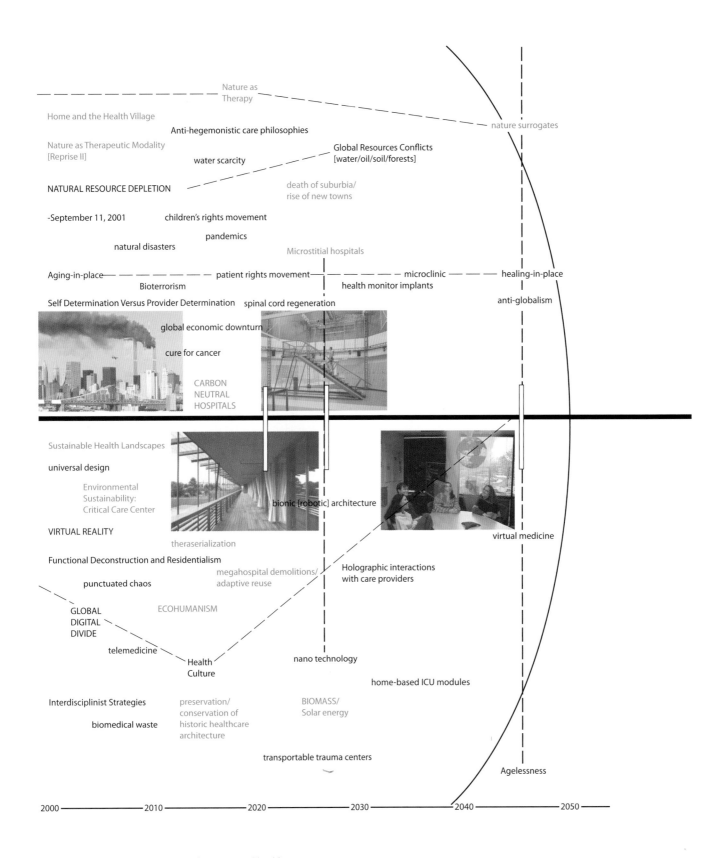

Nature as
Therapy

nature surrogates

Home and the Health Village

Anti-hegemonistic care philosophies

Nature as Therapeutic Modality
[Reprise II]

Global Resources Conflicts
[water/oil/soil/forests]

water scarcity

NATURAL RESOURCE DEPLETION

death of suburbia/
rise of new towns

-September 11, 2001   children's rights movement

pandemics

natural disasters

Microstitial hospitals

Aging-in-place ————————— patient rights movement — microclinic ———— healing-in-place

Bioterrorism   health monitor implants

anti-globalism

Self Determination Versus Provider Determination   spinal cord regeneration

global economic downturn

cure for cancer

CARBON
NEUTRAL
HOSPITALS

Sustainable Health Landscapes

universal design

Environmental
Sustainability:
Critical Care Center

bionic [robotic] architecture

VIRTUAL REALITY

virtual medicine

theraserialization

Functional Deconstruction and Residentialism

megahospital demolitions/
adaptive reuse

Holographic interactions
with care providers

punctuated chaos

GLOBAL
DIGITAL
DIVIDE

ECOHUMANISM

telemedicine

Health
Culture

nano technology

home-based ICU modules

Interdisciplinist Strategies

preservation/
conservation of
historic healthcare
architecture

BIOMASS/
Solar energy

biomedical waste

transportable trauma centers

Agelessness

2000 ——————— 2010 ——————— 2020 ——————— 2030 ——————— 2040 ——————— 2050

6.1   2000–2050 prognostications – architecture and health
considered in relation to geopolitical and environmental determinants

1 The growing importance of the home and the health village as being at the center of the healthcare equation

2 The ongoing influences of functional deconstruction of the tightly centralized modern hospital combined with the continued influences of residentialism in healthcare architecture

3 The growing importance of patient self-determinism in a knowledge-based healthcare landscape, and its implications for the healthcare provider in terms of improving access to care and its quality

4 The growing importance of sustainability across the healthcare industry

5 The therapeutic role of the natural environment in the healing experience

6 The growing need for collaborative and interdisciplinary approaches to problem solving with respect to built environments for human health.

These six trends are the foundation (and departure point) for an expanded discussion, a decade later.

1. The consequences of global climate change will pose daunting challenges, combined with a confluence of geopolitical hostilities over the exhaustion of oil and fresh water reserves, and exacerbated global population growth.

By the end of this century, the planet will heat up between 1.4 and 5.8 degrees Celsius, according to the *Intergovernmental Panel on Climate Change*. Six degrees may not sound like much, but it will be enough to radically transform the planet. Global warming is already a fact – the fabled snows of Kilimanjaro are melting away, the massive boulders of the Matterhorn, icebound for centuries, have begun to plunge in dramatic and dangerous rock falls, and the atoll nations of the Pacific are disappearing inch by inch under the waves. Scientific models demonstrate that climate change is an unprecedented challenge to societies around the globe, and is more than a routine swing of a slow pendulum. Coral reefs are already dying; polar creatures are losing their habitats. Some species may survive through migration, but countless others are doomed to extinction. With a three-degree increase, the American Midwest and the Amazon Basin – today the source of 20 percent of the Earth's freshwater – will begin to decay into arid, uninhabitable regions. Entire populations will become refugees as their land becomes uninhabitable, particularly along the earth's coastlines, in the face of rising sea levels. These changes will be pronounced by 2050. The great cites of New York, London, Mumbai, Shanghai, Tokyo, Los Angeles, New Orleans, and hundreds of others will be confronting at first periodic and, later, chronic flooding. In *Six Degrees: Our Future on a Hotter Planet*, Mark Lynas writes:

> In the four degree (temperature rise) world, with global sea levels half a meter or more above current levels, Alexandria (Egypt's) long lifespan will be drawing to a close. Even in today's climate, a substantial part of the city lies below sea level … by 2050 a rise in sea level of 50 centimeters would displace 1.5 million people … as the sea begins to encroach across ever wider parts of the Nile Delta, millions more will be evicted from their homes … beaches, wetlands, and agricultural areas will all be submerged, devastating an area that is the heart of Egypt's economy … farther to the east, Bangladesh will be losing a third of its land area, displacing tens of millions from the fertile Meghna Delta. In Boston, storm surge flooding from higher sea levels could inundate the central business district

… down the coast in New Jersey … three percent of the state [would be under water], including the most densely populated coastal areas … New York, London and Venice will only be saved if huge amounts of money are plowed into new and ever higher defenses against floods … Like today's New Orleans, coastal cities of the future may gradually become fortified islands, largely below sea level and under siege from all sides by advancing waters. Such a strategy would protect trillions of dollars worth of real estate, but it would also bring dangers: As New Orleans fatefully experienced [in Hurricane Katrina in 2005] one serious storm can bring down a vulnerable city in a matter of hours, putting many thousands of lives at risk. Rebuilding a city may be an option after the water is pumped out, as long as insurers are willing and able to cough up the necessary sums. But who will pay to build a city twice? Or three times? … the only solution will be for millions of coastal dwellers to retreat inland, as civilization's map is redrawn with constantly changing boundaries … inland cities will face a constant stream of refugees with thousands – and perhaps even millions – arriving all at once.[3]

What will happen to the healthcare infrastructure? Hospitals that are fully functional today will be rendered dysfunctional and uninhabitable. The effects of future wars over oil and water will have an impact on global healthcare. Climate change will alter patterns of travel and the spread of disease. The coming oil crisis will cause fewer people to travel from continent to continent. This crisis will lead to mass disruptions in oil production and distribution, resulting in less aid to poor nations, compromised immune systems, and millions of refugees with dire implications for an already delicately balanced network of hospitals and outpatient clinics. It will likely result in a healthcare infrastructure crisis. Water wars in the coming decades will have a similar effect on hospitals and clinics as the populations of parched cities and regions stream into places with adequate freshwater reserves. These reserves will have been secured through acts of war in an era of constant geopolitical tension over this most life-essential resource. Population growth will only compound the deleterious public health consequences of a crisis brought on by climate change, combined with the depletion of oil and freely abundant freshwater reserves.[4]

2. Global economic challenges will hamper multinational efforts and those of individual governments to make needed investments in environments for healthcare. Overdevelopment and its negative consequences – including unmitigated sprawl – exact their toll.

The global economic crisis that began in 2008 will persist in various forms. The near-collapse of the international banking industry will have unforeseen ripple effects for years to come. The culture of excessive consumption and instant gratification is being *reset*.[5] Economic recessions and intermittent periods of economic depression will likely cut into the amount of funding available for the construction and operation of healthcare facilities and the support infrastructure of laboratories and tertiary medical centers vital to advancing the fight against new diseases. Concurrently, it is likely that hyperconsumerism, the overconsumption of land, and deforestation, will continue. James Howard Kunstler writes:

> The dirty secret of the American economy in the 1990s was that it was no longer about anything except the creation of suburban sprawl and the furnishing, accessorizing, and financing of it … Nothing else really mattered … the economy of suburban sprawl was a systemic self-organizing response to the availability of inordinately cheap oil … Americans accepted [this] at face value as the logical outcome of their hopes and dreams and defended it viciously against criticism [but] it had no future … We [Americans] spent our wealth building an infrastructure of daily life that will not work very long into the 21st century … suburbia is the greatest misallocation of resources in the history of the world … [it] has a tragic destiny. More than half the U.S. population lives in it … [it] will lose its value catastrophically as it loses its utility … the loss of accustomed suburban logistics will be a nightmare for those stuck there. Will the collapse of suburbia as a viable mode of living tear the nation apart, both socially and politically? … If large numbers of people cannot unload their suburban McHouses and McMansions, then sooner or later many of these buildings will simply be abandoned, or become the slums of the future.[6]

In this scenario, hospitals, clinics, and other buildings for healthcare will face an equally uncertain future. Unchecked sprawl will lead to political destabilization in many regions. The massive speculative building boom in the city of Dubai in the Middle East came to a crashing halt in 2008. Rem Koolhaas and many other *Staritects* saw Dubai as an architectural sandbox in a place with few restrictions and an obsession with making its mark on the world stage. Kunstler and other critics of unbridled development view the underlying values of places such as Dubai and Las Vegas to be entirely fictitious, built on myth and little more.[7]

Transportation in the future will be very different from the culture of auto-dependency enjoyed up to now. Meaningful places and points of destination will need to be closer to one another.[8] Each year, the equivalent of hundreds of moderately sized cities are built on previously open, undeveloped land, although the parts do not add up to anything of lasting meaning. These non-places typically do not enrich people's lives from a civic standpoint. They are little more than loose aggregations of uncoordinated parts. Zoning laws, many obsolete, virtually guarantee an outcome characterized by a gangling array of meandering, overburdened roadways and diffuse non-relationships between buildings. This condition is avoidable if the basic ingredients – the houses, commercial establishments, office centers, civic institutions (including hospitals and other healthcare facilities), and roads – are assembled more intelligently. A healthy community – one that is both ecologically healthy and in terms of human health – includes clearly defined centers, short walking distances, pedestrian-scaled street networks, narrow versatile, streets which promote human interaction, mixed land and building uses, and the setting aside of key sites for renovated and adapted existing buildings and new civic buildings.[9]

Unlike the model of the traditionally evolved neighborhood, which evolved organically, sprawl is a dispassionate, idealized, artificial system. Unfortunately, this system is itself already unsustainable. Unlike the traditional neighborhood, sprawl is unhealthy growth and is essentially self-destructive. At a relatively low population density it consumes land at an alarming rate, while producing insurmountable traffic problems and exacerbating social inequity and isolation. If as much effort went into fewer in quantity but better quality infrastructure of civic buildings, including hospitals, clinics, and wellness centers, in and near to town centers rather than out on the fringes, more capital investment would be invested in a higher quality architectural built environment than is currently being built across America and elsewhere. Unfortunately, *smart growth* public policies remain rare. Fashionable suburban politicians continue to

attempt to build careers by attacking the sources of sprawl and advocating intelligent, smart growth policies and yet it is paradoxical, and dispassionate, environmentally, to continue to vote to build more roads to service new hospitals and clinics on sprawl sites while espousing anti-growth sentiments.[10] For example, ultra-aggressive, architecturally and environmentally destructive Wal-Mart megastores have only exacerbated matters. Wal-Mart's influence on the U.S. economy has reached levels not seen by a single company since the nineteenth-century rise of Standard Oil.[11]

3. The downsizing and redeployment of healthcare accelerates the functional deconstruction of the hospital. Care will be widely dispersed across an increasing number of small-scale microhospitals and clinics guided by smart growth planning principles.

By 2050, a higher number of smaller inpatient care facilities will be dispersed across the landscape; these places will continue to be required in the service of an increasingly acute patient population. They will be concentrated in large urban centers and their outlying neighborhoods, with some still needed in outer urban and fringe areas. Many small towns today have hospitals that themselves are dying financially and for lack of qualified patients and personnel. This situation has worsened over the past 25 years. Recent graduates of medical and nursing schools are often attracted by the higher salaries and amenities of urban life compared to the comparatively staid, tranquil tempo of rural life. In addition, the specializations found only in large urban medical centers and teaching centers today will become more decentralized. *Microhospitals* will have less than 50 beds each but every room will be acuity adaptable.

Dying hospitals will be renovated and reinvigorated for new uses, as thousands of these new *microhospitals* will be built in their place. This will occur in many regions, not only in advanced developed nations. Large tertiary urban *megahospitals* will still be needed, but they will have become the option of last resort for the sickest of the sick. These large institutions will by no means disappear – they will always be needed but there will be far fewer in number because they will have by then become too costly to operate except in the wealthiest urban centers. They will need to be more adroitly designed, located, and positioned than most are today. Microhospitals will need to be closer to where their patients live and work. These two extremes will define the endpoints of a continuum of facilities of varying sizes in between. Mixed-use, polyfunctional facilities will appear in communities of all sizes. This will contribute to the empowerment of the patient. Fewer will be able to afford the long pilgrimage to a Mayo Clinic, or an M.D. Anderson hospital if, through advanced high-tech telemedicine coupled with the newfound virtues and attractiveness of small scale communities, high quality care can be obtained closer to home, and provided more cheaply. This will influence all places where healthcare is received. New sources of inspiration will be explored, including the postmodernist sensibilities expressed in the contemporary hospice. Somewhat ironically, the spiritual dimensions of architecture for health will have experienced a full renaissance. The chapel, once a prominent feature of a hospital, will have all but disappeared in the megahospital by 2050. By 2000 it had often become next to impossible to locate a large hospital's chapel, as it had by then already been so shrunken in size. The capital resources invested in spiritual and nature-connected spaces and tectonic amenities in the microhospital will increase, with the hospice providing a particularly powerful source of inspiration.

4. By 2050, the home, not the hospital, will become the center of the healthcare universe. Health promotion (sickness prevention) will be inhibited only by global discrepancies between high-tech versus low-tech societies and the lacuna separating rich from poor.

Inequitable access, combined with the poor quality of healthcare for the poor and disenfranchised, will reach epidemic levels on an increasingly overpopulated planet. A network of microhospitals, as mentioned, will continue to be essential to care only for the sickest of the sick – the most acutely ill. Places other than microhospitals and the neighborhood clinic will have become the epicenter of the healthcare landscape. The patient and family (if resources and politics permit) will have universal access to health information anywhere, anytime. Our home will become a virtual clinic. Holograms and microimplants will monitor our health. The Institute of Physics in the U.K. reported in 2008 that smart holograms (holographic biosensors), which use materials called hydrogels that shrink or swell in response to local physiologic conditions, will be used to monitor many physical

ailments. These holograms will be able to check blood sugar levels, adrenaline levels, or even detect chemicals like anthrax after a terrorist attack. Moisture sensitive sensor holograms combined with these miniscule implants will be used to help us detect health threats before they actually occur.[12]

Holographic consult sessions with your caregiver will occur in the privacy of the family room or kitchen at home. Current advances in 3-D home entertainment will have led to holographic television. Imagine watching a sporting event on your full height wallscreen with the action exploding from the flat screen out into the room where you can view and be a *part of* the action from any angle, wearing 3-D glasses. Imagine showing your broken arm to your physician and from the physician's office he or she is able to instruct you to turn your arm for a full holographic examination in the same manner, or your nurse or therapist being able to project at full scale into your living room in 3-D (or vice versa) for a personal consult session. Commercial holographic TV and wireless Internet service will be widely available soon and this is when the really amazing possibilities will unfold.

In the hospital surgical theater, holograms will be used in a wide range of surgical procedures, including neurosurgery and cranioplastic reconstructive surgery. A Voxgram is a digital holography system able to provide a full size, transparent hologram of any part of the human body, enabling interaction in, around and through the image as if it were a real specimen of anatomy, not unlike that familiar childhood toy, the Visible Man and Visible Woman. This technology will go far beyond the 2-D CT or MRI scans that at present film in sequential slices. Voxgrams will be displayed in a viewing box and surgeons will have success in their use. As but one example of the thousands of possible applications, digital holography will be used to display congenital anomalies of the cervical spine, with holograms relied upon in pre-plan surgery protocols. The transparent nature of the image and the ability to fully invert (move) them to view the data from the opposite direction will aide in detecting unexpected relationships among the abnormally formed bones. Also, holograms will help parents better understand their child's problem. By 1997 more than 165-peer-reviewed scientific presentations had already been given at medical conferences by radiologists, physicists, neurosurgeons, orthopedic surgeons, and plastic surgeons touting the potential application of medical holography in the hospital surgical setting. Medical holography will also be used in a wide range of cancer treatments.[13]

5. The physical space at present separating the individual from contact with the natural environment will gradually dematerialize. Buildings for health will increasingly express anthropomorphic and organic forms, biophiliac, and anti-machine imagery.

Sensory immersion environments will very closely duplicate real, natural landscapes. Many hospices are currently employing these ecohumanist technologies, with positive results. A new field, design therapeutics, will explore these person-environment transactions. Artificial terrain tools and software packages will make it possible to fuse transparent linkages between human sensory modalities in the context of the human experience of natural environments. Nature immersion landscapes, many of which are already to be found in zoos and aquariums, will synthetically and seamlessly combine various elements of real and virtual natural landscapes, and will be geared to suppress any undesirable, i.e. counter-therapeutic, content. Theories of biophilia will guide the design of virtual systems fully controllable and monitored to create any desired therapeutic effect in the coming age of 'hyperreality' – a world where imitation will often be better than the real thing.[14]

Artificial landscapes will provide the recovering patient with a virtual, condensed version of world travel in which one can experience only the most interesting and edifying features of natural places. Experiences such as this will be well integrated into the planning and design of healthcare settings by 2050. The therapeutic effects of artificial landscape simulation in buildings will enhance the healing process. Sadly, the natural environment itself will have by then been widely contaminated in many parts of the world; all that will be left in many places will be faint recollections of what once was the real thing, for simulations, sad to say, will have become the norm rather than the exception[15]

Translucent, backlit curvilinear wall panels will have replaced the stoic traditional walls in the corridors and public areas of healthcare settings. These panels will span the color wheel, presenting dawn-to-dusk panoramic, theraserialized environmental progressions.[16] By 2050, hospitals in dense urban settings will be able to tune out all undesirable, i.e. countertherapeutic, stimuli (noisy traffic, smog, etc.). The condition of privacy as it is known today will have been completely redefined in the inpatient room. Active simulations will have been complemented by passive microimplants such as wall murals (a technique used at present in a number of institutions) and sophisticated biomorphic (robotic controlled) lighting. Modularized

inpatient rooms will incorporate active nature simulations and *theraserialization* will be the norm (see Chapter 3). Virtually every architectural feature of the patient room (and any room within or near to a healthcare facility, for that matter) will be fully programmable with successor gadgets to the current handheld PDA (Personal Desk Assistant) device. As for wall multiplexed wall panels, backlighting will be used to activate the nature scene and to provide ambient lighting, all entirely controllable by the patient (see Chapter 4).[17] Form-generative computer software combined with architectural nanotechnology and robotics will allow for these fluid form languages to be ubiquitous. Life scenarios will be played out in virtual *naturespace*. Artificial neural networking will yield perceptual modeling software to make it possible to plug in what/if scenarios with respect to an individual's person-nature preferences any time of the day or night. Moreover, the virtual stages of video gaming realms, together with holography, will have been adapted to virtually communicate health-related information between the patient and the caregiver, and between the client and the architect.[18]

As for buildings designed for health, the 'CO²' building, its nickname derived from its plan configuration, is an anthropomorphic community health and wellness center in Narita, Japan, near Tokyo. Designed by I. Kazuhiro (2000–2002) this anticipatory building provides a glimpse into the future as it intrinsically fuses nature and anthropomorphism in its parti'. Hospital architects will view the natural environment as itself therapeutic, seamlessly integrated into the formal language of healthcare architecture. In other words, the hospital will not only contain and relate to nature, but itself become inherently organic and biomorphic. In the CO_2 health center, nature provides more than stylistic or symbolic inspiration, a mere stage-set backdrop, or a glossy image for a slick marketing brochure. Here, actual trees from the actual site become part of the building's column structural system. These 'interior trees' anchor a white fabric membrane roof system, beneath which rooms are deployed around a pair of courtyards shaped by the irregular curvature of the structure. In this manner, nature is brought indoors as a means to protect and honor, and to 'save' it, ironically, from total destruction and to preserve its intrinsic beauty for future generations when deforestation will have nearly completely ravaged the earth's living forests. By 2050, biomorphic robotics, micromachine implants and tools, and anthropomorphism will emerge as vibrant movements. The cascading, wave-like formal vocabulary of the Balloch Children's Hospice, in Scotland (2003–2006), by Gareth Hoskins Architects, of Glasgow,

Scotland, elegantly reinterprets this timeless relationship between the ground, mid-building, and the roof plane in a way that strikes a compositional and aesthetic *lightness* similar to the CO_2 clinic in Japan.[19] Hospitals and other heterotrophic healthcare environments will express these and other emergent formal languages, extending far beyond the rigid orthodoxy of twentieth-century minimalism.

6. The digital divide will continue to separate the haves from the have-nots in the global healthcare landscape. The Internet holds the promise to significantly advance patient-centered care and sickness prevention but by 2050 the expert, empowered patient may exist only in cultures wealthy enough to afford the technology.

The continuing Information Revolution will elevate the patient and family to an unprecedented level of sophistication, but not all will benefit, not by a long shot. In poor societies the available options for access to the Internet will be tightly controlled for various political reasons. The most obvious being that information leads to empowerment and empowerment leads to a questioning of the status quo. That is why the leaders of Caribbean island nations are at present so fearful of having their vast compounds seen from the air by anyone, anyplace via Google Earth maps. A move is afoot to ban outright Google maps in many developing nations for this precise reason. This *digital divide* will continue to be an impediment to attaining healthcare equity between the privileged and the underprivileged in societies globally – those with Internet access versus those without. It will be little different than during the Middle Ages, when those who could afford to barter for privacy received their own room instead of a straw mattress in the hellish open ward.

A national health information survey in the U.S. in 2004 found that a 'tectonic shift' was already taking place in the ways in which patients accessed and consumed health and medical information. It was concluded that a high percentage of patients in the future would first acquire knowledge online before talking with their physician. Digital medical records are becoming the norm although some care providers and nations will be unable to afford the cost of conversion from paper to paperless systems. This will cause a schism internationally. Many care providers in even the wealthiest countries will remain wary of making large investments in hardware and software if they

believe that these purchases will be obsolete in a only few years.[20] Striking inequities in health outcomes will persist between racial and ethnic groups in the U.S., with many medically underserved groups experiencing significantly poorer health outcomes than members of the racial majority. Unequal access to online health information will continue to be a major underlying cause of this digital divide.[21]

The future of medically underrepresented populations in design decision making remains uncertain. If their voices are to flourish in the future this must occur in a way that truly reaches out to persons of all walks of life and socio-economic strata, not only the wealthy and the well connected. Unfortunately, as many as two billion of the uninsured will be locked out of the healthcare industry globally and concomitantly locked out of healthcare facilities.

It will no longer suffice for the designer to speak primarily with the top-end decision makers of a healthcare organization. The distance between the end user, usually at the bottom of the decision-making pyramid (the direct caregivers and the patient and family), and the leadership of an organization, nearly always at the top (the CEO), will have to be compressed and reconfigured. Patient–family empowerment in the planning and design process will cut across diverse contexts and healthcare constituencies. However, access to influence will remain difficult and a cause for much conflict cross culturally in the transfer of technology to areas where millions remain uninsured, and from the standpoint of transferring knowledge from universal health coverage system contexts to other contexts. This will be difficult to achieve unless cultural, political, economic, legal, and regulatory barriers are overcome. Even in countries with national health programs for all citizens, the pitfalls of the digital divide and the plight of underrepresented minority populations will remain unavoidable without built-in safeguards.

7. Progressive architecture for health will express the compatible values of both human *and* ecological health. Conservation will lead to new uses for abandoned hospitals and for carbon neutral healing environments. Ecohumanists will advocate for quality of life issues on a threatened planet.

Hospitals will no longer be among the worst polluters in their communities. They will generate no toxic waste, and institutions will be planned and built with high regard for sustainability and stewardship.[22] All healthcare providers will have long-adopted *net zero* policies. Hospital incinerators will have been long demolished, having outlived their original purpose. On the abundance of nuclear waste on hospital sites, Seanna Adcox writes:

> Tubes, capsules and pellets of used radioactive material are piling up in the basements and locked closets of hospitals and research installations around the country [the U.S.], stoking fears they could get lost or, worse, stolen by terrorists and turned into dirty bombs. For years, truckloads of low-level nuclear waste from throughout the U.S. was taken to a rural South Carolina landfill. There, items such as the rice-sized radioactive seeds for treating cancer and pencil-thin nuclear tubes used in gauges were sealed in concrete and buried. But since 2008 a new law ended all disposal of radioactive material at the site, leaving 36 states with no place to throw out the stuff. So labs, universities, hospitals and manufacturers are storing more and more of it on their own property in urban locations all over the country … and worries are growing … over the past decade, 4,363 radioactive material packages have been lost, stolen or abandoned.[23]

The biggest problem will remain excessive resource consumption. By 2050 the notion of 'healthy bodies equals healthy environment' will be widely accepted. But by then it may be too late. In the latest *Global Environmental Outlook*, the UN Environment Program points out that one of the three pillars of sustainable development, the environment, will be seriously listing because of the distortions placed on it by excessively insensitive human actions. Excessive consumption by the more affluent will have been reduced by force in some cases – the richest 20 percent will no longer account for 86 percent of all consumer consumption.[24]

In India there are currently more than 5,000 small and private hospitals and nursing homes. Increasing population will cause a rapid proliferation of health facilities there. India alone generates three million tons of medical waste annually and this figure is growing by 8 percent each year. Waste segregation at the source will remain the number one problem, a looming crisis by 2050, yet this concept will only have been partially ingrained in the nation's cultural psyche, and therefore will remain a low priority for hospital administrators.[25] Around the globe, ignorance, political malfeasance, and cultural indifference will continue to hinder progress. Reflective architects, armed with the results drawn from successful case studies, will work in interdisciplinary consortiums in public health education efforts. Architecture and the fields of community health and social ecology will eventually fold into a single *ecohumanist* entity, out of sheer societal necessity.

A new wave of best practices in sustainable hospital construction and historic conservation will be routine in professional practice. New ways will have been identified to integrate healthier healthcare facilities with *ecoparks* in towns and neighborhoods, and in materials specs on a 'fitness for purpose' basis.[26] In addition, zero waste protocols will be mandatory in many communities with respect to the demolition of old buildings (all materials will have to be rechanneled). If they cannot be saved and preserved, or adapted to new uses, buildings will be disassembled and redeployed, with recycled first generation 'new' building materials used only when absolutely necessary. Contractors will be daily participants in centralized waste co-op exchanges in order to stream old waste from healthcare and other types of facilities to new *wasteless* uses.[27]

Ecohumanism will adopt advanced robotic technologies to enable humans to attain greater ecologic interactivity with the healthcare setting. While the smart home will be a new concept (the Xanadu house prototypes were built back in 1979) intelligent buildings, including microhospitals and clinics, will be reconfigurable according to external conditions like wind and sun as well as to the movements of occupants inside. Active furniture is being developed; in 2008 Philips Corporation launched its *HomeLab*, an integrated home entertainment system with interactive devices. Perhaps one day we'll speak to our bio-homes and they'll answer us, or they will 'turn' their backs to block a windstorm.[28]

Ecohumanists will use bionic engineering, biomorphism, and redeployment in the support of occupants' daily needs. New building materials, assembly systems, and anatomical-operational systems will profoundly influence human well-being in post-disaster situations. Transportable *bionic hospitals* will serve the needs of disaster victims in the face of global climate change. These redeployable *smartbuildings* can be erected in a matter of days; in the coming years they will afford far more flexibility than standard fixed site, conventional hospitals. Mobile clinics will provide transprogramatic healthcare (see Chapters 7 and 8). The needs of the homeless will remain unmet in many parts of the world and will increase unless reflective architects rise to the challenge. At the end of the twentieth century a National Guard armory in New York City was in fact used as a gigantic hospital ward, with many inhabitants in this overnight shelter infected with TB by default in this reprise of a medieval open ward from the twelfth century.[29] Will this also occur in 2050?

8. A multifaceted discipline will fuse design and the health sciences. Current disciplinary barriers between architecture, interior design, industrial design, landscape architecture, ecology, biophiliaism, urban and regional planning, and the medical and social sciences will blur.

Since the late nineteenth century the field of architecture has evolved from a gentlemanly vocation with a singular, narrowly defined emphasis on professional practice centered on the making of buildings to a much broader disciplinary endeavor. This process has involved a continual search for greater professional relevancy to society while seeking to establish and hold onto its autonomy within the community of professions. Relevancy and autonomy, it has been reasoned, carry greater stature and prestige together than does one or the other alone. It has been further reasoned that the generation and legitimization of new knowledge through research carried out within a scholarly *discipline* of architecture would further propel progress toward attaining this aim. The medical and legal professions, for their part, successfully adopted this model over 100 years ago. In so doing, they catapulted to their present perches of relative societal esteem, visibility, and relevance.

By comparison, in recent decades a *discipline* of architecture has evolved at a snail's pace, pedantically accruing its own body of knowledge somewhat haphazardly. In addition, evidence-based research on built environments for healthcare lags far behind the medical and legal professions. Proponents and practitioners would have the public believe otherwise, 'We have our own journals, professional groups, awards programs, and our own certification programs and credentials for practitioners and researchers'. What they fail to realize is that the sheer vastness of the money spent on healthcare construction globally simply *dwarfs* that spent on research for design. This is the case regardless of whether it is defined by building type, i.e. schools, libraries, or by subject area, i.e. sustainability, historic preservation. Worse, it may be by a factor of as much as 50 to 1 when tallied as a percentage of the total annual healthcare construction expenditure in the U.S. versus the total amount spent on medical research.

Architectural theory is gradually evolving from a traditional reliance on historical precedent to a position informed by critical analysis and, to some extent, scientific method. Interdisciplinary activity in architecture remains rather fractured and diffuse, unfortunately. This is largely a function of the long-held practice of randomly borrowing from research paradigms in the social sciences, the humanities, and the engineering sciences. This random approach reflects a disinclination to meaningfully synthesize.[30] It is insufficient to simply assert expertise within *any* single discipline.

A clearly defined, coherent knowledge base that is trans-disciplinary will be prerequisite. In this regard, the profession of architecture has found itself at a disadvantage relative to other fields. Over time, unless it expands its scope its status as a viable profession will become more questionable. Before, the architect could simply be trusted to know about the building itself. The architect will be increasingly called upon to provide full empirical justification for the decisions about the building, and much more. However, the existing structure of this educational knowledge base and of theory within architecture does not easily incorporate new forms of explicit knowledge. Rather than simply being put in the responsive mode, reflective architects will by 2050 be more proactive in generating a full discussion of a widened palette of salient issues.[31]

The field of architecture for health will contribute to codified knowledge by aiming higher with the goal of eradicating fragmented efforts, attaining a new relevancy without necessarily sacrificing its complete autonomy. *Interdisciplinism* will denote an attitude of openness to the necessity of sharing, of collective problem solving. New professional consortiums will evolve with the allied design fields, global resource management, optical imaging and holography, human genetics and biomedical engineering, chaos theorists, nanotechnologists, community health agencies, public policy experts, gerontologists, other social scientists, and specialists in a host of fields. New hybrid interdisciplinary subfields will have emerged on the ethical dimensions of sustainable design for health, historic preservation, public health policy, and effective community-based participatory planning.[32] The agendas and methodologies of this hybrid discipline will be rendered on newly stretched canvases fusing biophiliaism with new formal/aesthetic languages.

9. Advanced health technologies and the agelessness movement will have an uneven impact globally on human health and well-being. Molecular nanotechnology will afford total control over the structure of matter, allowing the building of anything, even the reconstructed body.

Community development professionals have known for years that in order to engage effectively with disadvantaged groups one first must address head-on the power imbalances that persist between them. This practice is widely referred to as 'linking social capital'.[33] Advances in biomedical science will result by 2050 in what will become known as *agelessness* but it will have an extremely uneven impact. The debates are already reaching a feverish pitch.[34] The science of extrophy will have fused sweeping advancements in neurophysiology, neurochemistry, and human genetics, resulting in a cure for cancer and dementia. Prozac, Piracetam, Hydergine, Deprenyl, and other yet-to-be invented drugs will have modified our physiology, enhancing our concentration, and slowing the aging of the brain. Research in powerful modifiers will apply new tools from molecular biology, computer-assisted molecular design, and brain imaging. Health-monitoring machines will be bio-organic, self-modifying, intelligent. Artificial life systems, neural networks, and fuzzy logic will have added to an already vast arsenal of high technology for the re-engineering of the human body. Computers and their interfaces will have evolved to *fit* us: from mainframes and text-based interfaces to PCs and GUIs, tenth-generation PDAs, voice-recognition, and *knowbots*. Nanocomputers will have been implanted in humans to make us more 'intelligent'. It will be a strange new world with the transmutation of life itself in a bizarre quest for immortality.[35]

Some futurists believe that the abolition of aging and most involuntary death will have occurred by then.[36] Machine intelligence researchers, roboticists, and cognitive scientists foresee even more radical possibilities. We will be able to 'upload' ourselves, our psychological outlook, memories, emotional responses, and values. This will occur just as we now do with software, only from our biological brain to our synthetic brain. Powered by these devices our cognitive mental processes will then function hundreds of thousands of times faster than at present. This is the epochal world depicted in Steven Spielberg's futurist film *A/I* (2000). More attainable at a much earlier date than 2050 will have been the discovery of spinal cord regenerative medicine,[37] and the aforementioned fusing of robotics

with the design of the built environment, including the application of robotic personal assistants, or RPAs so, for example, residents will have 'helpers' in a long-term care setting. This is already occurring in Japan on a test pilot basis.[38]

But what good is it to extend the quantity of life if its quality will be significantly diminished? What if only people in wealthy societies have access to this new technology? New technologies are going to make new lifestyles possible well before and into our retirement. Our life expectancies have made tremendous gains over the last century, more than at any other time in history. People in developed nations already live longer, learn more, earn more, and consume more. The average life expectancy was around 22 to 25 years for most, from biblical times forward. Life expectancy started rising in the 1700s, moving toward 35 years by 1800 and then to around 47 years by 1900. Then in just one century it advanced *30 years*. The coming wave of genetic technologies will cause another wave of faster life expectancy inflation that will continue to occur to 2050 – when the average life expectancy could well advance to 110 to 120 years of age.[39]

The privileged (or unfortunate, depending on how one views it) will live longer, but will the quality of our life and health into these older age ranges improve dramatically?[40] The question remains, for whom? Will everyone share equally in a bionic-uploaded 'higher' quality of life in the face of this upwardly spiraling age trend? Will everyone equally reap the benefits of new forms of medical care? Will everyone have access to routine full body holographic scans?[41] Of course not. Health disparities will persist and only worsen if global access to healthcare resources remains disproportional, geared towards the 'haves'. Most indicators point to the stark reality that health disparities between the haves and the have-nots portend to only increase, magnifying, worsening the quality of life gap between the classes and races on an overpopulated planet.[42] The risk is that the poor will become further marginalized, only now across a longer lifespan and in greater numbers than ever before.[43]

Ecohumanism and the future of the hospital

Compassion is fundamental to human existence. Humans have withstood devastating diseases, epidemics, world wars, totalitarian rule, famine, apartheid, genocide, and catastrophic natural disasters.

Brazen, dispassionate rulers, acting with intense hatred and brutality, have left their stain upon the landscape of human history.[44] Despite this, through the centuries, acts of compassion expressed through architecture have expressed a sustained concern for the plight of others. Architecture is capable of uplifting the human spirit and nurturing the psyche. At its worst, it can be used to exact a deadening toll on human life.

The relationship between passion and compassion in architecture is complex, timeless, and contradictory. The modernists of the early twentieth century were no less passionate than those who designed and built the great civic edifices of Ancient Greece and Rome. An architect's 'signature' style may passionately express compositional elements, colors, materiality, and fenestration, the dramatic siting of one's buildings, and so on. *Passion* in architecture can invoke a building's developmental narrative as much as the physical end result.[45] A passionately conceived and executed building is typically praised for its aesthetic or tectonic innovations. In architectural discourse, compassion, on the other hand, is rarely cited as a laudable attribute. Often, it seems to matter little if the building explicitly speaks to issues of social empathy regarding those who have been disadvantaged or underserved by architecture. The compassion quotient expressed in a building or environment may therefore be glossed over, politely sidestepped, or dismissed outright.[46]

Compassion, by definition, remains somewhat oblique, and would appear to be subordinate to passionate qualities in architecture. The fact remains that many of the most enduring, timeless civic buildings constructed in history have expressed both sensibilities as a duality. A building is a cultural investment.[47] Architecture must first and foremost sympathize with the habitual inhabitant.[48] Empathic architecture, in a social and civic sense, is becoming rare in the ordinary everyday built environment.[49] This is because passion and compassion, in architecture, threaten to become divorced from one another. Most buildings in our everyday lives are banal, and this cuts to the heart of the problem. Professions generally seek to do good as they define it, often in ways to increase the power, status, and income of their members, through 'benevolent professional imperialism'.[50] This approach is not always in the best interests of the client or the end user.[51] Benevolent imperialism is impossible to hide in architecture. Anything-goes pluralism in popular culture and in the everyday built environment can cut both ways.[52]

Ecohumanism in architecture for health is rooted in the social sciences, the humanities, and in environmentalism. Environmentalism has been defined as the recurring and timeless tension between empirical science and human emotion, between preservation of the natural environment and patterns of human habitation.[53] Three architectural corollaries include the LEED rating system, historic preservation, and the adaptive reuse of buildings and places. These express social systems of interrelated hierarchies comprised of personal, institutional, and societal constructs.[54]

Architects are sometimes attacked for being insensitive, for being discompassionate. For the architect, two role models predominate – the 'egoist', and the 'pragmatist'. The egoist architect role model is the 'I-give-them-what-I-want' approach to practice, while the pragmatist is attitudinally described as the 'I-give-them-what-they-want' approach.[55] A third role for the architect, the 'I-give-them-what-I-can' modus operandi, is a middle ground, an in-between stance whereby the *facilitator architect* values both aesthetic autonomy (passion) and social engagement and equality (compassion). The egoist architect characteristically values the former highest and the latter much less.[56] The egoist's approach is paternalistic, whereas the pragmatist, on the other hand, is essentially an entrepreneur. By contrast, the midpoint perspective is that of reflective interpreter, aiming for an effective balance including one's own worldview.[57] In a study conducted by this author of the *Modern Healthcare* magazine annual design awards program, 2,047 submissions were examined over a ten-year period. It was found that buildings designed for public sector 'poorer' clients were rarely submitted.[58]

Conservative social theorists and politicians have a tendency to view the poor as deviant, arguing that they elect to pay little or nothing for housing, food, or healthcare. Further, they blame the poor's imprudence and lack of judgment for their inability to afford housing and other life necessities. The belief that the poor do not value housing in the same way as the middle class ignores the fact that the poor have much less income and opportunity. With less income, a poor person is not able to make the same choices as is a middle class person.[59] Shigeru Ban's 'Community Dome Project' provided a meeting place for victims of all classes and races in the aftermath of the severe dislocation caused by the Kobe earthquake in 1995. It was as much a public health intervention as an architectural intervention.

Architects around the globe must adopt a proactive leadership role.[60] Such efforts can place a spotlight on the emergency shelter healthcare and housing needs of victims of disasters and terrorist attacks.[61] The International Red Cross and the Pan American Health

Organization have published reports on disaster mitigation shelter and public health needs.[62] A prototype design for an HIV/AIDS mobile health clinic has been developed by the American organization Architecture for Humanity.[63] Fragmented government-sponsored initiatives to rebuild flood-ravaged housing in Bangladesh have been only somewhat successful to date, largely because they define the problem in overly narrow terms, as either a public health or a shelter issue, or because key experts from various fields of expertise are unable to coordinate, effectively, their efforts.[64] Architects need to soul search.[65] The medical profession has recently been engaged in its own soul searching. Medical schools and the health sciences professions have recently come under fire for physicians' insensitivities. So have architects and architecture schools. Ecohumanism in architecture is about having an equal concern for human *and* ecological well-being, and by its nature it touches on many uncomfortable truths.[66] The challenge now is to translate this unprecedented opportunity into action.

PART 2

Design

Designing for hospital-based care

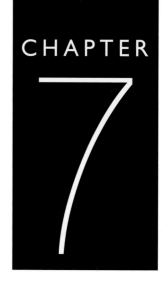

A hospital is a complex, contradictory building type, a system of systems. It is a dense aggregation of people, equipment, and supplies. There is no one definition that succinctly sums up the many types of hospitals, nor their diverse geographic contexts, populations served, or cultural determinants that shape and continually reshape them. However, established baseline principles and standards do exist for their planning and design. These criteria are shaped by local, regional, national, and increasingly by international building codes. According to the American Medical Association, a hospital in the U.S. is defined as an institution with at least six beds whose primary function is to deliver patient services – diagnostic and therapeutic – for particular or general medical conditions. A hospital must be licensed, have an organized physician staff, and provide continuous nursing services under the supervision of registered nurses. The construction and operation of a contemporary hospital in the U.S. is governed by local, state, and federal regulations, and third-party nationwide accreditation commission standards, as well as the aforementioned codes for their design and construction, fire protection, and sanitation.[1] Among the organizations with regulatory oversight, staffing and care delivery standards are set by the Joint Commission on the Accreditation of Healthcare Organizations.

Due to vast variations across cultures and across geographic regions of the world, it is virtually impossible to attempt to comparatively assess the efficacy of one region or locality's minimum planning and design standards compared to any other. Important determinants in identifying these highest ideals include:

- Local cultural traditions and demographic characteristics of the population
- Community attitudes towards sickness, disease and health promotion
- Identification of obstacles to the establishment of a sustainable healthcare environment
- An expectation in the local community that minimum standards will be set and exceeded for the design and construction of healthcare delivery environments
- Adherence to building codes and regulatory agency licensing protocols
- Building and sustaining strong community support for local healthcare institutions
- Establishing sustainable partnerships between not-for-profit and for-profit healthcare institutions

- Setting and attaining progressive yet realistic funding and budget objectives
- Establishing and periodically reappraising the organization's strategic future goals.

The compendium of planning and design principles presented below is an attempt to give architectural expression to the aesthetic, functional, symbolic, and spiritual dimensions of a hospital's internal elements, its connection to its immediate site, the role of environmental stewardship, and the importance of local culture and tradition. At the core is the intent to give expression to principles of sustainable architecture for health. Hospitalization is a nuanced, often stressful experience for the patient and family. Architects are well advised to first immerse themselves in the hospital experience, to explore its inner profundities. This is essential in order to fully appreciate the difficulty of caring for the sick, injured, and diseased on a day-to-day basis. The hospital as a type is not about to disappear anytime soon. They are growing in number as the earth's population rapidly expands. The global inventory of hospitals at present does not come close to meeting global demand. To confound matters, hospitals are disproportionately distributed across the globe. Wealthier regions and nations tend to have far more hospital beds per capita compared to poorer regions and nations.

This compendium is meant to be a vehicle to *elevate* the discourse on this building type. It is a reaction to the fear, uncertainty, and lack of control that so often is in the mind of the patient. It is a reaction against their isolation, marginalization, and dismissal. It is a reaction against any system or policy that would seek to isolate the patient from one's friends, family, loved ones, or community during hospitalization. Being hospitalized for most is a watershed moment in one's life. It is often a time of crisis. It is the loss of control over one's life and of those around oneself. The architectural environment must not be an additional source of stress or add to the feeling of being out of control. Architecture can and must provide therapeutic and curative support at this most critical of times. This support is generally of four types – instrumental, aesthetic, emotional, and spiritual. Instrumental support is personified in the degree to which the performance of the physical setting supports the day-to-day functional needs of its inhabitants. Aesthetic support consists of the abstract, largely interpretative role of built form and the meanings it possesses. Emotional support is the ability of the built environment to help expand inner horizons and to increase competency. Spiritual support denotes the support the built environment is able to provide as a stage upon which an individual is able to reflect and self-actualize.

This compendium consists of 100 design considerations (issues), presented as seven categories: 1. Site and context; 2. Arrival, public, and semi-public spaces; 3. The patient care unit (PCU) and inpatient room; 4. Diagnostic/treatment and trauma units; 5. Outpatient services; 6. Theraserialization and landscape; and 7. Administration/total environment. They are presented against the backdrop of these seven types of acute care settings:

- Acute care hospitals
- Rehabilitation hospitals
- Psychiatric hospitals
- Heart hospitals
- Women's hospitals
- Children's hospitals
- Hospital-based outpatient clinics

They are meant to be broadly interpreted for use by designers, planners, engineers, sustainability specialists, direct caregivers, including physicians, nurses, and others, fundraisers, administrators, Boards of Directors, federal governmental agencies, private foundations, community advocates, elected officials, health policy specialists, evidence-based design researchers, home health organizations, public health agencies at the local, regional and federal levels, and by patients and their families. This compendium is not to be misconstrued as prescriptive or dogmatic. The case studies in Chapter 8 are referenced as CS 1–28. It is hoped that others will build upon this lexicon of design considerations and view it collectively as a call to extend, to further improve the quality, scope, and efficacy of the built environment for healthcare.

1 Site and context

Community and neighborhood

Hospitals operate in virtually every site context – from urban core, surrounding older neighborhoods and districts, inner suburban, outer suburban, to rural settings. They exist in the densest of communities and in communities with comparatively low population densities.

and international patient constituency. Institutions grow and evolve over time. Large medical centers tend to face the most complex community relations challenges. Nevertheless, effective community relations are critical, as are effective lines of communication. The nearest neighbors are key stakeholders and therefore deserve a meaningful voice in matters pertaining to renovation, expansion, or relocation (Figure 7.1).

Hospitals and sprawl

Hospitals relocate from older urban centers to newer suburban and exurban locations for many reasons, including the quest for proximity and access to a larger patient pool, to fill a niche caused by unchecked population growth and sprawl, and for greater profits. Suburban fringe sites are often the most attractive sites from the standpoint of institutional relocation and market expansion.[3] In sprawl communities, a new hospital is a civic crown jewel, and its presence tends to fuel even more unchecked sprawl. Newly established medical centers tend to follow the same pattern as shopping malls, bland subdivisions, multiplex cinema complexes, and the like, as they similarly require large land parcels and large expanses of paved asphalt. Compared to older central city neighborhoods, the lower cost of land on the fringe is a powerful intoxicant to most hospital boards. This is one reason why so few completely new hospitals have been established in U.S. inner urban neighborhoods in the last decade. The Metro Health Village (2003–2006), built on a greenfield site at the edge of Grand Rapids, Michigan, typifies this pattern: it was built, at least in part, speculatively, on the assumption that Americans would continue to prefer to live in far-flung, disconnected suburbs where virtually every activity requires a car trip. The sprawl syndrome is by no means unique to the U.S.; it is happening on the edges of Cairo, Dublin, Taipei, Sydney, Auckland, Toronto, London, Mexico City, and many other places. When will hospitals become part of the solution – a carbon neutral building type – rather than continuing to be a part of the problem, as a wasteful, carbon intensive building type?

Climate change and the hospital

In the face of global climate change, carbon-reductive and net zero site planning and building design for hospitals and allied healthcare

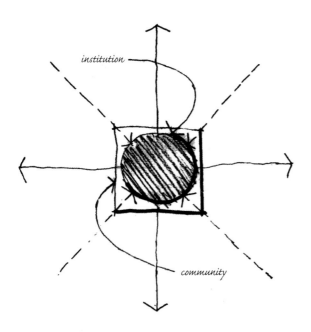

7.1 Sense of place is interwoven with community health

They exist in waterfront locations, on the open plains, in arid and semi-arid regions, in extremely cold climates, and in tropical forests. They exist below sea level and in high altitude communities. By definition, hospitals, visually, exert their civic presence by sheer virtue of size and appearance. The largest urban medical centers are by definition the most visible, unless surrounded by denser high-rise development, as in the case of the Northwestern Memorial Medical Center in downtown Chicago. By contrast, a hospital on the tundra on the edge of a remote village near the Arctic Circle may be visible from many miles away, as in the case of the Yukon-Kuskokwim Delta Regional Hospital (1976–1980), in Bethel, Alaska, by CRSS, of Houston.[2] Regardless, every hospital has an immediate site context and the people who live nearest are likely to be its nearest neighbors, patients, and often, its closest watchdog. Medical centers located in long-established residential neighborhoods may have less institutional autonomy because of this and matters can be further complicated insofar as the institution may simultaneously serve a local community, metropolitan area, region, or even a national

facilities should be informed by four basic climatic variants. In hot humid regions, employ linear building configurations, enhanced cross ventilation, transoms, ceiling fans and high windows that vent air, and roofs designed to capture and recycle rainwater, with expansive overhangs or sunscreens. In hot, dry regions employ more compact massing, courtyards, basement and subterranean spaces insulated by the earth, and roofscapes with broad overhangs. In moderate regions, employ a mix of pitched and flat roofs to capture rainwater and carry snow loads, with a combination of linear and centralized massing, operable windows, enhanced thermal insulation, overhangs, and sunscreens. In cold regions, employ a north–south exposure axis tempered to balance internal heat gain/loss ratios, flat and pitched roofscapes, operable windows and heavy thermal insulation systems. In addition, employ energy efficient landscaping and building materials. In hot humid regions, shield the hospital from excessive direct sunlight with shade trees in close proximity (especially to the south side) and trellises. In hot, dry regions employ trees and trellised walkways, screened and shaded patios, and semi-enclosed courtyards, operable windows, roof vents, and recycled building materials throughout. In moderate regions plant deciduous trees to the south and coniferous trees to the north face, and employ windbreaks to shield the hospital from harsh winds. Similarly, in cold regions, employ windbreaks and landscaping as screening devices without impeding solar gain.[4]

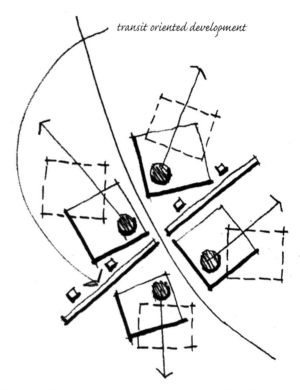

transit oriented development

7.2 Hospital/medical center at core of transit oriented development

Transit oriented development

In cities where the commuter rail station serves as a hub, the life of the surrounding neighborhoods gravitates toward this hub and it eventually evolves into the cultural epicenter of the community. Large urban medical centers in Tokyo, Amsterdam, London, Vienna, Prague, Mexico City, Moscow, and many other cities of the world are located adjacent to or very near to rail and bus transit stations. These transit hobs are in turn linked with a network of bus, light rail, pedestrian, and bike routes. Thus, a system of primary, secondary, and tertiary circulation arteries is created over time that function as the lifeblood of these places. Hospitals are often at the center of what planners refer to as *transit oriented development* (TOD) in these places. In these centers, it is possible to conveniently stop on the way to or from the rail station to pick up food preparations for the evening dinner, and then stop at the hospital's outpatient clinic for,

say, an eye examination, or a therapy session, and perhaps stop in to briefly visit a sick friend who is hospitalized. In the U.S., sadly, such places rarely exist.[5] In the past this situation was radically different: up until hospitals relocated en masse from city centers to more lucrative suburban sprawl markets, and especially from the 1960s on, most U.S. hospitals were located in dense urban neighborhoods, usually at a walkable distance from public transportation amenities. This pattern was obliterated in decent decades in the U.S. but continued to prevail in many other places. The Oregon Heath Sciences Center, in Portland (2002–2007) represents a genuine U.S. attempt to resurrect this traditional pattern within the context of TOD. It is an innovative case study in this regard (Figure 7.2).

Mixed use and urban infill

Large urban hospitals have often been described as cities within a city. Metaphorically, they are comprised of their own unique counterparts to streets, neighborhoods, districts, landmarks, complete with a housing realm, a governance realm, transportation amenities including auto parking and connections to public transit, and even a commercial-business realm. It is a vibrant tapestry, day in and out. The feeling of walking through a large, highly differentiated medical center can be exciting. The University Medical Center Groningen (UMCG) (1983–2003), in the Netherlands, is the largest university healthcare center in the northern part of the country and with 1,300 beds and 8,500 employees is one of the largest hospitals in the European Union (EU). The main 'city street' level contains a bank, stores, pharmacy, specialty health equipment stores, numerous outpatient clinics, a grocery store, café, and gardens. Sixteen fledgling companies in the biomedical and medical technology field have already been established on the UNCG campus. The UNCG represents one end of this spectrum. The Meyer Children's Hospital (CS 9) in Italy represents a midpoint condition with regards to the *hospital as city* metaphor with its mini-mall arcade on its main level. A freestanding community hospital with only one small gift shop represents the other extreme. However, even when a relatively small specialty hospital is located at or near an urban center, many opportunities exist to create an anti-sprawl, mixed use environment – businesses on the street level, with the hospital above or next door. Infill sites should be explored, together with adaptive use strategies where an existing building such as, for example, a former car showroom where gas guzzler vehicles were once sold, can be part of an infill/ mixed use strategy.

Edge sites on medical campuses

Many older medical centers purchased as much land as possible around their campuses and in many cases promptly destroyed the surrounding neighborhood and its infrastructure. In the U.S. this was frequently done through the use of local imminent domain powers. Vast parking lots frequently replaced intact, often historic, neighborhoods. Hospitals in long-established neighborhoods who downsize their bed capacity, and/or have increased their menu of outpatient services, may in time be left with unused and underutilized

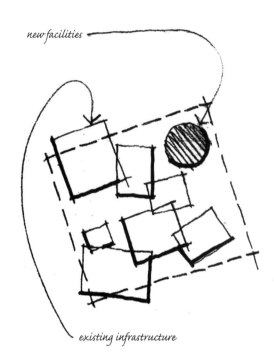

new facilities

existing infrastructure

7.3 Explore edge-site infill development

buildings and unsightly parking lots. It is prudent to seek adaptive uses for these structures and unsightly open spaces and to establish a mix of new infill development with re-used older structures, if land permits and such a strategy is pursued in tandem with local community groups and civic interests. A new facility type, such as a small freestanding specialty hospital, or a psychiatric facility, may opt to purchase a portion of the campus and build on it. New facility types can be introduced, perhaps built on an unused parking lot, combined with a new below-ground parking deck. New development can be linked with an agreement to share existing infrastructural elements, including the central power plant, laundry services, food services, materials management, and other support functions (Figure 7.3).

Historic preservation/adaptive use

More than 500 historic hospitals or portions thereof have been destroyed in the U.S. alone in the past 30 years. There are no global statistics on this trend although the number would likely be upwards of 5,000 demolished hospitals worldwide during this period. Most of these lost facilities were built in the early decades of the twentieth century (1925–1950) such as the Passavant Hospital in Chicago (built 1929; destroyed 2005). The current battle (2010) to save the art deco Charity Hospital (1938) in post-Hurricane Katrina New Orleans, and thoroughly renovate its core, points to the continued challenges preservation activists and preservationist-minded architects and their consulting engineers face (see Chapter 5). Clients and elected officials are often insufficiently aware of the myriad benefits of renovation versus knee-jerk demolition to make way for new construction and often, total replacement facilities. In the case of Big Charity, the Washington, D.C.-based National Trust for Historic Preservation strongly urged its retention and renovation. The site of Chicago's failed bid for the 2016 Summer Olympic Games called for the destruction of the Walter Gropius-influenced modernist nursing wings of the former Michael Reese Hospital, on the city's near South Side. A similar battle was fought (with some success, to date) to spare the neoclassical Cook County Hospital (1911–1914), on the city's near West Side. These examples point to the contentious debates that nearly always surround efforts to destroy such civic icons. Vintage hospitals deserve a far better fate in a carbon intensive world. Work to save historic hospitals and either renovate them or adapt them to new viable uses such as housing, dormitories (especially if on or near a medical education center as in the case of Charity Hospital) and other viable uses (see Chapter 2). Fight for time to explore alternatives and conduct due diligence. The public is often not educated to the point of being equipped with the knowledge to fully grasp the broader implications of what is about to be lost to the community's cultural heritage and collective civic memory until it is far too late – and these civic icons are permanently lost forever (Figure 7.4).

Striated adaptive use

Hospital boards and public governing agencies during the past thirty years have too often exhibited callous indifference to the

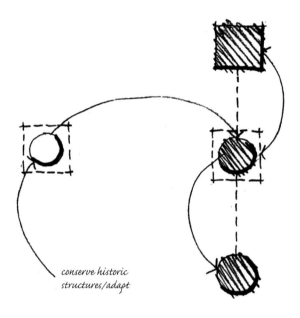

conserve historic structures/adapt

7.4   Explore historic preservation and adaptive use

preservation of historic yet timeworn healthcare facilities under their purview. Often, an obsession with 'the new' nearly always seems to take precedence. As mentioned above, time is not taken to conduct the due diligence that requires painstaking research on many levels, i.e. engineering, programming, and new medical technologies. Americans are particularly guilty of this syndrome. Instead, work together to save what is worth saving, and build new buildings to complement the existing fabric of the medical center. This is precisely the strategy that was taken in the planning and design of the recently built Martini Hospital, in Groningen, the Netherlands (see Chapter 3), at the Washington State Veteran's Center in Retsil, Washington (CS 16), and at the 1906 SERTC campus in southern Indiana (CS 20). Retain one or more core historic components and build next to them, around them, or as infill. Sometimes a striated strategy requires that the neighborhood simply can't be abandoned due to it being part of an existing medical center. In one extreme case a site was retained for this reason and a completely new building was built on the same parcel while the existing hospital on the parcel remained fully operational. This was the strategy taken in the case of Shriners Children's Replacement Hospital in Boston. It was rebuilt in four phases on its existing site. In the fourth phase the old facility was demolished and 'infilled' to complete the new facility. Would it not have been more prudent to find a reasonable way to retain the historic older facility and add on to it? Or, relocate nearby and adaptively reuse the old hospital?[6]

Brownfield sites

One reason why so many recent hospitals and medical center campuses have been built on greenfield and suburban sprawl sites has been the availability of land at a far lower cost compared to the urban core. The size of parcels required is a second reason, and a third has been that large parcels available in older urban centers are often former industrial sites that are now abandoned. Grayfield and brownfield sites nearly always require costly remediation to rid them of environmental contaminants such as lead and mercury. The Spaulding Rehabilitation Hospital, in Boston (2006–2010), by Perkins+Will, is a replacement facility (240,000 square feet; 22,300 square meters) built on a 2.6 acre site. It houses 150 beds and 300 below-grade parking spaces. The site is in the former Charlestown Navy Yard brownfield property, at the convergence of Little Mystic Channel and Boston Harbor. Besides site remediation, a green roofscape provides amenity for patients and families and harvests storm water for reuse on site. A public riverfront promenade connects the campus with the immediate urban fabric.[7] This strategy also promotes alternatives to automobile dependency: public transit is often in close proximity to these former industrial sites, and for these reasons brownfield reclamation is accorded priority within the parameters of LEED certification in the U.S.

Underground parking

First and foremost, a healthcare facility should promote alternatives to driving to and from it on a daily basis. It is an unsustainable assumption to require staff, patients, and others to drive excessive distances. Worse, upon arriving on campus, the parking garage looms directly ahead as if it were a huge spaceship – one mindlessly drives in and captures a tiny parking stall, proceeding to the main

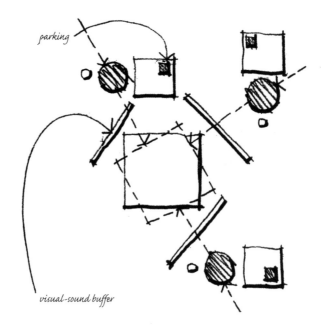

parking

visual-sound buffer

7.5 Incorporate screened and subterranean parking

entrance just like at an airport when trying to catch a flight. Too often, the parking deck is the first and last thing encountered on the campus. Surface parking lots are only slightly less intrusive, as they consume (together with parking decks) vast parcels of what would otherwise have remained unpaved green space, inhibiting proper drainage, contributing to urban heat island effect syndrome. The Graz-West Provincial Hospital in Austria parking deck is below the hospital (CS 22). The same strategy was taken at the Deventer Hospital in the Netherlands (CS 19) and at the Geriatriezentrum Favoriten in Vienna (CS 17). Create smaller clusters of parking, with a mix of stall sizes and provide incentives for the medical center staff to drive small electric, hydrogen fuel cell, and hybrid vehicles. Patients, staff and visitors do not need to see or hear vehicles on campus – particularly in patient rooms, therapy and treatment areas, dayrooms, meditative spaces, gardens, courtyards, and dining areas. Similarly, incorporate buffers such as berms, screened walls, shrubs, and trees to screen automobiles from direct view. Access drives should lead directly to the main entrance to drop off and pick up patients. Patients should be provided with alternatives to being forced to walk through a banal, lifeless parking deck, whether above or below ground (Figure 7.5)

Provisions for cyclists

The Netherlands leads Europe in the percentage of its urban citizens who cycle on a daily basis to work or school. China traditionally has led Asia in the percentage of its urban citizens who cycle daily to work or school. The difference between the two countries is that in the former, the number of automobiles on the roads has held fairly constant over the past decade, whereas in the latter more than 25,000 new autos were placed on the nation's roads each and every day in 2008.[8] The difference between Amsterdam and Beijing is striking in this regard. In Amsterdam a sustainable pattern of urban life remains intact; in Beijing, a thoroughly unsustainable way of life has taken root and shows no signs of retreat. China is rapidly adopting the unsustainable traits of the U.S. in terms of senseless sprawl: highways reaching out to far-flung suburbs sprouting up on former farmland and, by default, posing disincentives to cycling, and disincentives for continued use of public transit. Ever since the private auto became a high status symbol, it has been déclassé to be seen on a bike or standing in a commuter railway station in China. This pattern has been the norm, of course, in many places in the U.S. for fifty years. The result of the obsession with the auto and with driving everywhere are sobering, to say the least. To aid in abating this trend and its unfortunate consequences, the LEED rating system in the U.S. provides a credit for the provision of a bike rack on the site of a hospital or allied healthcare facility. An additional credit is obtainable if the facility is located near to a public transit stop or station. At this writing one major U.S. medical center has qualified for this credit (Oregon Health Sciences Center, in Portland). The stage is now set for many more hospitals in the U.S. and elsewhere to reconnect to pedestrian-scaled communities. Hospitals should become donor-sponsors for the construction of bike paths and trails connecting their campuses to the fabric of bike path networks in their surrounding communities.[9]

Community health promotion

In the U.S. the obesity epidemic has reached a crisis stage. As many as one-third of the population is obese, and the percentage of young children who are obese is dramatically rising. The causes for this trend are many and complex but Americans' love affair with their autos is a principal cause of this national malaise. The typical U.S. family now owns three cars and they are used excessively even on short trips where walking or cycling could easily substitute. Unfortunately, many recently built medical centers are primary contributors to suburban sprawl. Their location, often far from public transport links, bike paths, and walkable path networks, renders them inaccessible except primarily by private auto. Healthcare providers must seize this public health crisis as an opportunity to act in a leadership – even visionary – role as environmental stewards in this aspect of health promotion. On the campus, strive to promote wellness through the provision of bike paths, walking trails, linkages to public transportation, and the like. Beyond, connect these to the surrounding neighborhood. Create inviting, environmentally sustainable opportunities for staff and others to take public transport, to cycle, or walk to the medical center. Establish ride-share and carpooling programs. Many medical centers have achieved success with their smoking cessation campaigns. A focus now on wellness through outdoor physical activity is a next logical step.

Autonomous food production

In the past century, food production has become industrialized, globalized, and increasingly unsustainable. Fresh produce travels on average 1,500 miles from field to table in the U.S. while thousands of family farms have been consumed by mega-agribusiness, sprawl, and agricultural monoculture. Sadly, the farm-as-corporation paradigm has resulted in cost savings but has spawned food of highly questionable taste and healthfulness. Multiple pesticides, growth hormones, and other artificial additives are toxic to the body. Myriad health problems are traceable to diet and to the present food production system, including cancer, diabetes, hypertension, and Americans' biggest battle, obesity. A hospital can grow its own food at a minimal cost and also ensure its quality, for consumption on site. High quality food produced on campus will directly benefit the immediate hospital community as a beacon of sustainable public health policy. Benefits

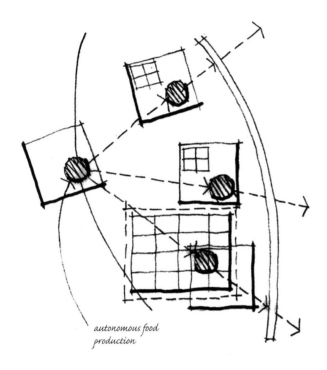

autonomous food production

7.6 Foster self-sufficiency in food production

include less energy use, cleaner air and water, and remediated soil (on grayfield and brownfield sites). Community benefits of an on-site garden at ground level or on a landscaped roof terrace include campus and neighborhood beautification, the establishment of an example for the community to emulate, and a more pronounced connection between care providers, care recipients, and the earth. A hospital is greatly empowered when it provides its own food. In Simei, Singapore, the Changi Geneat Hospital cultivates tomatoes on its roof. Access to water, sunlight, good soil, and proper drainage are prerequisites (Figure 7.6).[10]

Wind power

Hospitals around the globe consume vast amounts of non-renewable energy at the present time. Hospitals in the U.S. consume twice as much energy as office buildings per square foot and nearly $3 billion is spent on electricity alone. In the U.S., the federal government in 2009 committed $15 billion (USD) to develop the nation's alternative energy industries. In the U.K., a major investment is occurring in the wind turbine industry. A wind farm, to be known as the Greater Gabbard Offshore Wind Farm, is a $1.8 billion project that will produce 500 megawatts of power and will be the world's largest offshore wind farm, located 25 miles off the Suffolk coast in England. This wind farm, with its 140 wind turbines, will provide carbon neutral, renewable energy for more than 415,000 homes by 2011. The Antrium Area Hospital, a 220-bed facility in Northern Ireland, generates 50 percent of its peak electrical power from the wind. Explore governmental tax credits and grants for a wind turbine system; join a local co-op to partner to help build capacity. In what country will the world's first all-wind powered hospital open? It is a matter of intuitional will, governmental financing incentives, and technology.[11]

Geothermal, hydrogen, and methane power:

Geothermal energy systems are powering a growing number of medical centers in the U.S. The first U.S. geothermal powered hospital was the Great River Medical Center (1998–2001), in West Burlington, Iowa, designed by NBBJ Columbus. Its system featured a large retention pond.[12] Another viable alternative energy source with vast commercial potential is hydrogen, together with solar power technologies. It is only a matter of time before the first totally self-sufficient hybrid geothermal, wind, hydrogen, and/or solar powered hospital is built. Many possibilities exist on the horizon, especially for geothermal, hydrogen, and solar power. Hospitals have been moving in this direction since 2000. The Fachkrankenhaus Nordfriesland psychiatric hospital in Bredstedt, Germany (2004–2007) was one of the first round of case studies in the European Union Hospitals Demonstration Project. It has reduced its overall electrical energy demand by 57 percent compared to comparable German standards. This was achieved through the use of double skin facades, solar thermal mass walls, and a combined heat/power (CHP) plant, among its many carbon footprint-reduction features. In LaCrosse, Wisconsin, the Gunderson Lutheran Medical Center co-owns the local brewery's waste facility for its unused hops. This unused organic waste material is then converted to electrical power for 500 homes in the local community using excess methane waste.[13]

The zero waste hospital

In the near future, *ecohumanist* hospitals will be judged by how successful they are in helping to heal the earth as much as healing people. A regenerative hospital is one that is self sufficient in its energy use. The Embassy Medical Center in Colombo, Sri Lanka, uses an anaerobic digester to process and harvest its own trash for on-site electrical power. It operates its own wastewater treatment facility to recycle the water it harvests from the rain. The Royal Children's Hospital in Melbourne, Australia harvests all its rainwater for use in its plumbing system. Why remain dependent on the existing conventional power grid? Hospitals for a Healthy Environment (H2E) reported in 2007 that a small but growing number of leading healthcare organizations in the U.S. were approaching nearly 50 percent diversion rates in their operational waste streams. The GrassRoots Recycling Network's Zero Waste Business Principles are gathering interest as businesses explore ways to reduce their carbon footprint. The ten provisos are as follows: 1. Commit to a triple bottom line of social, environmental, and economic performance benchmarks, 2. Apply the precautionary principle before committing to any and all toxic or wasteful practices or systems, 3. Direct zero waste to local or regional landfill or incineration sites, 4. Assume all responsibility for take-back packaging and avoid all redundant packaging, 5. Purchase reused, recycled, or composted materials, 6. Prevent pollution and reduce the generation of on-site waste, 7. Opt for highest and best uses of available land and facility resources and constantly reassess policies and practices, 8. Develop economic incentives for customers, workers, and suppliers to help the organization achieve a zero carbon footprint, 9. Ensure that products and services sold or provided by the organization are not wasteful or toxic, 10. Adopt policies that promote nontoxic production, reuse and recycling processes.[14]

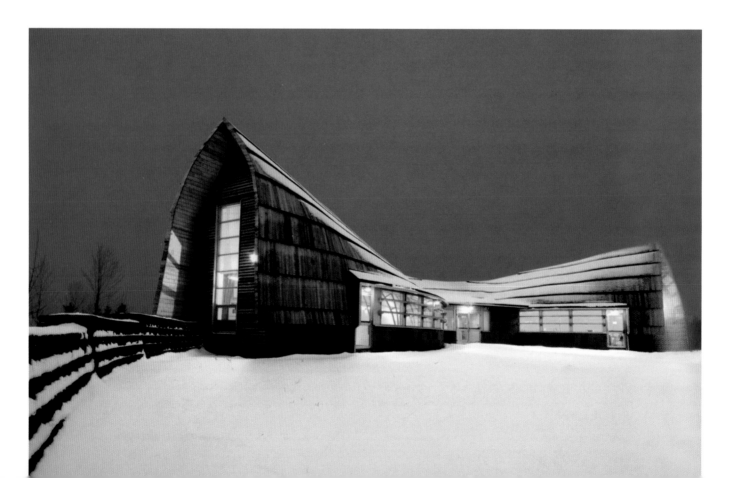

Critical regionalism

Postmodernism opened new avenues for a mainstream hospital's narrative to be about its specific location to an extent not imaginable during the modern movement in the decades dominated by the International Style. By the 1980s it became acceptable for monolithic hospitals to express local vernacular traditions. Materials, colors, and to a certain extent even methods of construction were soon incorporated. Examples included cutting-edge designs, in North America at the Hi-Desert Medical Center (1988–1990), in Joshua Tree, California, by Kaplan McLaughlin Diaz, in Europe; at the St. Mary's Hospital (1981–1991) on the Isle of Wight, by Ahrends, Burton and Koralek, London; in Africa at the Kaedi Regional Hospital (1985–1987), in Kaedi, Mauritania, by Fabrizio Carola and the AUDA (Association for the Natural Development of African Architecture and Urbanism).[15] Critical regionalism involves a conscious borrowing from precedent. It

is borrowing in a way that fuses locality with influences from afar. The Pictou Landing First Nation is a community of Mikmaq, an indigenous rural community on the East Coast of Canada. The Pictou Landing Health Center (2007–2008), by Richard Kroeker and Brian Lilly, includes clinics and consultation rooms, administration, and a large community meeting room. Language, oral traditions, and treaty agreements have defined this culture for centuries. The clinic was based on local materials, aesthetic vocabularies, construction methods, and a local tradition of skilled craftsmanship. Its design shields the severe north wind and encloses a medicine garden. The interior features natural light and local materials (Figures 7.7.and 7.8). The Grand Itasca Clinic (2003–2005), in Michigan, by Kahler Slater Architects, expresses the Midwestern Prairie school architecture of Frank Lloyd Wright. Extended overhangs, exterior wood cladding, and fenestration provide a striking silhouette on the open prairie (Figure 7.9).

7.7 Explore critical regionalist paradigms

7.8 Explore indigenous vernacular building traditions and aesthetics

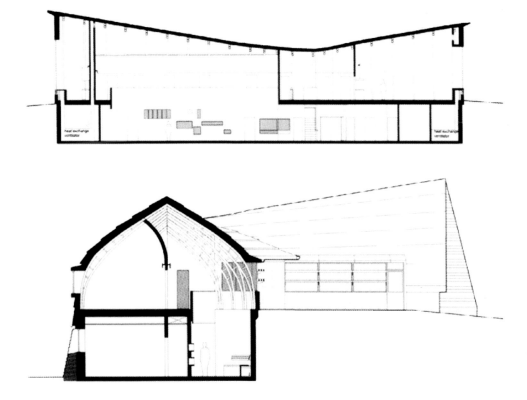

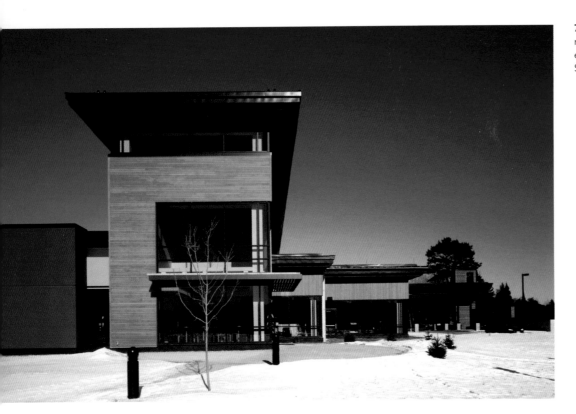

Health villages

A *health village*, architecturally, denotes a concentration of freestanding care providers sited in a small-scale setting. It is at times misconstrued with the term *healthy community*. The latter term is not apropos in an architectural sense, however, as the healthy community movement in public health is centered on the lifestyles and wellness of a population. As one tenet of postmodernism in healthcare architecture, the health village emerged at the end of the twentieth century as an aggregation of health-related services geographically located on a single campus such as a medical center, as in the case of the Freeport Health Care Village (1986–1989), in Kitchener, Ontario, by the NORR Partnership with McMurich and Oxley Architects, or as a loose affiliation of independent facilities located in close proximity yet non-contiguous to one another.[16] This has occurred around many community hospitals, frequently in small towns, where a variety of freestanding care providers are located across the street or around the block from the hospital, and this aggregation evolves over a period of years, i.e. an acute care hospital surrounded by an assisted living residence, later a primary care clinic, optometry clinic, a public library with a health information component, senior day center, wellness and fitness center, pediatric clinic, dental clinic, and so on. A suburban variant of this model has evolved near to the Patewood Campus of the Greenville Memorial Hospital System, in Greenville, South Carolina. Regardless, it is probable that the health village, as a type, will prevail well into the twenty-first century as a care delivery model because it expresses the functional deconstruction of the megahospital, is human scaled, is patient and family centered, is a one stop point-of-service care

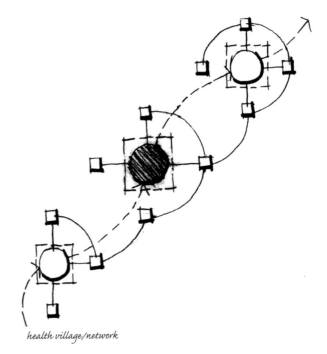

health village/network

7.10 Interweave small-scale health villages into the community fabric

model, and is an antidote to unchecked sprawl when the health village is located at the core of a population center, not on its periphery (Figure 7.10)

Virtual healthscapes

Of the many types of virtual healthscapes rapidly evolving at this time, two with particularly salient architectural ramifications center on telemedicine and specifically the *home as clinic*, and second, on virtual simulation as a *therapeutic modality* in healthcare diagnosis and treatment. The U.S. Department of Defense (DOD) has invested in this technology in physical medicine and rehabilitation with returned veterans injured in combat in Iraq and Afghanistan. Innovative research is occurring in artificial intelligence systems, voice recognition software, and in the emerging field of emotive computing. Interactive avatars facilitate back and forth interactive dialogue, enabling a physical therapist to dialogue with the patient in the patient's home anytime, anywhere as a supplement to face-to-face therapy in a hospital setting. Telemedicine has been used in distance surgery for a decade or more, and in physician-patient consultation and is continually being refined. The DOD's Center for the Intrepid, in San Antonio (CS 13) extensively uses virtual reality therapy in its treatment programs. Key equipment includes a virtual reality motion platform, an interactive device for the simulation of virtually any physical setting at any time of day or night in assessing gait and balance acuity. Flat panel LCD screens and high end gaming software employ gaming consoles to acclimate the patient to the post-hospital everyday physical environment. Current information technology allows for two-dimensional teleconferencing over conventional wireless and DSL bandwidths. Virtual *home-as clinic* software packages will soon allow both the caregiver and patient to be 'transported' via digital holographs back and forth between hospital and their kitchen or den (see Chapter 6).

2   Arrival, public, and semi-public spaces

Imagery and identity

The first few moments on a medical center campus foster indelible, lasting impressions in the individual. It is important that the built environment conveys a positive first impression versus an ambiguous, uninspired, or worse, negative impression. The grandly scaled hospitals of the nineteenth and early twentieth centuries featured civic lobbies, places of importance that impressed, not unlike a neoclassical railroad station, hot springs resort spa, or grand hotel of the era. These impressive spaces featured sculptures, foundations, terracotta ornamentation, and elaborate materials and tilework, such as in the lobby of the Spanish-influenced Hermann Hospital (1920–1922) in Houston. The neoclassical main facade of the aforementioned Cook County Hospital (1911–1914) on Chicago's Near West Side, designed by Paul Gerhardt, with Schmidt, Garden & Martin, of Chicago, left a strong impression on generations of Chicagoans.[17] Sometimes the hospital's most lasting visual impression is from afar, as is the case at St. Mary's Hospital (1971–1973) in Milwaukee, Wisconsin, by Bertrand Goldberg of Chicago. St. Mary's, with its undulating cast-in-place concrete patient tower set on a support pedestal, is perched on a bluff near to Milwaukee's attractive Lakefront. A narrow winding road leads from Lakeshore Drive up to the top of the bluff. By contrast, Evelina Children's Hospital (CS 11) in London, an infill hospital on a dense site, is best appreciated not from afar but from within its dramatic atrium. The eye is led vertically up through the space, and patients can see the city from its upper levels. At Evelina, the strongest first impression is experienced only upon entering, and then is reinforced repeatedly throughout the interior.

Arrival sequence

The porte cochère is a device that simultaneously serves three purposes: protection from the elements, a symbolic device to extend a 'helping hand' outward from the hospital and in so doing giving definition to the main entrance, and as a device to establish the institution's visual identity. The articulated wood canopy at the St. Francis Medical Center, in Virginia (see Chapter 3), functions as a human-scaled arrival portal and establishes a strong image of communality with its wooded site. Similarly, the arrival canopies at the Bloorview Kids Rehab (CS 7), and the Children's Health Center at Surrey Memorial (CS 8), both in Canada, establish a memorable image. The risk of an overly elaborate arrival canopy is that it will make the hospital appear to be an airport, rail station, convention center, or mall. The current tendency is to overdesign them, in an expression of irrational exuberance. An overscaled, obsessively high-tech canopy or one that shares little with the rest of the composition is therefore to be eschewed. Instead, it should be inviting, human scaled, and articulate without overpowering or

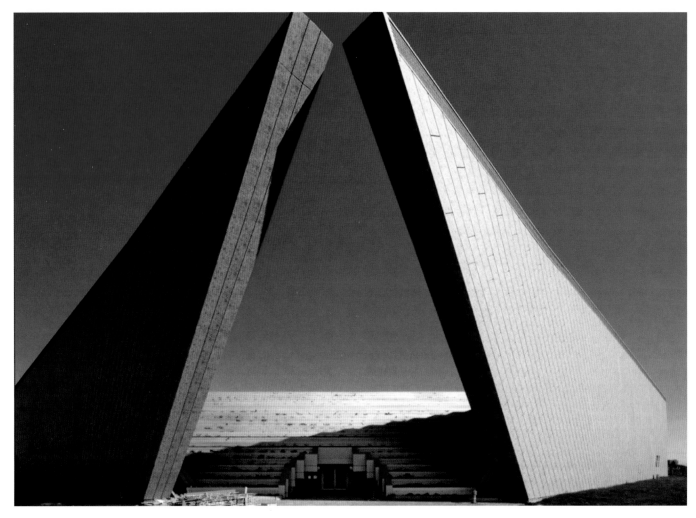

7.11 Articulate arrival sequences – scale, materiality, and image

becoming bombastic, as is perhaps the case with the main arrival portal at the New Mastre Hospital (2003–2008) in Veneto, Italy (Figure 7.11), by Studio Altieri S.P.A.

Lightness

A building that treads lightly on its site is a quality in architecture defined simply as *lightness*. It has been a key ingredient in innovative architecture throughout the modern movement, in Frank Lloyd Wright's best work, including Fallingwater (1934–1936), in Pennsylvania, in Mies Van Der Rohe's Barcelona Pavilion (1929) in Spain, and later, in Mies' Farnsworth House (1951) in Plano, Illinois, and at Crown Hall (1954–1956) on the campus of the Illinois Institute of Technology, in Chicago.[18] In both, the building floats, hovering in a delicate defiance of gravity. The effect is an atmosphere of repose, elegance, an almost dream-like, ethereal state, particularly at sunrise and sunset. It is a quality expressed in Australian architect Glenn Murcutt's best work. It is present in Andrew Metter's (of Epstein, Inc., Chicago) Serta Corporation Headquarters (2006–2009) in Hoffman Estates, Illinois. There, the composition appears to float ever so gently above the open prairie. The site was conserved/preserved, with the composition ever so lightly intervening, remaining as *undisturbed* as possible. It is a quality expressed in the REHAB Basel (2000–2002) by Herzog & de Meuron (see Chapter 3 and CS 12). It is a quality, when expressed in ecohumanist healthcare architecture, that expresses a supreme respect for treading lightly on the *health of the earth,* as an ecosystem comprised of human beings and all other life forms, inseparably intertwined.

Site connectivity

The austere hierarchies and mutual exclusivity that exists today in most hospitals between 'interior' and 'exterior' space needs to be reconsidered. As hospitals become *lighter* in both literal and in metaphorical terms a new universe of possibilities will emerge with respect to the transactive layering of space that can break down the present unnatural barriers between what *being* means indoors versus what being outdoors means (defined here as *theraserialization,* see Chapter 3, and below). The lone exception to the unfortunate state of much hospital design today is the public arrival realm.

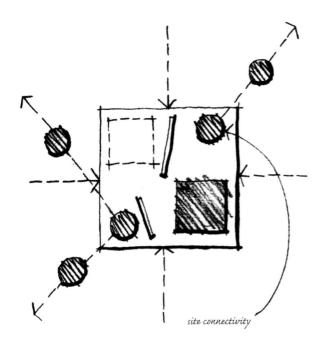

site connectivity

7.12 Layer site hierarchies – nature, aesthetics, universal design

indoors or out. It is inherently non-discriminatory and can create a seamless *barrier free continuum* of transparency between indoors and outdoors (Figure 7.12).

Spatial orientation

Some of the earliest research now referred to as evidence-based design research was conducted on the subject of wayfinding in hospitals. Studies in the 1970s revealed many large medical center campuses to be overwhelming to the patient and visitor. Problems frequently cited centered on their excessively long corridors, circuitous routes, labyrinth floor plans, and confusion caused by their monotonous appearance. It was difficult to discern one department from another. The old school method of painted stripes on the floor, and later, bold supergraphic color schemes were merely band aids that could not mask the fundamental problem: the hospital had become gridlocked because it was the equivalent of a muscle-bound heavyweight fighter who had lost his close range coordination and dexterity. A parade of additions over the decades disfigured many acute care hospitals to the point of unrecognizability. The initial (core) facility became lost in a maze of successive expansions. Wayfinding was cited by critics as a core failure of the modern hospital.[19] By and large, the movement to make the hospital more navigable and spatially coherent has been a success. Formerly blind corridors now provide views out, connecting circulation elements now afford transparency, inside-outside spatial orientation aids for occupants are now provided, as are landmarks in the form of works of art, water elements, skylights, and clerestories. In tandem, these function to establish identity and *genius loci*. Transparency that promotes spatial orientation and occupants' directional movement is achieved throughout the first level of the Banner Gateway Medical Center in Arizona. Global Positioning Satellite (GPS) technology also holds much promise in wayfinding applications on large medical center campuses. The wayfinder, upon arrival, keys into the destination and then proceeds on the journey. The route is punctuated by landmarks in the form of architectural elements (floors, walls, ceilings, formal devices, and so on), exterior views, and art, with a voice in the headset or PDA providing route directions.

There, tremendous progress has been made in the past decade in hospitals reaching out to their communities through the provision of generous, inviting, civically scaled amenities that both extend outward and draw inward. The dramatic yet understated arrival zones at the Katta Public General Hospital (CS 3) and at Thunder Bay Regional Hospital (CS 18), in Canada – one recessed and the other an additive, highly layered, transparent element – achieve simultaneous inwardness/outwardness. Unfortunately, particularly in the case of Thunder Bay, while its arrival and public atrium zone is somewhat captivating in its articulation and scale that is where any true possibilities for universal theraserialization end. Although skylights transmit daylight to bathe the radiation suites, thereby achieving a vertical connection with nature, the total effect remains episodic because the main hospital's massing is inward-focused. Relatively few openings allow for horizontal transactivity at the ground plane. Universal design, in theory, denotes an environment fully accessible to persons of all ages and virtually any type of physical limitation,

Art in hospitals

Art has been fundamental to the hospital experience since the earliest intuitions in the Far East, the temple-hospitals of Asclepius in Ancient Greece, Ancient Roman medical and bathing complexes, and the Mosque-hospitals of the Middle East dating back three millennia. Statues of pagan icons, such as the Greek god Athena, and later, Christian religious icons, such as the Virgin Mary and the Catholic Saints whose purview was the sick and diseased, were often installed in hospital public lobbies and courtyards throughout the eighteenth and nineteenth centuries. This trend continued into the twentieth century but the emphasis on religious themes dramatically lessened by mid-century. In the post-World War II decades tastes switched to more secular themes in art installations. By 2000, art in hospitals almost entirely had eschewed religious themes and iconography. A lone exception was in religious-affiliated institutions, but even there religious iconography lessened in its overt imagery and directness. With the emphasis now almost entirely on secular themes, art was to be perceived in more personal, spiritual terms against the broad backdrop of the widely recognized icons of a particular organized faith. In the U.K., the 'Vital Arts' program has in the past five years commissioned artworks for a number of healthcare facilities. A collective known as Peepshow created a bold and colorful alternative landscape that gave the Retinoblastoma Unit at St. Bartholomew's Hospital (Barts), London, a distinctive new identity. The Barkantine Vital Arts group worked with Tower Hamlets Primary Care Trust to develop artwork for the new Barkantine Centre on the Isle of Dogs. A series of vibrant, highly crafted pieces focused on nature and handcraftsmanship. At Barts and the London Breast Care Centre West Wing a series of site-specific commissions from leading artists was integrated with the architecture (all in 2006). At the Pathology and Pharmacy Building at the Royal London Hospital, artist Martin Richman created a lighting installation that transformed the building. The artists worked closely with the interior design team (2005). At the West Wing of Barts, prior to the start of its renovation, Julian Opie created a temporary light installation/billboard, working from the assumption that the typical hospital patient and visitor would 'rather be anywhere but here' (2002). To launch the new hospital construction program at the Royal London, artist Pae White created a temporary billboard of an American rural landscape (2002). In 2007, also at Barts, artist Lothar Gtz created a billboard based on the colors in traditional Korean wrapping cloths for gifts, and he also

created a permanent artwork for the hospital art collection. Vital Arts commissioned Liz Rideal (2007) to create a one-off temporary project on the fifteenth-century bell tower of St. Bartholomew the Less, to celebrate the coming of spring and the hospital's majestic architecture.[20]

Wayfinding and art

Positive first impressions in a hospital can be created when the patient and visitor, immediately upon arriving, see a lyrical, uplifting sculpture, painting, or photomural in the main lobby. It leaves a lasting image and can set the tone for the entire encounter. Art is fundamental to healing. Few would argue that art possesses therapeutic value in a hospital setting if properly selected and properly installed. Thematic artworks non-verbally connect with the occupant. The stirring World War II era imagery of the military-themed photomural at the Washington State Veteran's Center in Retsil, Washington (CS 16) works aesthetically and as a spatial orientation device. It is a landmark within the facility, i.e. 'Meet me at the mural at noon'. The exhibit in the main circulation artery at the Brigham and Women's Hospital in Boston, known as 'The Pike', is a 'talking wall' that presents a timeline chronology of its history. Community philanthropy can assist in this regard. The main lobby of the Children's Memorial Hospital replacement facility (2008–2010) in Chicago features a 'school' of aquatic life sculptures donated by Chicago's Shedd Aquarium. Art as wayfinding – spatial sequencing – requires the establishment of a familiar theme, intervals/nodes to instill thematic reinforcement, additional items to reinforce landmarks, and key corridor juncture design points. A serialized introduction of new themes subtlety reinforces the core theme, i.e. a new flower species encountered at each key decision point. The colorful light-well sculptures at the Meyer Children's Hospital in Italy achieve this effect (CS 9). The brightly abstracted human 'organs' at the Graz-West Provincial Hospital in Austria (CS 22) appear as if guiding wayfinders from the lobby to other parts of the hospital. The 'aquarium columns' at the 80-bed Red Cross Foundation Children's Hospital (2005–2008) in Darmstadt, Germany, by Angela Fritsch Architekten, are non-structural, and are a memorable interior landmark (Figure 7.13). The 17-level Prentice Women's Hospital (2004–2007) in Chicago, designed by OWP/P in a joint venture with VOA, features 1,100 artworks on display throughout the hospital. Thematic content can be universal

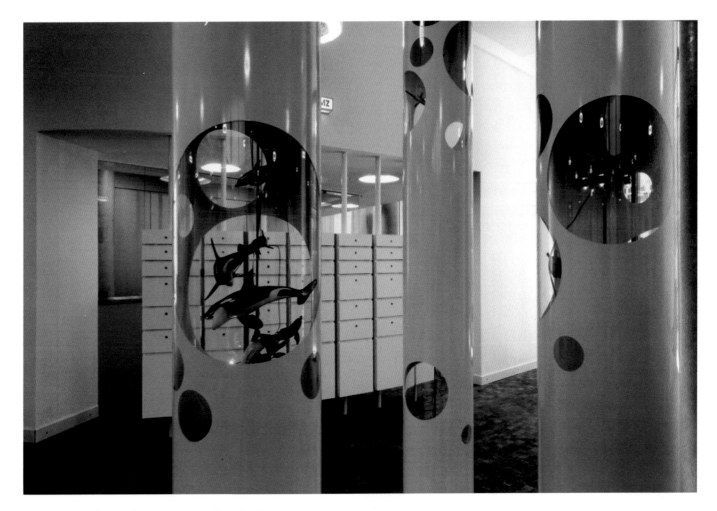

7.13 Correlate/fuse wayfinding systems with works of art

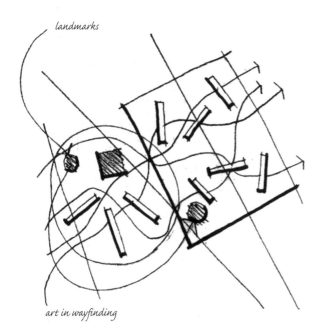

landmarks

art in wayfinding

7.14 Sequence thematic content in art/wayfinding systems

or place-specific (Figure 7.14). The California-based photomuralist Robin Constable Hanson has produced art installations in dozens of hospitals across the U.S. She first carefully studies local themes, places of historical significance, and the collective cultural memory of a community.[21]

Serialization

It is unsettling to abruptly 'fall' into a lobby of a hospital or allied healthcare facility that lacks spatial hierarchy. Neither is it effective to place an information/reception desk too near the entrance as this can be a cause of bottlenecks and confusion. A well-designed arrival station is a landmark, a place for people to meet, and a mission control center. The covered canopy at the main entrance and access drive should lead to this station point, preferably immediately visible from the moment one enters. It is, together with the lobby or atrium, the symbolic gateway. Given that many hospital directional wayfinding systems are notoriously confusing, it is critical that the facility itself provide the necessary orientation cues to facilitate effective navigational movement. At Bloorview Kids Rehab, in Canada

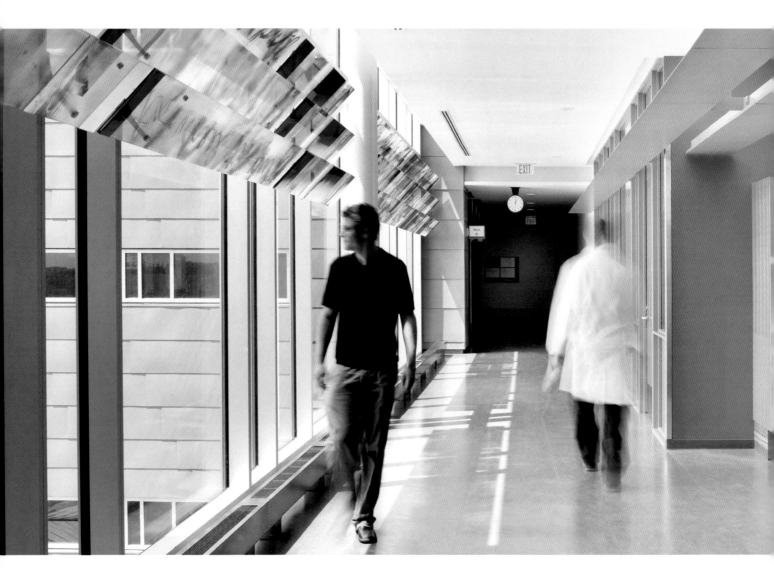

7.15 Choreograph navigation patterns

(CS 7), the spaces are carefully choreographed in this regard (Figure 7.15). It is axiomatic that the more sequenced and nuanced the formal composition of the building, the less need exists for compensatory directional graphics. In other words, a building that provides a clear and serialized sequence of spaces, carefully composed, without these elements contradicting or visually fighting against one another, is far more navigable. Navigable buildings provide memorable visual connections between their various parts (wings, pavilions), views to the exterior, spatial hierarchy, varied uses of colors, material shifts, daylighting, mass-void hierarchy, textures, proportions, and scale.

Atriums and lobbies

The atrium has made a major comeback in the past fifteen years. In most International Style hospitals the horizontality of the ground plane was often singularly emphasized. This preoccupation extended throughout the main level, creating spatial compression. In the era of austere minimalism it was often considered a costly extravagance to feature a large central lobby or atrium. The money was seen as better spent in diagnostic and treatment spaces and on their highly specialized equipment arsenals as opposed to a relatively 'useless' lobby. It was an appendage, albeit a necessary one, yet reduced to its purely circulatory function. People entered and passed through almost mechanically while en route to their eventual destination in

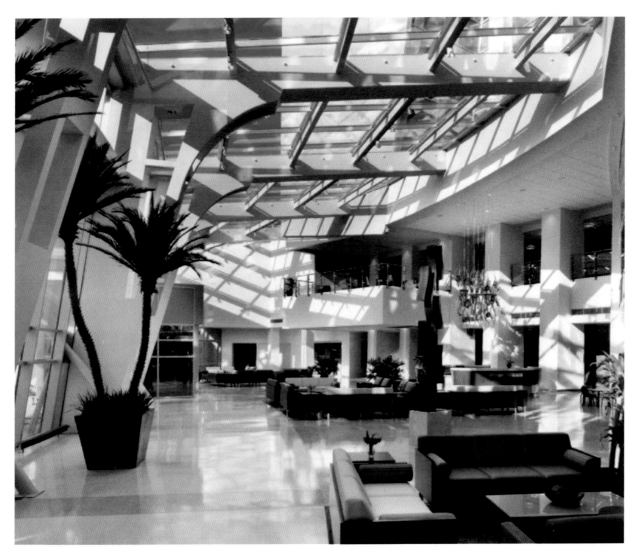

7.16 Articulate atriums, lobbies, waiting areas

the hospital-as-machine. This began to change in the 1980s in the U.S. when hospitals found themselves competing for patients in the open marketplace. These spaces were reconsidered for their *placemaking* potential – as a device to establish institutional identity, even uniqueness, and a place for people to enter and spend time rather than simply a space to rush through to reach another destination point. Many examples are noteworthy in this regard, including the atrium at the Dartmouth Hitchcock Medical Center (1988–1992) in New Hampshire, by Shepley, Bulfinch, Richardson and Abbott, and Pei Freed and Cobb's Mount Sinai Medical Center (1989–1992) in New York City.[22] Many recent hospitals feature an atrium as a place to stop and talk with friends, take a break near a fountain, or simply engage in people watching. This is a positive trend for the hospital

as a building type. The atrium at the Community Health Network Women's Center (2006–2008), in Indiana, by RTKL Associates. Inc., features a low-e glazing sloping wall-skylight-roof (Figure 7.16). The challenge is to cost-effectively design these semi-public places to meet the requirements of the carbon neutral/zero waste hospital of the twenty-first century.

Circulation options

Long, monotonous corridors are countertherapeutic. This contradicts the philosophy of patient and family centered healthcare. Worse, if there is only one way to get from Point A to Point B it can become

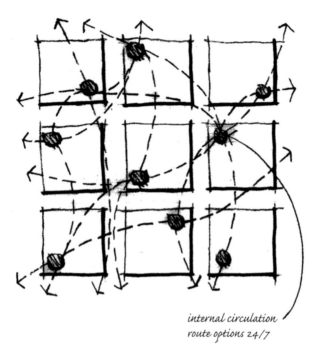

internal circulation
route options 24/7

7.17 Provide wayfinding route options – reduce stress

drudgery to have to use the same corridor, day in and out. It is no different from having the option of taking a different bike route to work once or twice a week. One can self-select one's route. This instills a greater sense of environmental control and hence the physical setting becomes more predictable and interesting. It may be that on certain days or times of day it is more interesting to take the path across a pedestrian bridge that leads past the dining room, where one can look out below over a space filled with people. At non-dining times this same path is likely to be far less interesting. The clustering of inpatient rooms in a PCU pavilion may yield shorter walking distances but if that is the only way to get to the inpatient rooms it can become tedious, regardless. Window seats, alcoves, and places to stop for an informal conversation contribute to the hospital as urban *streetscape*. Metaphorically, one should have many options for walking through its neighborhoods and its mosaic of public, semi-public, and private realms. Options in circulation paths in a hospital are preferable to having no route option (Figure 7.17).

Meditation and prayer

The archetypal medieval monastic hospital in Europe was a church-ward. The interior was, in effect, a chapel, with patients stationed, sometimes in bunks but usually in long open rows, as many as six in each bug-infested straw mattress. Every patient was at least able to hear, if not directly see, mass being recited from the center at the end of the long aisle.[23] From this era of chapel-as-hospital, the complete inverse had occurred by the late twentieth century, when the hospital chapel all but disappeared from the equation. By the 1970s the chapel had precipitously been demoted to a small room often no larger than a restroom or staff office. Its spatial and aesthetic appointments were little better, either. It became nearly impossible in many large institutions to even *find* the chapel. From this lowest of low points the situation has improved. In recent years it is as if the chapel has been rediscovered. This author, as a member of the design team, was responsible during schematic design of 'pulling' the chapel out from its previously deep burial within the bowels of the Department of Veterans' Affairs 900-bed replacement hospital, in Houston, Texas (1988–1990) and repositioning it squarely atop the main entrance to the hospital, clearly visible to all on the second level above the arrival canopy.[24] Nonetheless, often, the preferred strategy was to invest in other areas, combined with a general disinclination to emphasize the role of faith (versus science) in healing. It still remains somewhat unusual to place the chapel/meditation element immediately at or near the main entrance; many campuses now feature elements autonomous from the main composition, such as is the case with the *outboard* chapel/mediation 'building' at Legacy Salmon Creek Hospital, in Washington State (CS 2) or the semi-engaged cube at Banner Estrella Medical Center, in Phoenix (see Chapter 3). The former is autonomous, the latter partially engaged (see Chapter 3). Both are set in nature, versus oppositionally. The *inboard* chapel at the Orange City (Iowa) Area Medical Center (2004–2006) by HGA and Cannon Moss Brygger Associates, features dramatic circular sloping stone walls and a high, spiral ceiling (Figure 7.18).[25]

Noise abatement

A hospital is a noisy place. The constant hum (at worst, drone) of people and supplies ensures there are few lulls in activity. Nevertheless, it is imperative to buffer unwanted sounds from filtering into rooms

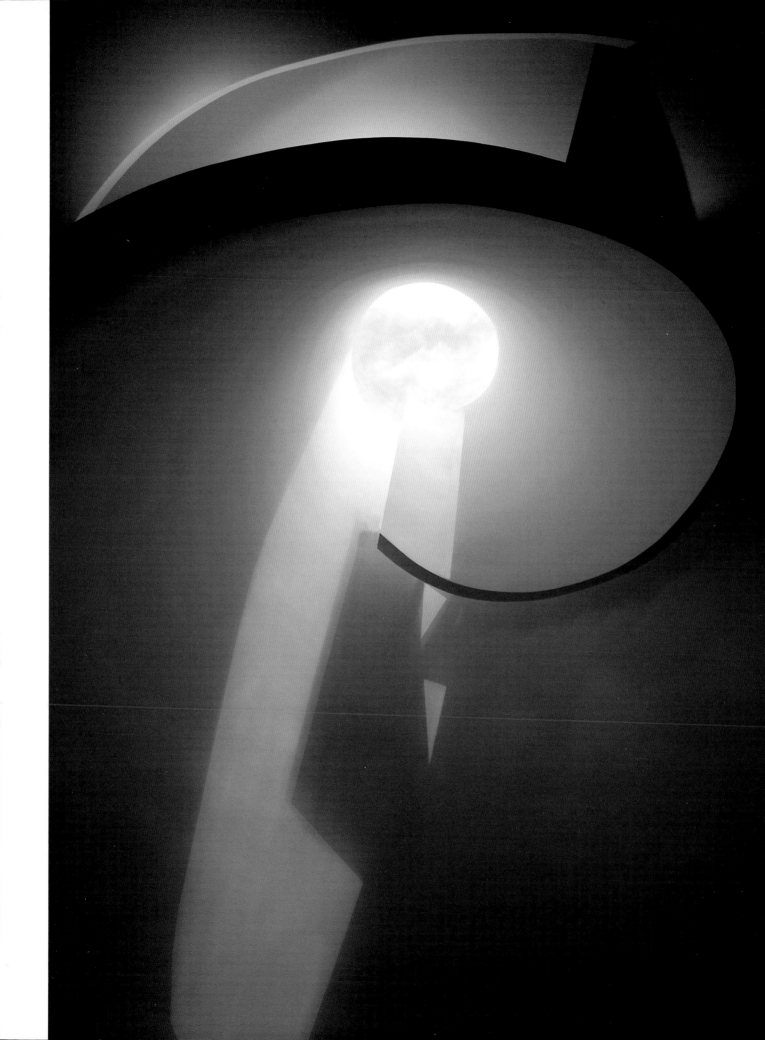

and zones where quietness is to be maximized. Excessive street traffic, corridor traffic, alarms, the sound of equipment, all are sources of environmental stress. Particularly upon first arriving at a hospital, the first night for the inpatient is often the most jarring in this respect. Nurses are coming and going on an hourly or more frequent basis, the equipment, coping with their own situation, being with family and others – this can be too much to cope with. Recent evidence-based research has revealed noise to be a continuing major source of stress to patients. A period of time is required on the part of the inpatient and the family to adjust to the elevated noise levels in the hospital environment. The patient, already under undue stress, may be unable to sleep or relax at all, causing irritableness, tenseness, and anxiety and it would therefore be prudent to install sound-absorbing materials and finishes on walls, ceilings and floor surfaces for this purpose. Thickened walls, double-insulated windows, and locating the bed away from the corridor can help in this regard. Hard, sound-reflecting (rather than absorbing) chairs and window seats also contribute to sound attenuation and echoing. Landscaping, screen walls, and setbacks in the building composition, recessed door thresholds, and the judicious orientation of windows, doors and furnishings all function as buffering devices.

Dayrooms

The dayroom, or waiting room, in most hospital PCU settings is actually a multipurpose room. It may be used as a dining area, a place to celebrate a birthday, or a holiday. It affords respite from the inpatient room when things are not going well. This, both from the perspective of the patient as much as the family member, depends on the situation. This space may at times be crowded and in need of further spatial definition. It would be prudent to create niches or alcoves within this room yet off to the side, or above, accessible via dedicated internal circulation. It does not suffice merely to provide a simple, unadorned room with a few tables and chairs. Architects and their clients need to challenge conventional thinking and reconsider the role and importance of the dayroom within the praxis of patient *and* family centered care. This space can open onto a balcony or terrace. Provide a space for media and entertainment options, and a place to check one's email or surf the Internet. It can be an adjunct to the inpatient room and to the overall PCU environment. In outpatient clinic waiting rooms these criteria do not apply to the

same extent, although it is equally prudent to provide an alcove for the mother who is in need of breastfeeding her infant, a space for media and Internet access, a space for use by young children, and direct access to the outdoors in the form of perhaps a nearby semi-enclosed play space or courtyard.

Dining areas

The dining experience in a hospital is an important opportunity for social interaction and exchange, but it is rarely seen in that light. To most, eating is purely perfunctory. Hospitals in the U.S. have realized this for more than a decade and many now provide the equivalent of a shopping mall food court. A variety of foods can be sampled. The options are short order and for fast consumption. A dining room is often provided in upscale for-profit institutions as a somewhat more leisurely dining option although most hospitals globally continue to operate cafeterias that are profoundly institutional in their appearance. These are noisy places, rather unsuitable for lingering over any meal let alone a five-course meal. Dining options includes informal food courts, conventional cafeterias, and dedicated formal dining rooms. In the PCU realm dining options include the dayroom, in an alcove or window seating area off of a hallway, in the inpatient room, and/or in an informal family room that may be provided adjacent to the central nursing station. It is therefore prudent to provide eating places that are flexible in an attractive atmosphere, with options similar to those at home, i.e. views to the outdoors, residential lighting types, contact with nature, and general options for the patient and his or her family members and other visitors to be able to control ambient conditions.

Children's activity rooms

It is still considered taboo to bring young children into a hospital in many parts of the world. In the U.S., the curfew time of 8:00pm remains widely enforced. When a young child and later as an adolescent, this author can recall being shooed out of more than one hospital room by a stern nurse, while visiting a sick friend or family member with my parents. Acute care hospitals tend to make poor accommodations for child and adolescent visitors. No wonder they (we) were non-gratis. No spaces were provided specifically for

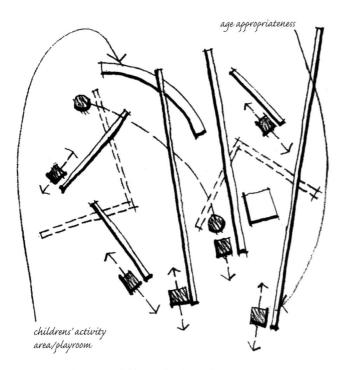

age appropriateness

childrens' activity area/playroom

7.19 Places for young children to be themselves

their (our) use. Activity rooms provide children with a place to get away and simply let off steam and excess energy. This type of space has become more common in libraries, the workplace, shopping malls, churches, temples, and in many other places. Even IKEA stores provide this type of room for kids. It is important to provide places for all young persons, however, not just the very young. These are ideally located near enough so parents can supervise their children, without being too near to the patient rooms in the PCU. Design considerations include acoustics, physical hazards, boundaries, shade, scale, soft, absorptive wall and floor surfaces, durable materials and finishes, and visual connectivity with adjacent spaces to minimize supervision problems. Therefore, make every effort to avoid accidents caused by a combination of poor design compounded by inadequate supervision (Figure 7.19).

Color palettes

Color in the hospital environment remains a much-discussed but little-understood phenomenon. Hospitals in ancient Islam featured colorful tile murals. These panels depicted scenes of everyday life and celebrated local social celebrations and customs. Ancient Roman public baths featured bright earth tones and red accent hues. Nightingale called for the nursing ward to be painted all white as it to her was the purest and most antiseptic of all, most easily showed dirt and grime, and therefore would compel the staff to regularly scrub the unit clean. By the late nineteenth century the Kirkbride psychiatric hospitals were all white on their interiors, augmented by natural wood frame windows and doors with transoms above.[26] By the twentieth century this attitude was firmly ingrained in the minds of most hospital superintendents. It lasted until the late twentieth century, when postmodernism in the 1980s fueled a reconsideration of the functions of color in all types of healing environments. It continues to be generally assumed that warm colors promote social interaction, and cool colors to a somewhat lesser extent. Colors that tend to agitate, such as intense reds or purples (in a psychiatric facility), and somber, dark hues of brown and grey (in a skilled nursing facility), are to be eschewed. All surfaces – walls, ceilings, floors (carpet and otherwise), stairs, finishes, and objects – are subject to being rendered in a full spectrum of color. The upper floor of the exterior of the Mildred Sheel House (2002–2004), in Dresden, Germany, by Behnisch & Partners, has bright, playful color spots and bands (Figure 7.20). A clinic in Seekirchen, Germany (2006–2008) by SEHW Architects, features a facade nearly entirely covered in a perforated steel mesh screen, depicting a uniform pattern of leaves and foliage. The screen panels are cut out to only reveal windows and entrances (Figure 7.21). Too little variation in the color palette (understimulation) is as dangerous as too much variation (overstimulation) in color. Case in point: a hospital dining room wall bathed in natural daylight may in the design phase be considered a nuanced effect. However, and unbeknownst to the architect, the client later changed the paint color scheme to have this same wall painted an intensely bright red. Unfortunately, the room became unusable on sunny days because the wall caused too much glare.

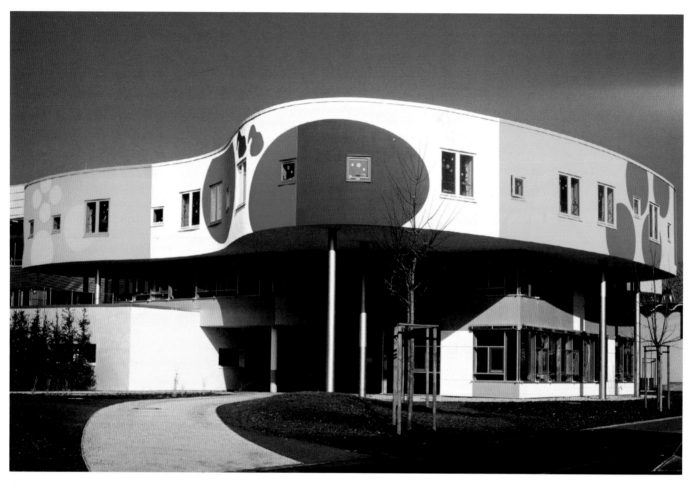

7.20 Color as a therapeutic modality

Virtual resource library

Traditionally, hospitals did not provide a library for patient or family use. They were strictly for use by the medical staff. This became standard practice in teaching institutions around the world. The library for staff remains a valuable resource, but it can be shared with patients and family or a separate resource room can be provided on each PCU. Decades ago, medical journals lined the shelves, now, a complement of magazines and reference books are preferred, with full access to the Internet provided. It may be preferable to locate this space at the end of a hallway, an alcove with a door either in or near to the dayroom, in a dining area, or at the center of the unit near the nursing workstation. The acquisition of health-related reference information by the patient and family member should be a personal activity, yet of a completely different nature than the input and routine retrieval of information by staff in their daily duties. Parents of young patients in a pediatric PCU can work from the patient room, if workspace is provided along a wall in the form of built-in desk, perhaps with bookshelves and drawers provided (see Chapter 4). These spaces should be relatively quiet. Therefore they should not be near to a children's activity room or outdoor space with high pedestrian or vehicular traffic volume.

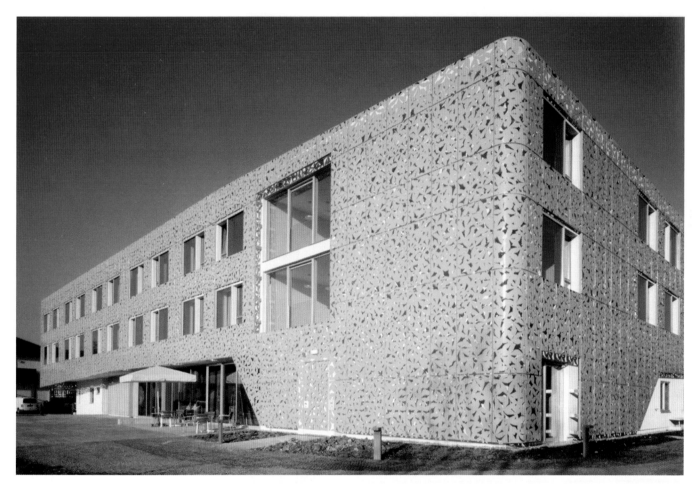

7.21 Innovative and evocative materiality

Fenestration and ornament

The ornate monastic hospitals of the Middle Ages in Europe often featured grand, stained-glass windows. These provided filtered light to the interior, which was usually a wretched place filled with inpatients whose prognosis for recovery was next to none. Nonetheless, patterned light gently filtered down to the floor. The leaded tracery set the brightly colored glass off from surrounding dark stonewalls of the Hôpital des Fontenilles (1277–1293), in Tonnerre, France. The high, pointed arches of the ward-chapel building at the Hôtel-Dieu (1437–1445), in Beaune, France, appears nearly exactly in scale, articulation, and craftsmanship as comparable churches of the period.[27] Contemporary hospital architecture may be on the cusp of a renaissance in ornamental fenestration, as evidenced in two recent hospitals, one in the U.S. and the other in South Korea. The difference now is that these amenities are located in the main public arrival areas rather than in the patient housing realm. They are designed for maximum visual effect and particularly so at night, when illuminated with dramatic interior lighting. The courtyard of the Banner Gateway Medical Center (2005–2007), in Arizona, by NBBJ Seattle, features a curtain wall mosaic of tinted aqua and grey glass panels (Figure 7.22). The Cha Women's and Children's Hospital (2005–2008), in Seoul, Korea, by KMD Architects, features a highly orchestrated, layered, superimposed curtain wall composed

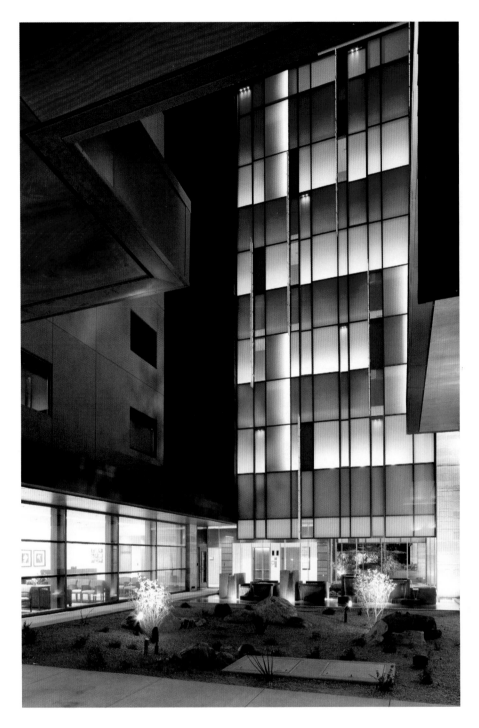

7.22 Innovative fenestration and ornament

with a number of overlapping elements (Figure 7.23). The panels appear to be suspended, achieving lightness, yet engaged with the interior space, and feature operable windows. In both examples, a memorable first impression is established.

Spatial distortion

It is not uncommon for a twenty-first-century hospital to feature a skewed, folded, or sloping glass wall in a public space. Distortion of walls or ceiling planes alters spatial perception by means of unconventional, unexpected, even jarring treatments of prosaic, conventional elements. It is a formal compositional strategy for establishing a strong, memorable image, a device to assist in heralding the building's civic presence as a unique *place*. This strategy is particularly effective when accentuated with dramatic natural or

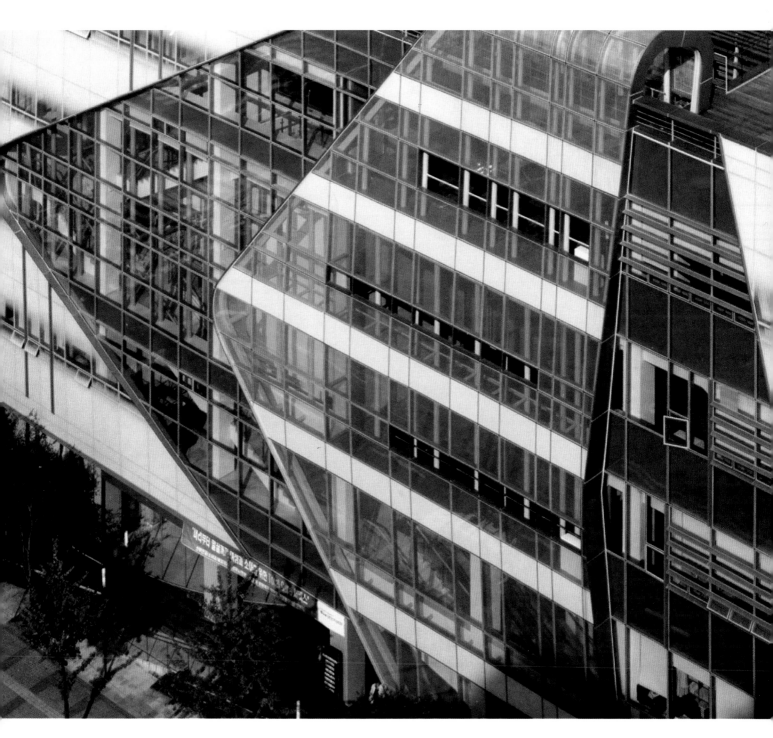

7.23 Superimposition, layering, collage

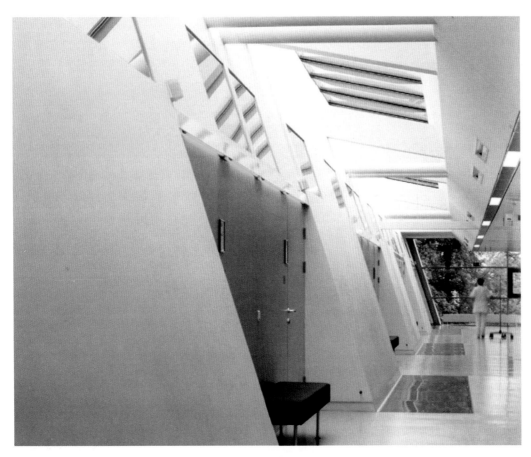

7.24 Spatial irony fused with sustainability

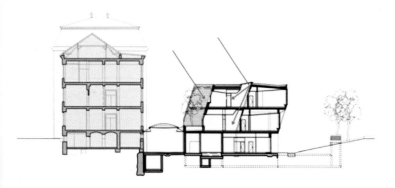

7.25 Daylighting, nature connectivity, and irony

thereby ensuring direct access between the inpatient treatment areas and the outpatient clinics. The treatment rooms on the upper two levels open onto a tree-planted roof terrace viewed through glass panels. In the lower 'platform' level, the space between new and old buildings is enclosed with a translucent membrane roof. Daylight is transmitted into the interior rooms and circulation spaces through distorted, angled walls and roof planes, with unconventional yet interesting results in a manner that does not sacrifice the building's functional integrity (Figure 7.24 and Figure 7.25).

Formalism and sustainability

Aesthetic/formal invention need not be considered as mutually exclusive from invention in sustainable hospital architecture. The two must be thought of as one and the same from the very earliest phases of conceptual design. The situation remains, however, that in the eyes of its critics, sustainable design, and in the U.S., LEED certification specifically, has had a tendency of inadvertently watering down, even suppressing design invention. For too long the idea of sustainable design has carried negative connotations of materials, techniques, and processes, and somehow holding designers back from achieving their best work. Designers need to draw inspiration from the challenge of the carbon neutral

artificial lighting. It is a formal compositional device to create, above all, a memorable, aesthetic *event*. In a museum, a sloping wall is equally dysfunctional as a surface for displaying a painting as is a diagonally sloped headwall in an inpatient room. However, the sloping glass wall in the atrium at the Feldkirch State Hospital (1992–1994) in Germany succeeds in this regard. Core volumes are rarely distorted in healthcare architecture. Similarly, this strategy was used at the Knittelfeld State Hospital (2005–2008), in Austria, by Fasch & Fuchs with Lukas Schumacher, although to a more dramatic degree. A three-level building was built to the immediate north of the existing hospital,

hospital. It is important that product manufacturers work closely with designers to develop products in tandem with those who will be applying them in actual buildings. The U.K. interior design firm Fitch has developed a program with a number of its clients, including the department store chain Marks & Spencer, to incorporate green practices in its entire supply chain and network of retail outlets. Clearly, opportunities exist to fuse formal languages with the language of net zero buildings and interiors. Environmental stewardship need not preclude design innovation. It is a two-way street: leadership in the design community matched by leadership in client boardrooms. The general public benefits from competitions and exhibits of exemplary recent projects.[28]

3   The patient care unit (PCU) and inpatient room

The patient care unit

In the megahospitals of the post-World War II era (1945–1990), the patient housing realm was often located in a tower atop a platform that housed all other functions of the hospital. These functions included the arrival, intake, accounting, administration, medical records, laboratories, diagnostic and treatment services, emergency department, surgery, dietary support, materials management, and outpatient services. This arrangement can still be found on many medical center campuses. The unit was configured in plan as a rectangle, square, radial pattern, sawtooth, L-shape, triangle, and myriad variations thereof. Recently, the prevailing trend has been to locate the patient housing realm beside (as opposed to on top of) the other component parts of the hospital. This horizontality has allowed for the patient care unit to be closer to the ground, configured as a wing rather than a tower, typically up to four levels in height. In a subsequent construction phase, additional levels can be stacked atop existing ones. Frequently, the interior remains completely cut off from the outdoors except for its windows and views. One can see outside but not *be* outside. An alternate strategy is to create an internalized health village whereby patient housing units are configured as pavilions with umbilical cord linkages to various support functions. Each pavilion is semi-autonomous, with exterior space interspersed in-between, i.e. as transitional and semi

private spaces, with these *in-between* exterior spaces themselves functioning as meaningful places.

Articulated thresholds

In most hospitals the relationship between the patient room and the adjacent corridor is abrupt, awkward. As one approaches the room, the corridor exerts its overwhelming visual dominance. This is often why so many think of hospitals as forbidding, institutional places, places to not be in unless one has to be there. Long, drab corridors perhaps did more in the post-World War II decades to give hospitals this poor reputation than any other single architectural attribute. Unfortunately, it was a reputation well deserved in most cases. Corridors in medical/surgical patient care units were typically devoid of color, artwork, niches, views to the outside, effective wayfinding signage, and were characterized by excessively hard surfaces, i.e. tile floors, plaster walls, and suspending acoustical tile ceilings with harsh fluorescent light fixtures. The entry sequence to the room need not be a source of anxiety. The area immediately around the door, on the corridor side, can feature artwork, a different floor pattern or texture, space for a plant, and a recessed light above the door. When multiplied by the total rooms on the unit, the effect can be transformative. Recessed doors off of a corridor help in the transition from home to the hospital. Floor and ceiling differentiation, i.e. color, texture, lighting are particularly effective interventions. The door itself should have a window, either a full height or top half window, with a louvered blind operable from the inside of the room, whether from bedside or otherwise.

Window seats

These provide semi-private, autonomous places to retreat to for a short period without having to completely retreat from the patient care unit. Respite is especially important during inclement weather or when attempting to cope with a difficult issue related to a patient's health status or prognosis. As the family may be experiencing a difficult time, personal space is extremely important and in hospitals this is often very hard to find. These semi-private nodes are best placed strategically along corridors, at the end of a hall, in an alcove adjacent to a dayroom, or in the patient's room. They can also be

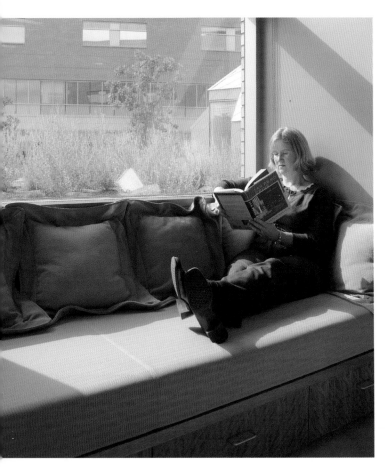

7.26 Window seats at the periphery

stationed between patient rooms, particularly in semi-private suites. They afford opportunities for interactions with staff in a consultative format, away from the patient room, if and when such interactions are deemed necessary. The overnight bed at the Legacy Salmon Creek Hospital (CS 2) in Washington State, doubles as a window seat (Figure 7.26 and Figure 7.27). The risk remains that window seats, other than those in the inpatient room, may add excessive square feet to the overall unit and would therefore be rejected by the client. If built in, off-the-beaten-path window seats or alcoves are not possible, a simple freestanding bench placed at the end of a corridor can yield sufficient privacy.

PCU circulation options

An inviting ambiance cannot be established if there is one and only one way of reaching a given patient room after one has entered the realm of inpatient care unit. It is prudent to avoid long, monotonous corridors whenever possible: the shorter the distance, the less imposing is the circulation path. Short walking distances with multiple options for circulation within the unit can help to express a philosophy of patient- and family-centered care. This is achievable through the judicious clustering of patient bedrooms and support spaces, with window seats, alcoves as places for respite and social interaction, views to the outdoors (being outdoors without leaving the unit), visual reinforcement through floor, wall and ceiling treatments, and preferred colors. These measures can help break down the scale of the unit and make it a less stressful environment. Inpatient rooms should be differentiated from other areas within the PCU. Paths informally bisecting the center of the unit, near the nursing station, preclude the individual having to traverse many extra steps.

Layered spatial zones

The inpatient room is a complex sequence of superimposed, functional layers. Five (and perhaps six) zones exist in an empathically designed room of this type. First is the space in the corridor immediately next to the room and whether the patient can be easily viewed from the corridor whether the door is flush with the corridor wall, or recessed. This layer may include a satellite nursing perch for data entry and retrieval. Second, the staff-patient zone is the space

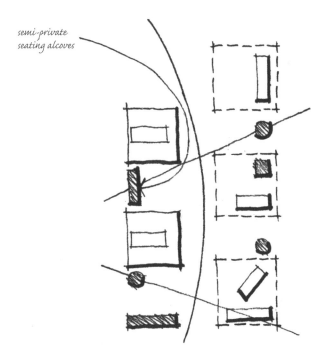

semi-private seating alcoves

7.27 Semi-private alcoves – getaways within the PCU

146

devoted for the staff to access and attend to patients' needs. The third zone is defined by patient bed size, positioning, and amenities. It is the heart and soul of the room as it symbolizes the center of the hospitalization universe. The fourth zone is the bath/shower room, and its relation to the patient's bed. Fifth, a family and visitor zone may contain table and chairs, a desk, and storage space for personal belongings. A sofa bed for overnight accommodation, or a window seat is often provided. Some patient rooms have a sixth zone, the provision of outdoor space, i.e. an exterior balcony, terrace, or patio, accessed via a door in the inpatient room, such as the Katta Public General Hospital in Japan (CS 3) and at the REHAB Basel Centre, in Switzerland (CS 12). Many options exist for layering these zones in relation to the most important one – that occupied by the patient. Ample space can be provided for family members' and patients' personal artifacts, and the display of cards, flowers, and gifts. In an acuity adaptable room it is necessary for personalization to remain a priority in its appearance and functionality. It would be counterproductive for personal space to diminish or disappear as the level of acuity intensifies. The loss of space for gifts, cards and the like may have a subtle yet deleterious psychological impact as acuity support intensifies. Patient rooms should therefore accommodate an increase in acuity intensity with a continuous (even heightened) level of amenity with respect to room personalization measures.

Acuity adaptability

The capital investment of constructing a patient room is significant. For this reason most hospitals today in general build as few patient rooms as possible. In this scenario, each room must perform to its maximum potential for the widest range of patients and acuity levels. Two terms are used to describe this concept – acuity adaptability, and universality – although broad consensus on the definition of each does not yet exist. A common definition of *acuity adaptability* is a room that is sized and designed for the full spectrum of patient care. Some define a *universal room* as able to support labor, delivery, recovery, and postpartum (LDRP), space for portable computed tomography (CT) or magnetic resonance imaging (MRI) in support of more invasive bedside procedures. In the U.S. these rooms are now nearly always designed for single-bed occupancy. Therefore, it is prudent to provide identical patient rooms equipped and staffed to support a continuum of step-up/step-down progressive levels

of care. It is imperative from the outset of the planning process to define a 1:1 correlation between the institution's staffing model and the design of the PCU and patient room. Most contemporary PCUs in developed countries have a 6:1 ratio (6 beds per registered nurse). The typical acuity-adaptable patient room in the U.S. has a 4:1 ratio, while the typical intensive care (ICU) room has a 1:1 or 1:2 staff-to-bed ratio. The ramifications of this are profound in terms of the delivery of nursing care. The appropriate size, internal amenities, proximity to the nursing station, and provisions for family and visitors are all co-dependent with the PCU staffing model. This information should be made available to the A/E design team at the outset of the planning process. The absence of these data may result in critical miscalculations in size, orientation, and design.

Storage options

Most patients and their families arrive at the hospital with relatively few personal belongings. But regardless of the patient's length of hospitalization, space is needed for the proper and safe storage of personal items and artifacts. It is prudent to provide a full height closet for the patient, and a second for family members' use. Storage should be flexible to serve dual purposes. Some families will require more storage space than others, particularly those who travel long distances from home to hospital. These families may need to, in effect, *move in* for a period of weeks at a time. Extra storage space is provided for this purpose for patients' families at the Bloorview Kids Rehab in Toronto (CS 7), and at Deventer Hospital in the Netherlands (CS 19). Similarly, for staff, certain supplies are needed on hand in the room on a 24/7 basis. It is recommended that a small lockable cabinet or drawer is provided for these items. In semi-private rooms and suites, a portable, nomadic storage unit on wheels can be relocated, as needs change, adaptable to occupants' preferences, and aid in housekeeping and infection control. A room can be partitioned into two sides without the construction of permanent walls. Infection control is related to the design and location of spaces for storage.

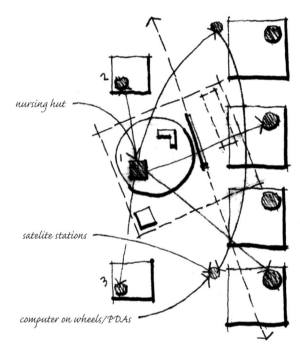

nursing hut

satelite stations

computer on wheels/P.D.As

7.28 Reappraise/reinvent nursing station typologies

Nursing station typologies

The days are long gone when all nursing was administrated from a central nursing station. The term 'station' itself is a vestige from the Nightingale era when the nurse could view every patient in the ward from a single vantage point. Surveillance was critical in tracking each patient in the ward, prior to the invention of electricity. Today, a variety of high-tech surveillance, nurse call, and health status protocols are in use. Digital technology has enabled the nurse and his or her support staff to perform duties virtually anywhere, anytime, within the PCU with a greater degree of precision compared to any time in history. The advent of the paperless PCU has given rise to within-room, room-adjacent (in the corridor or an alcove outside the door to the patient room), and core-centric (central) workspace. It is recommended that multiple workstations are provided for nurses, in decentralized (hub and spoke) networks. Make provisions for satellite workstations to afford visual contact (window) with

two rooms simultaneously. Laptop computers on wheels (COWs) mounted on portable stands have become standard equipment and allow for increased flexibility although these are likely to be used in tandem with, or eclipsed, by the use of hand-held PDA devices. The core-centric nursing workspace should consist of one or more conference-sized tables and chairs plus one or more private consultation rooms and related support amenities. Make provisions for natural light to bathe the space from a skylight, clerestory or nearby window (Figure 7.28).

Medications

Recent research indicates medical errors can be greatly reduced through automated medication dispensing systems. Make provision for an alcove in the core workzone, in a manner that does not block either circulation, space needed for cart storage, or the dispensing of medications. Automated systems, such as Pyxis' *MedStation*, aid in nurse and pharmacist productivity by simplifying workflow in the distribution of patient therapies, reducing turnaround time and errors, protecting against diversions, improving data archiving, and security. In the central pharmacy, innovative robotic technology, such as the *ROBOT-Rx* system, automates the storage, dispensing, return, restocking and crediting unit-dose, bar-coded inpatient medications. A robotic arm operates on vertical and horizontal rails and is programmed to retrieve medications and deposit them into patient-specific cassettes. A technician delivers the patient-specific envelopes to the PCU nurse's central workstation for distribution to the patient. The system can stock 40,000 doses of 771 types of medications, and is able to dispense between 6,000 and 7,000 doses per day. Advantages include it lowers pharmacist and tech support labor by 65 percent, slashes expired medication costs by 90 percent, curtails missing medications by 60 percent, trims inventory by up to 20 percent, reduces tech labor by 50 percent, increases pharmacist interventions by 200 percent, and improves picking and checking protocols for transport to decentralized medication dispensary stations. This system is currently used in more than 130 U.S. hospitals.

Lighting options

Research on lighting indicates a preference on the part of patients and family members for a variety of lighting types within the room. This allows for personal control of the ambient conditions and foot-candle distribution within the five principal zones – room threshold/entry, caregiver area, patient bed, family area, and bath/shower room and outdoor zone (if one exists). A mixture of full spectrum fluorescent and incandescent light fixtures is recommended because different lighting is preferred at different times of the day and night. For example, an over-bed fluorescent light source is recommended for staff use and also in the bath/shower room to facilitate safety, observation, and assistance. Above-bed recessed ceiling configurations allow for these uses without being visually intrusive (see Chapter 4). Wall-mount and tabletop lamps create a residential ambiance and help to extend an ambiance of home into the hospital environment. Incandescent task ambient fixtures may pivot on an armiture, allowing light to be redirected based on individual preference. The patient should be able to control all light sources and their intensity from the bedside control panel.

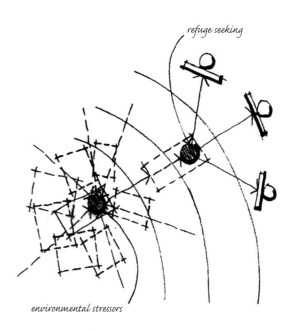

refuge seeking

environmental stressors

7.29 Prospect-refuge preferences and behaviors

Prospect-refuge

The patient and family prefer options to control social interactions with other patients, families, and visitors. As it is, the hospital experience can be extremely disruptive and chaotic for the patient (and family) depending on the patient's level of acuity. The prospect-refuge theory of human involvement with the built environment, as put forth by the British geographer Jay Appleton in the 1970s, is applicable.[29] It is important to distinguish unwanted interactions with others from controllable or otherwise desirable (prospect) interactions. The latter types are those where the patient may actively seek to engage in a conversation, or perhaps watch a television program with others, by choice. Similarly in semi-private rooms it is important to provide the option to greatly reduce contact with others (refuge). This can be achieved through the judicious design of pull curtains, well-positioned and easily deployed wall partitions, proper orientation of the bed, wall recesses and nooks for personal artifacts to be both stored and retrieved, such as a chess board that can be readily accessed, and proper orientation of the door and windows to the room. In addition, the patient room should be zoned for social space,

flexible, and adaptable to diverse activities, including sleeping and quiet rest periods. Make provision for comfortable chairs, a table, window seats, and an identifiable carpet or floor pattern that sets this space apart from other zones within the room. Layered interactivity between a family area, the patient's bed, and an entry-threshold area is ideal as this provides options for prospect-refuge behaviors (Figure 7.29).

SmartBeds

The bed is a high-tech machine. In Nightingale's era it was a steel or wood frame, mattress, bedding, bedpan – and little more. The tectonics of the patient bed have evolved to where *SmartBeds* facilitate physical modulation through the use of information and pneumatic technologies, i.e. Hill-Rom's *CareAssist ES bed*, Huntleigh Healthcare's *Electric Profiling Hospital Bed*, and the *Stryker LD304 Birthing Bed*. The patient can control all IT media, room lighting, temperature, humidity control, web access, bed configuration from a handheld remote or touch screen PC monitor, and curtains and LCD window opacity. Nurse call is by touch screen, button, or voice activation. Metropolis Magazine in 2005 asked four teams of designers to redesign the standard bed. The *Patient Couch* bed (by Constance Adams) consists of seven segments that support the body's basic pressure points. It is adapted from the seating inside NASA's X-38 crew return vehicle, designed to minimize debilitation caused by prolonged sitting. The positions range from upright seating and wheelchair position to supine, using a sophisticated *servoelectric* mechanism and drivetrain processor to adjust positions and transport the patient. It can accommodate children to extra-large adults. An onboard Patient Infortainment Control System (PICS) can be integrated into the room. The *Mobile Bed* (by Rockwell Group) requires, upon arrival, that the patient is assigned an RFID bracelet that programs their personal data, along with a mobile bed that also serves as an interchangeable bed/chair/gurney. It reclines, docks, and undocks from a spherical pod and also folds. Once docked, the pod syncs data from the bracelet, projecting medical data as well as personal photos and messages on hanging screens, construable within the pivoting spherical dome-hood above the bed. A privacy curtain inflates to form a semi-grid shell, housing screens and pockets. The *JetFlu Bed* (by Eric Lifton) borrows heavily from first-class-section seats in airliners, with its multiple stowaway trays, screens, and storage units. The fourth designer, Jason Miller, simply depicted a Hill-Rom *VersaCare Bed* set within his own apartment in order to convey just how out of place, excessively mechanized, and inhumane they continue to be. He argues 'Make the hospital itself more humane, and the beds will have to follow'.

IT choreography

Opportunities for engagement in the world beyond the walls of the hospital are profoundly greater than ever before. The challenge for the architect and interior designer is to sensibly harness this arsenal. It requires that each medium/media be carefully weighed for its usefulness in healing. In the patient room the bedside panel or remote handheld device is mission control. This device activates a flat screen panel monitor/TV comprised of one of more apertures (see Chapters 3 and 4). In a multi-panel arrangement various screens can be orchestrated, with one or more apertures for Internet use, others

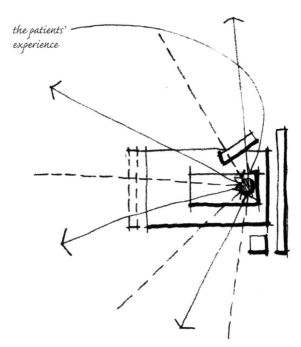

7.30 Choreograph bedside media technology

may depict views of the outdoors, or a film or conventional television programming. The *Vocera* is a handheld device that facilitates direct voice contact with a caregiver rather than going through the nursing station. By curbing phone calls and overhead paging, *Vocera* helps reduce noise levels. Information overload can be minimized if a DVD or similar room-user's manual is available for viewing by the patient and family on their first day in the room. This occurs in the Adopt-a-Room prototypes in Minnesota, and resulted from interviews with patients, staff, and family members (Figure 7.30). Media technologies in the inpatient room are expanding exponentially in the Information Age, i.e. wireless handheld devices such as telephones, iPhones, Blackberrys, and handheld DVD and game devices. Holography will make it possible for a hospitalized child to see and converse in simulated 3D, from the bed, with a parent who may be far from the hospital. The Philips Corporations' high-tech prototype, 'Simplicity Event: The Ambient Hospital Room' (2008) has been viewed on *YouTube* thousands of times at the time of writing.

Headwalls and footwalls

The *headwall* is the wall plane behind the patient's head. The *footwall* is the wall plane facing the patient bed. These two surfaces are typically parallel to one another. A footwall may be angled to the bed, stepped away from, or subdivided by other elements within the room such as cabinets, a desk, overnight bed, TV monitor, light fixtures, and so on. The headwall houses all medical gases, lighting, IT and electrical support, and may completely or partially conceal some or all of these items. An option is to provide a door that slides up or down, housing the blood pressure cuff and suction canister. The headwall is the nursing *nerve center* within the room, and the concealment of headwall elements requires a frame or aperture; this can be as deep as a foot or more. The headwall may have a recessed panel to display a work of art or house a light fixture. Supplies used by staff, such as gloves, sharps, and universal precaution equipment, are stationed within or on the headwall. These items can be concealed yet are immediately accessible as needed. Clinical handwash sinks are preferably located in close proximity on the headwall. Wood grain panel sheathing and translucent acrylic panels allow for an inviting aesthetic, blend in with room furnishings, and house multiple lighting effects (see Chapter 4).

Ceiling lifts

In U.S. hospitals, back injuries account for 44 percent of lost workdays for nursing staff.[30] Performing manual lifting and the transference of patients (an increasing percentage of whom are extra-large) is the source of a large percentage of inpatient room injuries. Mechanical patient-handling devices are increasingly being installed in the ceilings of inpatient rooms as a means to eliminate this type of accident. Ceiling lifts are preferred for their convenience and relative ease of operation. A Pebble Project research study conducted at PeaceHealth Sacred Heart Medical Center in Eugene, Oregon (in 2007) documented the costs associated with these types of injuries and the savings incurred after patient lifts were installed and full staff-use compliance was attained. The lift should be designed to be unobtrusive in its appearance, and embedded within a ceiling alcove or concealed in a specially designed compartment in the ceiling directly above the bed. Their particular functional requirements render them at this time ideal candidates for the attention of industrial designers because

these assistive devices are yet to be fully aesthetically integrated into the overall design of the inpatient room. Industry observers predict these devices will gain wide acceptance in reducing staff and patient injuries.[31]

Bath/shower placement

Adequate space for personal hygiene in a hospital is essential for the patient and family. Particularly for the patient, the bath/shower room is an indispensable amenity because it is used on a 24/7 basis. It must be near to the bed and the room itself must comply with and exceed minimum universal design specifications – that is, able to be negotiated with success by a diverse spectrum of individuals with an equally diverse range of mobility and sensory capabilities. The most fundamental decision in terms of overall facility design and the configuration of the PCU is whether this room is located on the interior/corridor side of the patient room, in midsection, or located along the outer perimeter of the room and building envelope. The first condition is referred to as an *inboard* condition, with the third referred to as an *outboard* condition. A decision must be reached early on as to whether this space is to be semi-private, i.e. available for use by patients in adjoining rooms (multiple patients), or private (one patient). An inboard or midsection bath/shower room placement allows for an unbroken perimeter wall, and for the transmission of additional natural light and air. The full availability of the perimeter wall of the envelope also allows for a glass door connecting to an adjoining balcony or terrace, plus a window seat/bed for overnight accommodations.

Bath/shower aesthetics

Most bath/shower rooms continue to be institutional, drab, strictly utilitarian spaces and this is because aesthetic attitudes towards this space have evolved surprisingly little over the past fifty years. There is no reason for this to continue to be the case. Sinks, water closets, grab bars, emergency alert devices, mirrors, seating, bathing/shower units, overhead lighting, materials, floors, doors, walls, ceiling surfaces, and color palettes are in urgent need of reconsideration. Continued inattention to the functional nuances and aesthetics of this space is particularly unjustified in the context of the evolving inpatient room. An aesthetic/functional disconnect persists between the design of the patient room and the bath/shower room with the former far ahead of the latter. In private rooms, this space is nearly always a single volume, whereas in semi-private rooms some compartmentalization may be warranted. This usually consists of wing wall separations between two (or more) water closets, and between two (or more) shower or hydrotherapy units. If located on the inboard side of the patient room or suite, or at midsection, windows are typically not possible. In a one-level facility, provide a clerestory to allow daylight to transmit, or install a flat pane monitor screen or artwork of surrogate representations of nature or other preferable view content, as 'windows ' where there otherwise would be none. In outboard conditions, endeavor to provide natural light and ventilation. Conventional doors in bath/shower rooms are the cause of many injuries and falls due to their bulkiness and weight. For this reason, consider the option of a lightweight sliding one or two-panel door versus a single 36 or 42 inch wide single panel swing door.

Bed orientation

A *same-handed room* in a PCU is one where every inpatient room is oriented with the patient's right side (for nurse access) closest to the door, as this is the preferred side for addressing the patient during an examination. Every inpatient room in this type of PCU is orientated identically (see Chapter 4). Same-handed rooms differ significantly from mirror-image rooms, where the beds are typically positioned (in plan) A/B, A/B down a corridor, because this precludes the back-to-back placement of headwalls and the housing of medical gases, electrical outlets, and related amenities, including plumbing, in a shared wall. The underlying assumption in a same-handed room is that all amenities needed by the caregiving team are located in the same place in every room. Benefits of standardized all-single-handed rooms therefore include a potential reduction in staff errors because the staff are trained to work in one room condition rather than having to shift back and forth constantly in mirror-image room configurations within the PCU. Critics of this trend contend that all-single-handed PCUs are more costly to build although this may be contingent upon local construction industry practices. Cost savings may be attainable through the standardization of room components during fabrication and installation. Additional evidence-based design

research is needed and this will be possible when more PCUs of this type are built and post-occupancy building performance assessments are completed.

Semi-private rooms/suites

In the U.S., the all-private-room hospital has become the norm in new construction. Some variations are still considered acceptable, in limited situations, i.e. patients admitted for observation. The case for the private room has been advocated most forcefully by evidence-based researchers and advocates of American consumers' cultural obsession with privacy at any cost (similar to the privacy of one's own automobile), who cite recent research on infection control and patient safety (see Chapter 4). Cultural privacy-rights advocates, for their part, claim that this makes the hospital more hotel-like, more attractive, and therefore more marketable. Meanwhile, in most other countries multiple occupancy remains the standard in the form of semi-private rooms, suites of 3–4 beds, and small wards of 5–8 beds, where single-bed rooms are set aside only for patients requiring isolation. However, even here, since 2000, privately insured patients in Europe and other parts of the world have increasingly sought privacy in upscale hospitals. This is the case at the Graz-West Hospital in Austria (CS 22), and confers a higher socio-economic status on the part of the patient and his or her family, or because this is a route to faster access to treatment. As throughout recorded history, unfortunately, those who can pay the most receive the greatest amount of personal privacy. The evidence in favor of the all-private-room hospital remains inconclusive, however. Too few studies have been reported in the scientific literature in support of this position, and no studies have sought to scientifically replicate the studies that have been reported. In Chapter 4, this debate is discussed in greater detail and various case studies presented in Chapter 8 feature semi-private patient rooms and small-scale wards. As such, the debate continues on a global scale.

Theraserialization in the PCU

This consists of layering, collage, superimposition, and the eroding of physical barriers that isolate nature from the healing experience in humans. It requires rethinking the total building envelope in

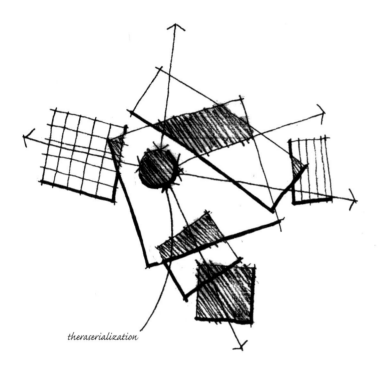

theraserialization

7.31 Theraserialization in the PCU

in Japan (CS 14) and the balcony/terraces at the Geriatriezentrum Favoriten, in Vienna (CS 17). Examples in closely related yet non-PCU settings include the meditation room at the Banner Estrella Medical Center, in Phoenix, theraserialized by means of foldaway walls (see Chapter 3). This concept is inherently interdisciplinary, and as both encompasses and supersedes what is widely referred to at present as the *healing garden* (Figure 7.31).

Transprogrammism and the PCU

The interstitial movement of the 1960s and 1970s was in large part premised on the unencumbered flexibility and utopianism of the superstructure. The entire movement would later be called into question, as interstitial hospitals required up to an additional 40 percent in front-end construction costs. Ironically, the initial goal of the first generation interstitial systems, which perhaps reached its apotheosis in the McMasters Medical Center in Hamilton

terms of openness, and lightness. Interactivity is achieved in a two-way manner whereby space is conceived from interior to exterior with nature connections at the forefront (see Chapter 3). Space is layered sequentially, hierarchically, with various zones of transition representing opportunities to pull/push the therapeutic properties of nature deep into the building envelope. Theraserialized space is both horizontal and vertical, that is, from side to side and from bottom to top. For the architect, landscape architect, and interior designer, this denotes transparency, spatial hierarchy, landscape, indigenous materials and local methods of construction, water, light, air, sound, and the revealing or peeling away of the building's outer envelope through a combination of additive and reductive means. Case study examples (see Chapter 8) of this concept in the PCU realm include the terraces of the Bloorview Kids Rehab, in Toronto (CS 7), the courtyards at the Dell Children's Medical Center in Texas (CS 10), throughout the REHAB Basel Centre in Basel, Switzerland (CS 12), in the perimeter balcony/terraces at the Kokura Rehabilitation Hospital

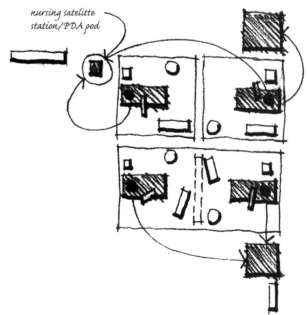

nursing satelitte station/PDA pod

7.32 Transprogrammism in the PCU

Ontario (1969–1972) by the Zeidler Partnership, was to create transprogrammatic space – space whose function and physical attributes could be changed as facility requirements evolved over time. Curiously, since then, the patient care unit has remained an inflexible, static domain. Units are typically configured as 'towers', with little inherent flexibility due to stacked plumbing chases, standardized anatomical support, and circulation requirements resulting in their placement on top of one another but is often still the most expedient method to achieve additional bed capacity in later expansions. Yet recent technologies make it possible to revisit the issue of walls that can be reconfigured, added, or subtracted. It is important to revisit the possibilities for flex PCUs and inpatient rooms, including nursing and support staff work spaces that can be reconfigured as functional needs evolve, and for patient rooms to be expandable or contractible, perhaps cantilevered beyond the column grid as at the Martini Hospital, in the Netherlands. Martini's structural frame allows provisions for removable walls, breakout walls and panels, and flexible, re-deployable bath/shower room fixtures able to transform a private room into a semi-private room or suite, and vice versa (Figure 7.32).

Overnight accommodation

Families, in many cases, are required to travel long distances from their home to the hospital. In the case of specialty hospitals, such as regional trauma centers, the family may need to be as near as possible for many nights because a family member may require a lengthy period of hospitalization. The patient room remains the most preferred location for the provision of overnight accommodation for family members. Consider providing a lift-up or pull-out bed from a wall cavity or as a pull-down Murphy bed from an adjoining wall. In other cases it may be preferable for a bed to be brought into the room. Chairs that can transform into sleeping units are also widely accepted. This type of chair should be used as a supplement, not in lieu of a pull-out, pull-down, or lift-up bed unit. Where space permits, having both options in the room provides additional amenity for the family as well as the patient. In cases where families travel too far to return home each night, consider providing apartments on the campus or within the hospital itself. An overnight unit may be shared between two families in a suite arrangement, communally, as in a hostel, or in autonomous quarters, as in a hotel. Whether private or

semi-private, the intent is to provide a place as near as possible to the patient (see also the section on medical tourism below).

Natural light and ventilation

The era of the hermetically sealed, minimally fenestrated PCU is over. Its demise occurred with the rise of sustainable design principles. Energy cost reduction strategies increasingly emphasize hospitals' reduced dependency on mechanically provided air and mechanically provided light. It is a strategy that has not been considered acceptable in hospital architecture since the 1930s. The transmission of fresh air and natural daylight into the interior is therefore once again seen as integral. This translates into operable windows in patient rooms and in adjacent spaces, larger window apertures, the use of low-e glazing types, new full spectrum light fixtures, multiple lighting options for the patient and family including a mix of both incandescent and florescent light sources, skylights, clerestories, and other means to bring light into the interior realm with the intent being twofold – to simultaneously engage the patient in the natural environment as part of the healing experience, and to reduce the facility's annual energy expenditures. All but *two* of the built case studies reported in the following chapter feature operable windows (see Chapter 8). These examples feature narrow footprints to facilitate the transmission of natural light and air. It is an international trend expected to become more widespread in subsequent years.

Intensive care units

The intensive care unit (ICU) is devoted to the care of critically ill and injured patients. Critical care units first appeared as ventilator units for polio victims in Copenhagen in the mid 1950s. By the 1960s, ABC (air, breathing and circulation) protocols for mechanical ventilation and cardiac defibrillation were developed. The ICU monitors and cares for patients with potential severe physiological instability requiring technical and/or artificial life support. This translates into a typical nursing ratio of 1:2 patients. The 2006 *AIA Guidelines for Construction of Health Care Facilities* requires a 13-foot clear headwall and larger clearances than in a typical room. A minimum of 200 square feet of clear floor area is required, and for Intermediate (Step Down) Care rooms a minimum of 150 square feet of floor area exclusive of bath/shower rooms, closets, lockers, wardrobes, alcoves, or vestibules. Rapid movement of the bed is essential, as is the need for in-room fluid disposal, and openness and clear visibility throughout. Remote monitoring has lessened the nurse's need for continual direct view of the patient. Bath/shower rooms are optional. Studies since 2005 support the increased involvement of the patient's family in the ICU but this remains a topic of some controversy. The NICU at the aforementioned Prentice Women's Hospital in Chicago (2009) is configured as a series of pods in cubicles of six or twelve to a ward. Each has telescopic glass dividers along its side and a retractable curtain, allowing the family privacy during visits, plus space for family personal artifacts and a recliner/sofa bed, because a baby's average stay is 14 days. The incidence of infection in ICUs is among the highest of all care units in U.S. hospitals.[32]

Birthing units

Labor/delivery/recovery (LDR) suites are major income-generators in many community and urban hospitals in the U.S. These units came into the vanguard in the 1980s in residentialist acute care settings, i.e. Cottonwood Women's Hospital in Utah, and similar LDR units and freestanding facilities in other countries. Until the mid twentieth century most births occurred at home. The midwife or the family physician was at the side of the mother. As medical practice became centered on the hospital this changed. Virtually every freestanding women's hospital in the U.S. now features an LDR unit. The Sharp Mary Birch Hospital for Women is San Diego's only hospital devoted entirely to women's care. Its facility provides pre-birth testing, labor assessment, delivery and recovery amenities. Private suites are provided during delivery, with a private bath/shower room. Recliner/sofa beds are provided for overnight accommodations. Wireless IT communications and close family/baby interactions are emphasized. Its 18-bed perinatal SCU is for babies born prematurely. Other babies with complications are treated in a 61-bed NICU. Evidence-based research findings have aided in the renovation of many older med-surgical units into LDR units, in the past decade. A quantitative study conducted at one large hospital in Texas undergoing renovation utilized staff and patient movement patterns to develop recommendations for its new LDR suite with respect to its configuration, the quantity of beds, and preferred amenities.[33]

Psychiatric units

The era of the psychiatric ward with its cinderblock walls and relentlessly shiny, oppressive surfaces is over. New opportunities exist without compromising the patient's personal safety or that of the caregiver team. The number of patients in state and county mental hospitals in the U.S. declined from 337,691 in 1970 to 49,443 in 2002, and the number of hospitals decreased from 315 to 232. Many organizations are currently in the process of building replacement facilities and just as in the nineteenth century, the specialists who provide mental health care are anxious to build their theories into the walls of their new buildings. The ideal now is to emulate the post-hospital everyday milieu to the maximum extent. Recent facilities feature inviting dining rooms, courtyards, atriums, natural light, color, and human scale. Security is balanced with personal autonomy and dignity. The image of a village, neighborhood, and private dwelling is preferred, with provisions for direct access to landscaped courtyards and nature. Prospect-refuge seeking is encouraged although this must be balanced with the probability of self injury (particularly suicide). The design of the 8-bed adolescent psychiatric unit (APU) at Kelowna General Hospital in British Columbia involved the caregivers and the families of inpatients. Patient and staff safety was of highest priority, without compromising a residentialist aesthetic or atmosphere. The new unit included special security glass, breakaway curtains, reinforced wall construction, special blinds, dual door swings to preclude patient and/or staff entrapment in high risk areas, careful selection of ceiling materials and smoke detectors, sprinkler heads, and light fixtures (with tamperproof screws), a staff duress call system, sharps storage, designated 'writing walls' for patient graffiti-like use, and tamperproof furnishings.[34]

Rehabilitation units

Physical medicine and rehabilitation (PMR) units were founded in the basements of hospitals at the end of World War II when many returning veterans were in need of therapeutic treatment for injuries sustained on the battlefield. These have evolved into one of three types: in-house, semi-autonomous on a medical center campus, and freestanding autonomous facilities on independent sites, often adjacent to or near a medical center. The Sutter Acute Rehabilitation Institute (2005–2008) at Sutter Roseville Medical Center, in Sacramento, California, by HGA Architects, is a 106,500 square foot facility on a medical center campus, for patients disabled by spinal and brain injuries or illness. It is a Level II trauma center. The institute houses 40 beds and shell space for an additional 16 beds. The second level houses a 30-bed ventilator unit and ancillary support functions. The PCU is adjacent to central gym, dining, and recreation spaces, with natural light and views. This close proximity between inpatient sleeping area and support space minimizes staff travel distances. Three courtyards/gardens are in close proximity to these areas and provide a visual buffer from a nearby parking structure. Interior circulation is a central *Main Street* that connects a two-level arrival atrium with the aforementioned PCU and related amenities. A second example, the Tokyo Bay Rehabilitation Hospital (2005–2007), in Chiba Prefecture near Tokyo, by RTKL, is a freestanding 90,000 square foot, 160-bed inpatient facility built near the Yatsu-Hoken Hospital. The facility features balconies directly accessible from the inpatient rooms, therapeutic gardens on two levels, and prefabricated bath/shower rooms. Prefabricated building materials and systems in Japan are of relatively high quality. The parti' is circular, with spaces opening up onto a central atrium. Colors are of therapeutic amenity for the patient, uplifting and positive without being overbearing or incessant. A third example, the Children's Specialized Hospital in New Brunswick, New Jersey, by HKS, Inc., features bold, playful color palettes throughout.[35]

Palliative care units

Palliative care has evolved over time to a position of relative stature within acute care and specialty hospitals globally. An interdisciplinary care team tends equally to the needs of the patient and the family. In-house PCU settings are generally of two types. An inpatient unit is either *centralized* on one floor or wing of a hospital, or is a *semi-autonomous* unit located on the campus but not in the main hospital. Centralized units differ from the typical medical-surgical PCU in numerous ways. First and foremost, their patient rooms are larger by as much as one-third in order to meet the sleeping needs of families and their storage needs, and support the four (and the fifth) spatial zone in the PCU. Second, nursing stations tend to be more informal. Some units dispense entirely with formal nursing stations in favor of a decentralized nursing model. The NTT Hospital Palliative Care Unit (1988) is a centralized unit housed on one floor of a large medical

center in the heart of Tokyo. In Japan, a roof terrace and ground level courtyard is provided for patient and family use, with direct access through a door from the bedroom. The Seirei-Mikatagahara Hospital Hospice (1995–1997), in Shizuoka Prefecture, Japan, by the Architects Collaborative for Public Facilities, Tokyo, was the first hospice program in Japan (1981). This 27-bed semi-autonomous facility is residential, connected to the hospital by a covered walkway. Bedrooms are arrayed on two sides of a landscaped garden court. This facility is one level in height. A second example is the 20-bed Sakuramachi Hospice (1992–1994), in Tokyo, by Hasegawa Takashi Architects. This two-level facility was built on the grounds of a 275-bed medical center. Both were built at the edges of their medical center campuses, and both convey warmth and domesticity.[36]

Grieving and bereavement

The modernist hospital, the machine for healing, provided few places for grieving with dignity. Death was (and still to a large degree remains) a medically unacceptable option. Hallways and waiting rooms are entirely unsuitable places for grieving. The medical profession has only grudgingly accepted the view that death does not symbolize utter failure. The architectural profession has been equally uncomfortable with the subject of death and dying: how many hospital morgues have been considered noteworthy in recent years? Death and dying is relegated to a strictly back-of-the-house, low stature. The corpse is usually whisked away without a word immediately following death, to some unknown place. Loved ones are instructed to wait in the corridor or down the hall in the waiting room. Visual contact and touching is awkward although this of course varies from culture to culture. In many cultures bereavement begins prior to the moment of death. Western culture generally does not accept this view, with an attitude of denial usually predominating until the actual moment of death. Compassionately designed hospitals provide semi-private and private spaces for grieving and bereavement. These places are a key ingredient within the hierarchy of public to private space. It is unnatural to postpone this process to the wake and funeral, which may be a number of days away. Within the family zone of the inpatient room consider providing space to be near the deceased's bed. This zone should allow for a small number of people to gather, regardless of time of day, prior to the body being transported to the morgue. Consider providing an adjacent exterior space such as a balcony or terrace. Such amenities are integral to the philosophy of hospice care. Acute care hospitals can be more compassionate places than most are at present, in this regard.

4   Diagnostic/treatment and trauma units

Operating theatres

Operating theatres in the nineteenth-century hospital were equipped with a skylight or oculus for use when the sunlight directly bathed the operating table. Since the invention of electricity, surgery has shifted almost entirely to windowless operating rooms. Technical requirements and equipment, required patient pre-operative staging area, and post-surgical areas must be antiseptic, hermetically sealed from the outdoor environment and all other units within the hospital, with all surfaces and the indoor air free of contaminants. Clean and soiled linen support, sterilization equipment room, staff prep areas, and general storage requirements are highly specific. The functional deconstruction of the hospital resulted in the redistribution of hundreds of surgical procedures to thousands of outpatient surgicenters. These procedures required a somewhat less rigorous level of technical support in terms of facility specifications and design. As for hospitals, the conventional approach to surgical theatre design is for the operating room to be windowless and entirely inward focused, as is the case at the Grand Itasca Clinic (2003–2005) in Grand Rapids, Minnesota. A recent, alternate strategy is to allow natural daylight into the operating room not unlike in the pre-twentieth century hospital, as is the case at the Brandenburg Clinical Center (2004–2008), in Brandenburg/Havel, Germany, by Heinle, Wischer and Partners. There, the theatre is equipped with a full height window and horizontal screens (Figure 7.33).

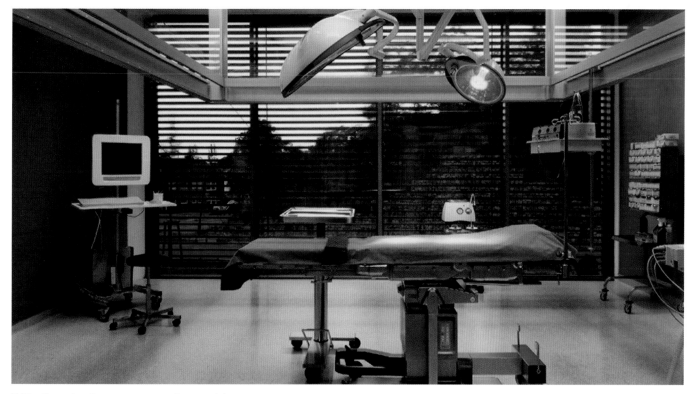

7.33 Operating theatres, nature, and sustainability

Pre- and post-operative units

Pre- and post-surgical areas are usually dreary, windowless places lacking in design attention. The patient is placed in a stark 'holding bay' with thin curtains, bland in color, with the entire space bathed in *Twilight Zone* lighting. Pre- and post-op patients are often semi-conscious from the effects of anesthesia. In the past decade two trends have impacted the design of Stage 2 pre- and post-operative areas. The first was their merging into one shared unit allowing for sharing staff and a more efficient use of space. This yielded more balanced concurrent utilization of every bed station. The pre-op zone is most heavily used during the early part of the day and is relatively quiet in the afternoon, while the Stage 2 recovery area is just the opposite. In order to address concerns about privacy in adjoining stations, a second change was introduced in many hospitals: they became either semi-private, typically three-sided rooms, or fully private, typically with ICU-type breakaway doors. The PCU has usually remained independent of these merged pre-op/ Stage 2-recovery suites, due to the criticality of the patients. The PCU is often designed to be side-by-side or very close by to facilitate staff and patient movement. Kaplan McLaughlin Diaz designed a prototype at the Hoag Memorial Hospital Presbyterian (2004–2006), in Newport Beach, California (fully private room), and at the John Muir Medical Center Concord Campus (2006–2007), in Concord, California (three-sided room). In each, a 120-square foot minimum space was provided per bed.[37]

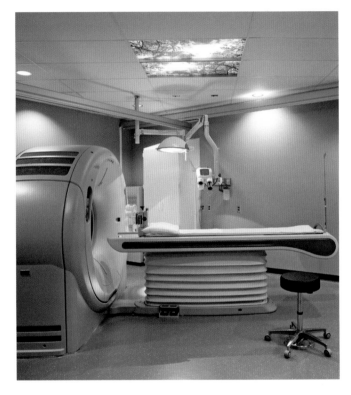

7.34 Diagnostic imaging, nature, and well-being

Imaging suites

Diagnostic imaging has highly technical performance requirements. These rooms are usually bland, with white walls and tile floors and acoustical tile ceilings with recessed fluorescent fixtures. CAT scan units are in the center of the room to allow unobstructed staff access to the patient. Recent advances in the design of these spaces has centered on the introduction of color and the provision of surrogate representations of nature – scenes of forests, waterfalls, rivers, lakes, mountains, sunrises, oceans – in illuminated apertures and placed on the ceiling above the procedure station so the patient can see the view from a supine position. The performance criteria guiding the selection of representational content is for this information to be perceived as soothing and calming. Colors are soft and life affirming

and have been selected based on evidence-based research on this subject. Music is also used in some hospitals to complement and reinforce the desired effect of the visual stimuli presented to the patient. Technical requirements of the high-tech equipment are stringent, and mandate that these rooms remain free and clear of all other objects, as any other objects are considered to be extraneous to the success of the testing procedure. The CAT scan suite at the Banner Gateway Medical Center (2004–2007), in Gilbert, Arizona, by NBBJ Seattle, features a nature-themed ceiling mural (Figure 7.34).

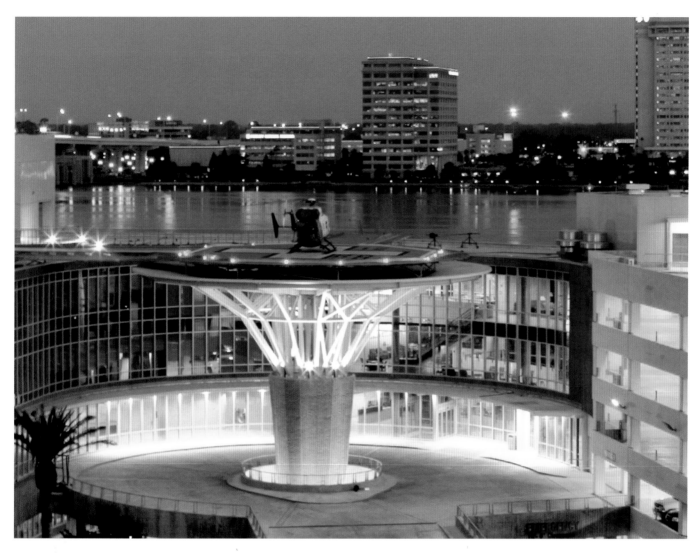

7.35　Emergency departments and regional trauma centers

Trauma center intake

Most trauma centers have highly prescriptive routes for the arrival and transport of patients. Unfortunately, architects have devoted remarkably little design attention to the reconsideration of these areas, including the initial entry portal through which the patient arrives at the trauma center. Modes of patient transport to hospital trauma centers include emergency EMS ambulance, and helicopter. Emergency Department (ED) entry points are located at grade level or a raised platform, and in the case of helicopter access, a helipad. Airlifted patients are routinely transported to the helipad site and into the trauma center's triage area. If located on a rooftop, the patient is transported from the helipad to dedicated vertical transport and to the ED entrance. If the helipad is atop an adjacent parking deck, transport occurs from this area via a dedicated staircase or elevator then to the entrance of the ED. A ground-level helipad, of course, allows for direct horizontal transport to the ED entrance. At the Baptist Medical Center (2003–2005), in Florida, the helipad is positioned in a highly visible location at the center of the campus atop a slender pedestal (Figure 7.35). It is clearly

visible and simultaneously serves as a beacon-sign, proclaiming its role as a Level 1 Regional Trauma Center. Iconic exterior signage, clearly visible from a distance, enables the ED to be seen by day or night, as is the case at the Banner Gateway Medical Center in Phoenix. There, a large 'EMERGENCY' sign in red letters is on the roof above a one-level entry vestibule.

Disaster preparedness

Emergency care systems typically consist of pre-hospital emergency services, hospital emergency departments (ED), freestanding urgent-care centers, and transportable MASH-like emergency response units deployed in pre- and post-disaster response scenarios, such as in the aftermath of Hurricane Katrina in New Orleans in 2005. In the U.S. the demand for emergency healthcare grew by 26 percent between 1993 and 2003, while the number of hospital-based ED units declined by 425 and the number of hospital beds declined by 198,000 in this same period. As a result, hospital-based ED and trauma centers are overcrowded and the majority of emergency and trauma patients (78 percent) are walk-in patients.[38] Over utilization of fixed-site care settings has occurred and is worsening due to a combined shortage of nurses, physicians, and hospital beds. In the U.S., ED waiting room times often average six to eight hours. The aftermath of natural disasters, manmade disasters, and the outbreak of new viruses, such as the H1N1 (Swine Flu) virus in 2009, can push a system beyond the breaking point. When a pandemic occurs, an already overloaded emergency response system cannot effectively respond.[39] Consider providing emergency and trauma care settings whose internal spaces are re-deployable – with flexible and moveable walls to provide maximum amenity in post-trauma situations such as during mass decontamination episodes. Include provisions for expanded triage capacities and staging areas for patient transport to nearby hospitals.

Redeployable trauma centers

The effects of climate change and sea level rise are threatening coastal populations around the globe. The increasing occurrence of natural disasters of greater magnitude will place unprecedented strains on existing conventional healthcare systems and fixed-site physical infrastructures. The tragic post-Katrina plight of the historic Charity Hospital (1935–1938), located in the center of New Orleans, is a cautionary tale for communities elsewhere who may in the future be confronted with health services breakdowns in the aftermath of natural or manmade catastrophe (see Chapter 5). The World Health Organization (WHO) promotes the development of transportable, redeployable trauma centers in post-disaster contexts. Portable, flexible facilities that can be transported to a remote site via airlift, rail, ship and/or roads and configured 24–36 hours after arrival are generally of three types: private sector civilian, public sector governmental, and military. In the military sector, the U.S. Army's transportable DEPMED hospital units were most recently deployed in the Iraq War (2002–). New, anticipatory prototypes are needed in the private and not-for-profit governmental sectors, such as mobile medicine hospitals funded and built by consortiums of European Union (EU) nations and operated by the International Red Cross. In post-disaster contexts, transportable trauma centers will likely become more important in the repertoire of first responders' 'tools' because fixed-site, permanent hospitals will simply be unable to meet the critical demand alone (Figure 7.36).

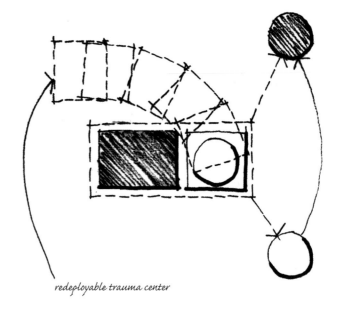

redeployable trauma center

7.36 Transportable trauma centers as adjuncts to fixed-sites

5 Outpatient services

Network aesthetics

The era of a hospital as a one-stop-point-of-care was transformed in the U.S. after 1983, with the enactment of TEFRA (Tax Equity and Fiscal Responsibility Act) and DRG (Diagnostic Related Group) cost containment legislation enacted by the United States Congress. Almost immediately, the industry's emphasis shifted from resource intensive inpatient care to an unprecedented emphasis on less costly outpatient care. Facing severe cost containment pressures, care providers and third-party insurers turned to less costly alternatives. Many thousands of freestanding clinics were built in communities served by a hospital *mothership*. Provider organizations evolved from a single community hospital, such as the Ochsner Foundation Hospital, in Jefferson Parish, Louisiana, founded in 1952 and evolved, by the late 1990s, into a multi-nodal hub and spoke network of sixteen specialty clinics functioning in consort with the original acute

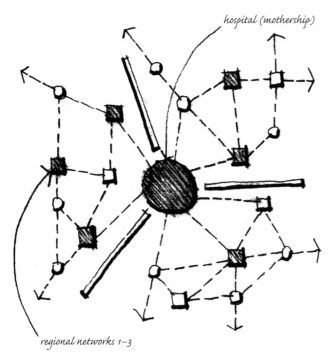

hospital (mothership)

regional networks 1–3

7.37 Coordinate neighborhood health centers with acute care centers

meetings over the years, invitations to speak to local charitable groups, annual fundraising events, and the use of its facilities for the meetings of community organizations who lacked meeting space of their own. Consider the provision of a community room and office space for not-for-profit and volunteer organizations in the mothership hospital as well as in every outpatient clinic throughout the care network. This will result in shorter travel distances, and greater grass-roots engagement on the part of local residents in the well-being of the institution. Consider the function and appearance of these outreach amenities, from the earliest phase of a capital improvement initiative.

Image and identity

Hospitals have run outpatient clinics since the Middle Ages. Non-overnight care was for patients either considered not ill enough to warrant an overnight bed with the other 'in' patients, for individuals who were considered social outcasts, too poor to pay, or for whom there was no available bed on a given night in the hospital. A small wooden door opened directly onto a stone-paved city street. Hospital-based ambulatory care clinics include emergency care, pediatric, mental health, general internal medicine, outpatient surgery, ENT, and oncology/women's health. The outpatient pavilion at the Brigham and Women's Hospital in Boston (1990–1993) remains an example of an outpatient clinic that functions as a midpoint facility, linking the city and local neighborhood with an acute care hospital.[40] Its architectural vocabulary bridges the residential vernacular of a traditional working class neighborhood with the high-tech world of an advanced medical research institution. It established a clear image and identity and immediately became the new front door and its mall-like naturally day-lit atrium the 'living room' of the campus. Older hospitals will likely continue to renovate spaces formerly used for inpatient care, sometimes even entire wings of aged hospitals, for the expansion of their outpatient services. This remains an architectural and facility planning challenge in terms of the ability to readily establish a new image and identity for itself without relinquishing that which is worth holding onto.

care facility (which had been greatly expanded in the interim). This pattern was replicated in cities and in suburban areas across the U.S. Carefully consider the aesthetic vocabulary of these care satellite centers as complementary, rather than autonomous, disconnected, or remote from the mothership's aesthetic vocabulary while integral to the institution's overall *organizational culture* (Figure 7.37).

Community rooms

The outreach activities of a healthcare provider organization are integral to its overall mission. These function as a primary means of communicating with the local community and the core constituencies with whom the hospital/medical center and outpatient care network interacts on a frequent basis. The Children's Hospital in New Orleans has prospered from its efforts over the years to establish an effective rapport with the residents of its immediate neighborhood in the historic Uptown section. This has required innumerable public

Docking portals

Mobile medical units are widely used in ambulatory diagnostic assessment and treatment at remote sites. These vehicles are equipped to be staged throughout the community and are often docked on medical center campuses when not deployed in the field. Heart screening, blood donor programs, immunizations, nutritional education, mammography, and magnetic resonance imaging are frequently provided. *Startracksmedical* is a U.S. manufacturer of custom mobile medical units. They manufacture a number of unit configurations, including a multipurpose 40 foot dual-side, 35 foot clinic with slide out room, a Class A mobile pediatric clinic, a Ford F550 37 foot 4 x 4 unit, Fifth Wheel clinics pulled by trailer cabs, and a 39 foot dental clinic with rear diesel engine. Audiometric units are designed to abate sound, for use in hearing screening clinics. These units feature either multiple small test booths or larger sound test rooms. Another U.S. company, *LifeLine Mobile,* has also produced mobile units since 1987 for medical imaging, mammography, community health clinics, laboratories, and dental clinics. Their Internet home page provides a detailed walk through of the design and manufacturing process. A docking portal to a permanent facility enables the mobile unit to assist when the fixed-site facility is experiencing a high level of utilization, and it is also a means to replenish its equipment and supplies prior to redeployment in the field.[41]

6 Theraserialization and landscape

Therapeutic gardens

These places can empower the patient and the patient's family, and regenerate an individual's attitude and spirit. In urban hospitals it is particularly important to provide far more than a mere *outdoor room* where trees and ground plantings are clearly visible and invite use, and instead, to establish an unbroken continuum between the exterior and interior realms. Exterior landscaped spaces on the grounds of healthcare facilities have become widely referred to as *healing gardens*. Theraserialization – achieved through a two-way continuum of layered transactive transparency and superimposition – can be created with structural and non-structural glass in a seamless visual transition from the interior to the exterior space of a garden.

These spaces afford respite, and a hiatus, however brief, from the day-to-day stresses of the hospital. They were at first developed primarily for use by patients, but more recently therapeutic gardens have been created for equal use by patients, family members, visitors, and staff. Consider providing a space for contemplation, rest, activity, and social interaction. Numerous well-designed spaces of this type have been documented. Among the case studies (see Chapter 8), the Dell Children's Medical Center, in Austin (CS 10) and the Providence Newberg Medical Center (CS 1) are noteworthy.

Vegetable gardening

Hospitals are beginning to set aside plots of land or space on their roofs and trellises for the cultivation of plants and vegetables. Rooftop gardening is a means of landscaping an otherwise harsh roof surface, thereby reducing heat gain while activating space that would otherwise be unused. The 800-bed Changi General Hospital (1985–1988) in Singapore cultivates tomatoes on its roofscape through the use of drip irrigation container trays that are elevated slightly above the roof membrane. The provision of gardens and vegetables is seen as life affirming. Plant hydroponics on the rooftop provides food for the hospital and also absorbs heat gain, thereby cooling interior spaces below. More than 190kg of cherry tomatoes were harvested in 2008. A recent survey by Ngee Ann Polytechnic students found that in four suburban areas of northern Singapore – about one-tenth of the total urban land mass – apartments and commercial rooftops were already cultivating vegetables using inorganic hydroponic techniques. By extension, approximately 1,000 hectares of rooftop space could be cultivated in this manner in Singapore alone. In Ohio, the ProMedica Health System network of clinics used a Toledo hospital roof to grow more than 200 pounds of vegetables in stacked buckets filled with a ground coconut-shell potting medium. The tomatoes, peppers, green beans, and leafy greens were served to hospital patients. Many hospitals globally will become community leaders in this facet of environmental stewardship.[42]

Patios, balconies, terraces

Opportunities to be outside in nature yet near to one's place of work or, in the case of a hospitalized inpatient, near to one's room, can be of immeasurable therapeutic benefit. There is no reason why a hospital cannot provide patios at grade level, balconies on upper floors, and roofscapes atop the facility and/or at intervening rooftop levels. The roof terraces at the Katta Public General Hospital (CS 3), in Japan, allow for the patient and family to experience the outdoors vis-à-vis the door provided in each patient's room without having to settle for peering out through the window aperture, as so often was the case in the post-World War II hermetically sealed International Style machine hospital. Such conditions are equally untenable in terms of reducing a facility's carbon footprint and in terms of the occupant's social, psychological, and spiritual well-being. The balconies at the REHAB Basel Centre (CS 12) in Switzerland, and at Kokura Rehabilitation Hospital (CS 14) in Japan, both also accessed directly, provide respite from the monotony of indoor confinement. Similarly, the rooftop terraces at Bloorview Kids Rehab (CS 7) in Canada, at the Meyer Children's Hospital (CS 9) in Italy, and at the Women's Pavilion at St. Olav's Hospital (CS 23) in Norway, are frequently used by patients and their families, and safety is of utmost importance.

Small courtyards

In the modern machine hospital, courtyards were often reduced to narrow, poorly lit volumes, and at worst, obscure light wells. As urban hospitals in dense neighborhoods built out their sites, nature was expunged from the equation. Patient rooms, while required by building codes to provide light and view, were often insufficient in this regard. However, large, ill-defined courtyards are little better. These spaces (as opposed to places) lack in spatial definition, shade, and in the intimate places to obtain solace and refuge. Intimately scaled courtyards promote social interaction, and when adjoining the inpatient's bedroom, or a small grouping of 2–4 rooms, or a dining area or dayroom, can draw people together. The patient wings at the Children's Health Centre at Surrey Memorial (CS 8) in Canada are scaled to promote use by patients and families. Ground level connections to the outdoors are echoed on upper levels by balconies, which overlook the landscaped space below. Consider providing a door for direct access to these spaces. Use low partition walls, level modulations, roof extensions, trellises, seating, trees, perhaps a small fountain, artwork, and landscaping to screen semi-private 'outdoor rooms' from direct view.

Water as therapeutic modality

Fountains, ponds, and small waterfalls – successful examples of all can be found in recently constructed hospitals. The rushing sound of a fountain or waterfall, the sight of fish in a pond, the reflection of sunlight across a pool, all can potentially provide positive, memorable, sensory experience. A waterfall in an atrium, or the act of walking over or around a pond, can create a memorable first impression. Provide comfortable seating and interesting station points and sight lines to achieve the maximum sensory impact of these amenities. The rock-waterfall at the Boulder Community Foothills Hospital (CS 4) provides visual and auditory amenity in this regard, as does the fountain in the exterior forecourt of the St. Francis Medical Center in Virginia (see Chapter 4), the reflecting pool at the Zhangjiagang First People's Hospital, in Zhangjiagang (CS 24) and the indoor and outdoor therapeutic pools at the Sarah Lago Norte Center in Brazil (CS 15).

Nature immersion modules

Healthcare settings for the aged, including assisted living facilities and hospices, provide rooms that allow the patient to become immersed in the soothing, restorative powers of nature. These rooms simulate natural settings – a seascape can be projected three dimensionally, complete with the sounds of seagulls and the swirling sound of the wind, as can a forest scene, with sights and sounds of wind rustling through the trees. It remains rare for an acute care setting to provide this type of therapeutic space although these modules are more likely to be found in psychiatric and in rehabilitation hospitals. The nature immersion module is a capsule-like device – a vehicle for simulated transport – a virtual journey, and is a key component in many hospices. A recent example in a rehabilitation setting is the virtual reality simulator at the Center for the Intrepid (CS 13), in Texas. At Intrepid, the rehabilitation patient can virtually experience activities of daily living, learn to walk virtually along a city street, across fallen leaves, climb a set of stairs, walk along a beach at sunset, and experience the process of re-assimilation into society. In an acute care setting, a recovering patient can accrue the benefits of virtual landscapes through the use of light, sound, color, imagery, holography, and the application of advanced innovations in visual and soundscaping technologies. It is, ideally, chameleon-like, ever

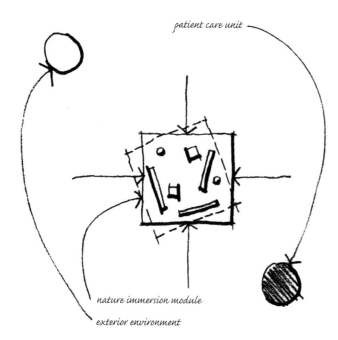

patient care unit

nature immersion module

exterior environment

7.38 Nature immersion as therapeutic modality

changeable, and adaptable. It is particularly recommended in extreme climates, either in northern zones that experience long periods of darkness, or in warm climates that do not experience a significant change in seasons (Figure 7.38).

Ground textures and illusion

The floor surfaces in most hospitals are monotonous, institutional, and a source of glare. Carpet ameliorates this condition although it too can become monotonous, if overused. To counterbalance this, consider providing an orchestrated palette of ground surface textures: grass, sand, stone, pavers, and pebbles are effective in simulating naturescapes, as they symbolize a break from harsh, monotonous surfaces. The clever application of unconventional materials can achieve illusion, such as a blue stream running through a corridor – without the actual physical presence of water. The effect is accentuated

with dramatic lighting. Consider providing a footbridge over an imaginary riverbed, or provide contact with actual water that one can walk over or in a mobility assistance device such as a wheelchair. In therapeutic gardens it is recommended that a mixture of hard and soft surfaces be provided, affording access to all, regardless of age or physical capability. Consider the ground plane as a blank canvas upon which an interwoven tapestry of forms, materials, colors, plant species, level changes, and paths function in consort.

Children's playspaces

Hospital waiting rooms can be tortuous places for a young child. Having to sit still, quiet, for a long period can be nearly impossible. It is becoming common in acute care facilities to see children's play rooms, equipped with a TV/VCR, books, games, table and chairs, bright color palettes, perhaps lower ceilings, an object for climbing or crawling through, and soft floor cushions. An outdoor area, adjacent to an indoor playspace, can be supervised by the hospital's volunteer program. The sight of small children can uplift a patient who, for example, is undergoing strenuous chemotherapy treatment and this can take one's mind off of one's personal situation and the challenges ahead. Children who visit the hospital as outpatients or otherwise need to engage in imaginative play, especially in children's hospitals. A child seeks out movable play objects, as these stimulate the imagination. Several points are worthy of mention: this space must be easily visible and accessible from the indoors via a connecting door, it must accommodate a range of ages from 2 to 14 years of age, accommodate a range of cognitive and gross motor abilities in the child, provide shade, safe and clean places to sit on the ground, and a table and chairs for art activities. Materials and finishes must be able to withstand rigorous use. Again, safety is of utmost priority.

Wood

Wood is of the earth, a tree grows with time, and its age rings symbolize this process. A tree, a renewable, precious resource, can symbolize life even in a transformed state. Wood is timeless, and has maintained a central, enduring place in human healing. Not by coincidence, wood is a material widely used in progressive hospitals and allied healthcare facilities. It possesses organic properties, reaffirms

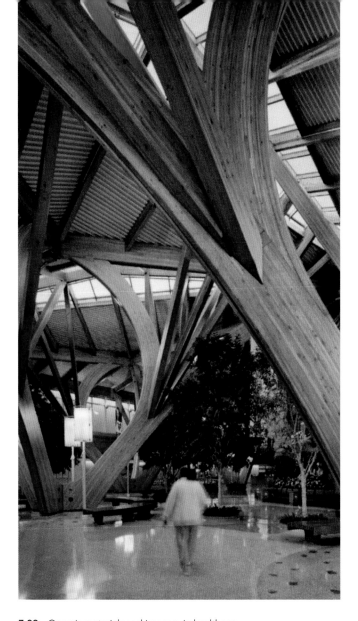

7.39 Organic materials and imagery in healthcare

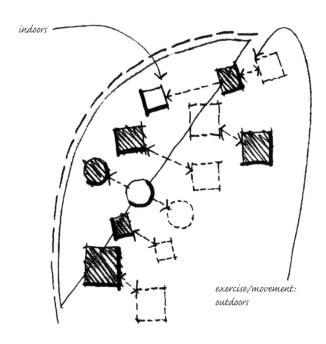

indoors

exercise/movement: outdoors

7.40 Physical exercise, built form, and health promotion

Movement and exercise

life, and holds positive associational meanings. Increasingly, wood is used in structural and in non-structural applications in healthcare facilities, i.e. in beams, columns, trusses, interior and exterior cladding, finish panels, door and window frames, flooring, ceiling finishes, exterior decks, balconies, in built-in cabinetry and finish millwork, and furnishings. Its therapeutic benefits resonate when used in the interior spaces of a hospital, no less so than when incorporated in exterior landscape design. It is a material that was, in effect, banished from hospitals for nearly half a century. The Credit Valley Hospital, in Mississauga, Ontario, Canada, by the Farrow Partnership Architects, is exemplary in its application of this material (Figure 7.39). The main public lobby of its 320,000 square foot cancer center features massive tree-like columns fabricated of laminated wood. These columns slope as they rise upward in a flourish not unlike the graceful movements of dancers.

A wellness center on a hospital campus can provide an opportunity to be indoors while engaged in physical fitness activities. This place can provide a source of respite, exercise and, depending on one's physical abilities, a source of social interaction. Activities available at progressive hospitals, in this regard, include weight lifting, treadmill machines, climbing walls, spa-pools, saunas, and aerobic classes. These typically occur in a wellness center available for staff, patients, and their families. The health promotion of persons of all ages is the goal. It is not enough to provide only an indoor space, however. Exterior space adjacent to an indoor wellness center can function as a therapeutic adjunct. A landscaped courtyard, semi-enclosed lawn, or partially covered space can provide a sense of protection and sufficient enclosure. Patients in particular do not want to feel as if they are on display while exercising. A trellis adjacent to interior space represents a midpoint condition – part inside/part outdoor zone – or an outdoor pavilion within a therapeutic garden, can provide semi-enclosure while still being outdoors. If large enough this pavilion can be used in inclement weather, such as during a sudden afternoon downpour on a summer afternoon (Figure 7.40).

Outdoor works of art

In a hospital setting, works of art that do not cognitively connect with the viewer can exacerbate an already stressful personal situation. Abstract sculptures with bold, jarring forms, colors and imagery may not *connect* with persons in need of meaningful, non-stressful connections with their surrounding world. Abstract art perceived as unduly challenging or difficult to interpret can be a source of further stress to someone who is already experiencing stress.[43] In a setting already as stressful as an acute care hospital it is worth the time and effort to commission works of art that do not cause further stress or a negative response such as avoidance. It is not that these artifacts are required to be universally interpreted as 'happy' or unambiguously positive – such as the Ronald McDonald icon – only that they do not invoke hostile or antagonistic interpretations. Obscure, museum-quality art is likely to fail in a therapeutic garden, atrium lobby, or courtyard. Patients prefer representational content depicting nature and closely related scenes. In one U.S. hospital it was reported that abstract figures of birds installed as an exhibit in a courtyard eventually had to be removed. This was because the artwork was disliked and viewed with apprehension by the cancer patients housed in an adjoining oncology unit.[44] Children's hospitals, in seeking to establish playful imagery, may unwittingly cause fear and apprehension in young children – when an 8-year-old encounters, for example, a real locomotive engine at the main entrance, or a real sailboat perched above the entrance. By contrast, the thematic content of the art was well received by patients and families at the Women's Oncology Center (2000–2002) at Mount Sinai Hospital, in San Francisco. There, small-scale garden sculptures complement an adjoining interior corridor lined with art produced by patients, facing the courtyard.

7 Administration/total environment

Environmental stewardship

Hospitals have acquired a well-earned reputation as being among a community's chronic polluters. They generate voluminous amounts of toxic materials and then often do not take the measures needed to properly store, remediate, or dispose of these materials. It no longer suffices for the administration to merely construct elaborate public relations campaigns. It is now possible in the U.S. to access online the Environmental Protection Agency's (EPA) Energy Impact Calculator to determine the carbon footprint profile for any given zip code in the nation. A hospital can no longer lag behind in terms of environmental best practices and must demonstrate stewardship in recycling programs, sustainable land uses, health promotion programs, and the adaptive reuse of historic buildings. Dozens of initiatives exist for the undertaking. Healthcare facilities must be purged of their toxic contaminants: lead and mercury must be removed from the food chain and stricken from hospital campuses. When the Hackensack University Medical Center launched its 'greenness' campaign in 2008, it took out an eight-page advertisement supplement in *The New York Times*. Leading-edge institutions have realized the marketing potential and sheer good will that can be fostered in the community through sound practices in environmental sustainability and stewardship – and the positive ramifications for an institution's financial bottom line.

Sustainability certification

In the U.S., LEED is both a point-based and metric tool to guide best practices in sustainable design and construction, and a third party certification system to verify compliance with its criteria for certification. A rigorous registration, documentation, and review process is applied to a building seeking a rating at one of four levels: certified, silver, gold, or platinum. This program was launched in 2001 by the USGBC. Soon, the USGBC began accrediting professionals and by 2009, 81,155 professionals had obtained LEED accredited professional (LEED-AP) status in the U.S. and Canada.[45] By 2007 more than 90 LEED-related initiatives had been enacted by local, regional state and federal regulatory agencies in the U.S. and Canada, further embedding LEED as the standard bearer for sustainable practices. The LEED-affiliated *Green Guide for Healthcare* began in 2003. It is a joint project of the *Health Care Without Harm*, and the *Center for Maximum Potential Building Systems*. A self-certification tool was established. Its point system closely parallels the LEED system but it pertains specifically to the complex issues associated with an acute care hospital. In 2002, the *Green Building Council* of Australia launched its *Green Star* rating system. Its rating tool assesses the sustainability quotient of new and renovated healthcare facilities. Its Energy Calculator Guide was released in 2006 to support the use of the *Green Star Healthcare-PILOT*. Healthcare organizations globally are embracing these certification systems in ever increasing numbers. In the U.K., the *National Health Service* (NHS) initiated its assessment tool (NEAT) as a self-assessment software tool in new construction and retrofit improvements; it is guided by ten criteria: management, energy consumption, transportation issues, water resources, materials management, land use and ecology, pollution, the occupied interior environment, the socio-cultural ramifications of sustainability, and operational waste storage and recycling 'best practices'.[46] To some, however, this *green certification industry* is seen as controversial due to the rising cost of the process and because it is feared it will lead to a have/have not dilemma, similar to the global *digital divide* (see Chapter 6).

Patient Safety Infection control

It is of critical importance that hospitals reduce medical errors. Hospital acquired infection, i.e. nosocomial infections, are a leading cause of death in hospitals. The evidence-based research literature strongly points to the design of the physical environment as impacting all three major transmission routes – air, human contact, and water. Hospital acquired infections in the U.S. in 2002 numbered approximately 1.7 million, and the number of associated deaths reached 98,987.[47] According to the *Centers for Disease Control and Prevention* (CDC) the cost of treating these patients is estimated to be $5 billion per year. Many hospital-acquired infections are drug resistant and difficult to treat and eradicate. Patients are particularly vulnerable when they are immunocompromised or otherwise weakened by age, medical or surgical treatments, or collateral underlying disease. The international trend toward an increasing intensity of patient acuity portends a future of greater

patient vulnerability to hospital-acquired infections. A review of the state of knowledge on this issue in the planning and design of hospital environments was provided in a 2008 report by Roger Ulrich and colleagues.[48]

Patient and family empowerment

Staff personnel referred to as end users, or *primary user constituencies* – work on site on a daily basis. The hundreds of roles assumed include lab technicians, physicians, nursing personnel, administrative staff, social workers, psychologists, chaplains, IT specialists, buildings and grounds staff, dietary services personnel, volunteers, and pharmacists, to name but a few. Secondary and tertiary constituencies include off-site administrators, community advocates, the board of directors,

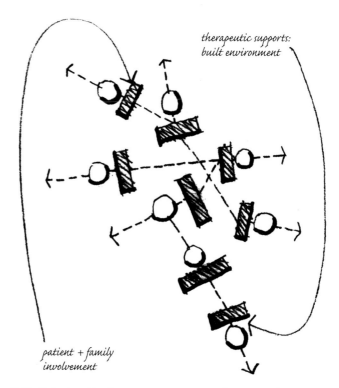

therapeutic supports: built environment

patient + family involvement

7.41 Patient and family empowerment – supportive care settings

fiduciary advisors, neighborhood organizations, and elected officials. A representative from each key constituency should be invited, from the earliest date, following board approval to proceed with a capital improvement initiative. Subcommittees, pursuant to information provided by the board, are constituted to ensure a voice in site selection, design goals, the size and composition of the services to be provided, staff recruitment and retention, master planning strategies, transportation, external review board approvals, landscape design, interior design, building design, internal configuration, equipment, and project scheduling and phasing. The Dell Children's Medical Center in Texas (CS 10) and the Dublin Methodist Medical Center in Ohio are two recent exemplars in this regard. At the Prentice Women's Hospital in Chicago (2005–2007) the design team interviewed representatives of 125 user groups, including direct caregivers, families, and volunteers who staff the main information desk, and queried on everything from the hospital's color palette to the design of the NICU (Figure 7.41).

Life cycle design

Life cycle design (LCD) is premised on a facility's long-term use, and is part of the earliest planning and design phase. In terms of total life-span use and occupancy, this consists of materiality systems, construction methods, energy use, site factors, growth and retrofit options, health ramifications, waste disposal, daily use, and routine operations and maintenance. The goal is to create a building that treads as lightly as possible on the earth. These benchmarks will in the future emphasize a greater degree of carbon neutrality and autonomy in terms of energy conservation, and a net zero healthcare facility and campus. Additional benchmarks will include flexibility, the establishment of regional and local performance criteria, cooperative agreements, and the control and monitoring of all inflow-outflow protocols. These include food, medical waste, supplies, impacts of human occupancy and patterns of use, and the continual reappraisal of all input-output systems for their environmental conservation affordances.[49] This protocol needs to be assessed in direct relation to the organization's goals, priorities, and aspirations with respect to environmental stewardship. In the future these measures will be critical to the degree to which an organization is judged as a success (Figure 7.42). The innovative yet ill-fated Gaviotas Hospital (1982–1986) in eastern Columbia

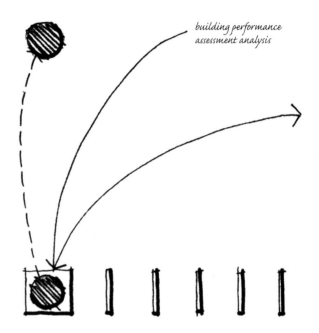

7.42 Building life cycle and sustainable design

remains an early yet enduring precursor of energy independence in a healthcare facility.

Theraserialization/total environment

Most hospitals today still need to reinvent themselves with regard to their operative assumptions about the built environment – as large undifferentiated boxes filled with internal departments and services jammed together. It is no longer necessary for *every* department to be directly adjacent to every other relevant department. This attitude reflects a pre-Information Age mentality, and is anachronistic from both an administrative and procedural standpoint. As large hospitals continue to functionally deconstruct their constituent parts, their reassembly in new ways continues. An unprecedented degree of both literal and figurative breathing room is now possible between its dozens of complex and at times contradictory parts. New types of umbilical connections are linking these constituent parts. New types of spaces in-between these elements need to be accorded equal architectural attention with conventional internal space. This will facilitate person/nature connections and places for respite and regeneration. Internal realms can nurture and inform these in-between or *transitory* realms, and vice versa. This was achieved to a certain extent in a number of the case studies, including the Jiaikai Amani Hospital in the United Arab Emirates (CS 6), at Bloorview Kids Rehab in Toronto (CS 7), at the REHAB Basel Center in Switzerland (CS 12), and at the Sarah Lago Norte Center in Brazil (CS 15).

Evidence-based design

The evidence-based design movement is at present (2010) premised on three assumptions: first, patients should be able to devote their energies to healing and recovery without having to cope with an unsupportive built environment; second, healthcare providers should be able to perform their duties without becoming ill themselves or being injured due to an unsupportive built environment; and third, non-carbon-reductive and high energy consuming buildings for healthcare are tantamount to an unsupportive built environment. This movement aims to reverse the role of built form as a contributor to medical errors, drawing upon an earlier parallel initiative in the U.S. medical profession and a growing wave of parallel efforts in a number of other professions and sectors.[50] To advance these core aims, an accreditation and certification process was recently launched to develop a cadre of industry professionals through education and assessment, in the field of environmental design. This protocol, *Evidence-based Design Accreditation and Certification* (EDAC), was funded and sponsored by the Robert Wood Johnson Foundation (New Jersey), and The Center for Health Design (California). A set of three study guides were published in 2008: *An Introduction to Evidence-Based Design: Exploring Healthcare and Design; Building the Evidence Base: Understanding Research in Healthcare Design;* and, *Integrating Evidence-Based Design: Practicing the Healthcare Design Process.* It is an interdisciplinary effort and EDAC is for healthcare providers as well as for design, planning, and engineering professionals in the field.[51] However, some view this push for certification in the U.S. as premature and it therefore remains the source of some controversy.

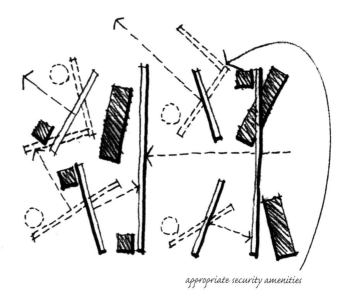

appropriate security amenities

7.43 Security, therapeutic support, and well-being

Campus security

Hospitalized patients often experience severe emotional trauma. Upon arriving, particularly in the immediate aftermath of trauma, they are in critical need of a safe, secure, and predictable treatment environment. Lockable doors, secure windows, safe places for the storage of personal items, and an overall sense of refuge and personal safety are essential in the PCU. This is particularly important in urban hospitals, where the threat of theft and bodily harm may exist in the immediate vicinity of the facility. The threat of being violated via theft, or worse, can exert fundamental disruption to one's well-being. Consider the provision of buffers between the street, the main entry, and semi-private and private areas on the campus, as well as throughout the facility. Security measures should include video surveillance technology in public spaces only, and electronic card access, and wireless controls at all access points. However, advanced security and surveillance technologies must be balanced with their unobtrusive appurtenance. It must be *invisible*: the greater the invisibility factor, the better. Safety and security measures need not create a fortress-like or institutional ambience. Therefore, members of the design team should guide the selection and *design* of all campus security technologies in the earliest phase of the planning and design process, to preclude bulky, unsightly equipment from being poorly installed after the fact (Figure 7.43).

Health information technology

As discussed above, the Institute of Medicine in the U.S. and other organizations have reported that fragmented, disorganized, and inaccessible medical records data can adversely impact the quality of care and compromise patient safety. In the U.S. at this time the federal government has awarded states and private sector healthcare organizations grants to transition from traditional paper-based medical records systems to digital medical records systems. The core argument for the Health Information Technology (HIT) initiative is that digitization is a more cost-effective and consistent method from the standpoint of the patient. Proponents of this strategy assert that medical errors will be greatly reduced as a result of the higher degree of continuity of care available to patients, particularly to those who relocate to a new geographical region. This will also reduce the need for voluminous records rooms. Vast records rooms housing conventional paper files, in the future, will otherwise needlessly continue to consume valuable capital improvement resources. These resources can be more prudently invested in other places within the medical center. However, there will still remain a need for a certain percentage of paper records, particularly in disaster response conditions where electrical support is unavailable, and in field-based operations where paper records are initially used and later digitized, with the paper records recycled.[52]

Medical tourism

The planet's population is increasingly falling into one of two groups – the haves and the have nots, not dissimilar to the wide digital divide which continues to isolate Internet users from Internet non-users. As such, those who can afford to receive care beyond the borders of their home country are availing themselves of care options overseas. In 2008 alone, more than 6 million people traveled to India to receive healthcare, in some cases at one-tenth of the cost of comparable healthcare treatment in their home country. In the case of the Max Hospital, in New Delhi, India, a full-scale hotel is available

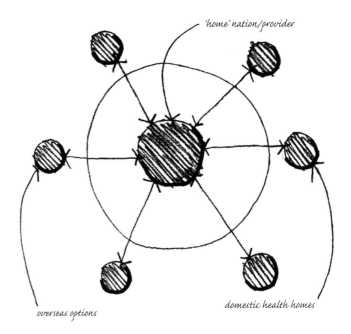

'home' nation/provider

overseas options

domestic health homes

7.44 Globalism and health in the twenty-first century

for the family and support space is provided on the campus in the form of dormitories, in response to the torrent of patients arriving from overseas. Within the U.S., a number of prominent institutions, including M.D. Anderson, in Houston, St. Jude's Children's Hospital, in Memphis, the Cleveland Clinic, in Ohio, and the Mayo Clinic, in Rochester, Minnesota, have for years solicited patients from across the country, and beyond. The world-renowned Texas Medical Center (TMC) in Houston has more than 40 hospitals, research institutes, and educational organizations. Thousands of patients travel to Houston annually for specialized diagnostic care and treatment. The M.D. Anderson Cancer Center is but one of many at the TMC that attract international patients and patients from across the U.S. Hospital administrators need to assess their institution's role in anticipation of medical tourism in the coming years, as this trend is expected to increase (Figure 7.44).[53]

Ecohumanist facility management

Core operational functions of a typical hospital include the administration, admitting department, medical records, central pharmacy, accounting, dietary operations, materials management, and facility management. These will continue to be essential although new technologies are transforming the relationship of these units to the hospital's physical infrastructure in an age of diminishing environmental resources. Software developed through HIT initiatives can greatly advance the control and transport of materials and supplies within the hospital, thereby contributing to a reduction in medical errors. Medical centers employ highly trained facility and grounds managers. More and more, these specialists have post-secondary credentials in the field of Facility Management. The *International Facility Management Association* (IFMA) has a large subgroup of members (450, ranking 7th in membership out of the 16 councils that comprise the IFMA) who specialize in the management of healthcare environments. Constant wear and tear on a physical plant exacts its toll and sophisticated, holistic, ecohumanist facility management skill sets are needed in the appropriate management of alternative technologies such as geothermal energy, carbon neutral material assemblies and building systems, digital media technologies, natural lighting and ventilation monitoring systems, new types of plumbing and HVAC systems, roof rainwater harvesting and landscaping systems, the proper maintenance of cisterns to capture rainwater for re-use on the campus, seasonal upkeep of gardens, water elements including ponds, fountains, and waterfalls, to name but a few examples where new skill sets will be required.[54]

PART 3

Case studies

Case studies

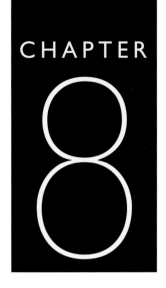

The projects

Autonomous community-based

1 Providence Newberg Medical Center, Newberg, Oregon:
   Mahlum Architects, Seattle, Washington

2 Legacy Salmon Creek Hospital, Vancouver, Washington:
   Zimmer Gunsul Frasca Partnership (ZGF), Portland, Oregon

3 Katta Public General Hospital, Shiroishi City,
   Miyagi Prefecture, Japan:
   Taro Ashihara Architects/Hideto Horike+Associates, Tokyo

4 Boulder Community Foothills Hospital, Boulder, Colorado:
   OZ Architecture, Colorado/Boulder Associates, Inc., Boulder

5 Vivantes Clinical Center, Neukölln, Germany:
   Schmucker and Partners, Mannheim, Germany

6 Jiaikai Amani Hospital, United Arab Emirates (UAE):
   *Katsuya Kawashima, Nikken Sekkei, Ltd., Tadao Matsubase,
   Shimomai Architecture Design Office, Ltd., Tokyo*

Children's care centers

7 Bloorview Kids Rehab, Toronto, Ontario, Canada:
   *Montgomery Sisam/Stantec Architecture – Joint Venture,
   Toronto and Vancouver*

8 Children's Health Centre at Surrey Memorial Hospital, Surrey,
   British Columbia, Canada:
   Stantec Architecture, Vancouver

9 Meyer Children's Hospital (Ospedale Pediatrico Meyer di Firenze),
   Florence, Italy:
   *Anshen + Allen, San Francisco/Centro Studi Progettazione
   Edilizia (CSPE), Florence*

10 Dell Children's Medical Center of Central Texas, Austin, Texas:
   Karlsberger Architects Planners Designers, Columbus, Ohio

11 Evelina Children's Hospital, London, U.K.:
   Hopkins Architects, London

Rehabilitation and elderly care centers

12 REHAB Basel Centre for Spinal Cord and Brain Injuries,
Basel, Switzerland:
Herzog & de Meuron, Basel, Switzerland

13 Center for the Intrepid – National Armed Forces Physical
Rehabilitation Center, San Antonio, Texas:
SmithGroup, Washington, D.C.

14 Kokura Rehabilitation Hospital, Kokura,
Kyushu Prefecture, Japan:
Yasui Masahiro and Associates, Tokyo

15 Sarah Lago Norte Center for the Seriously Handicapped,
Brasilia, Brazil:
João Filgueiras Lima (Lelé), Brasilia

16 Washington State Veteran's Center, Retsil, Washington:
NBBJ, Seattle

17 Geriatriezentrum Favoriten (Favoriten Geriatric Center)/
Franz-Josef Hospital, Vienna, Austria:
Office of Anton Schweighofer, Vienna

Regional medical campuses

18 Thunder Bay Regional Hospital, Vancouver, Canada:
*Salter Farrow Pilon Architects, Inc. (successor firms: Farrow
Partnership Architects, and Salter Pilon Architects), Vancouver*

19 Deventer Ziekenhuis (Hospital), Deventer, the Netherlands:
De Jong Gortemaker Algra, Amsterdam

20 Southeast Regional Trauma Center (SERTC), Madison, Indiana:
RATIO Architects, Inc., Indianapolis

21 Shugaung Hospital, Shanghai, China:
*SmithGroup, Washington, D.C./CNA Architecture, Bellevue,
Washington*

22 Provincial Hospital of Graz-West (LKH Graz-West), Graz, Austria:
Domenig Eisenköck Gruber Zinganel, Graz

23 St. Olav's Hospital, Trondheim, Norway:
*Medplan AS arkitekter/COWI Denmar/Frisk Architects (Women
and Children's Centre)*

24 Zhangjiagang First People's Hospital, Zhangjiagang, China:
*Meng Jianmin, Hou Jun, Wang Iijuan, Tai Renji, Peng Ying, Wu
Lianhua, Xia Changsong, Mu Li, and Mai Xuanwei, Shanghai*

Prognostications

25 ER One, Washington, District of Columbia:
HKS, Dallas/Pickard Chilton, New Haven

26 Apex Prototype, Six All India Institutes of Medical Sciences,
Jodhpur, India:
Heinle, Wischer and Partners, Berlin

27 Core Hospital Prototype, Rotterdam, the Netherlands:
Itten + Brechbühl AG/Venhoeven C.S./BM Managers, Bern

28 Transportable Trauma Center Prototypes for Global Deployment:
*Tulane University Rapid Response Studio/Clemson University
Architecture + Health Graduate Program Studio/Project
Coordinator: Stephen Verderber*

In this chapter twenty-eight case studies are presented in relation to a five-part architectural typology (rather than based on geographic location). This set of case studies represents a cross section of public and private sector healthcare environments. All are medically based programs, with some providing a more robust residential/inpatient component than others. Aside from a high level of overall architectural design *consistency*, the criteria upon which each case study was chosen for inclusion were as follows.

First, the facility had to have been built recently (all opened in 2003 or later) or a work-in-progress; second, its design intent had to possess broad ramifications for other hospitals and closely allied building types elsewhere; third, it must express innovative principles of sustainable site planning and architectural design; fourth, it must exhibit design excellence in its own right. Beyond this, each case study engages the philosophy of hospital-based care in interesting social, technical, and formal terms, or in a few cases, as non-mainstream, radical, speculative propositions relative to the hospital and allied building types. As a result, these twenty-eight case studies resonate within and between one another. Diversity and imagination is celebrated. The five facility categories are:

- *Autonomous community-based*: these hospitals are based in and provide services for a specific local community. They are independent in terms of day-to-day operations although some are owned by local government while other case studies of this type are owned by a regional or federal government agency, as in the case of the Katta Public General Hospital in Japan, and the Amani Hospital in the United Arab Emirates (UAE).
- *Children's care centers*: these five case studies are children's specialty hospitals that provide care for infants through to patients eighteen years of age. Two are located in Canada, one in Italy, one in Great Britain, and one in the U.S. They are all located in urban settings. Two are situated on campuses with historically significant architecture: Meyer Children's Hospital in Florence, Italy, and the Evelina Children's Hospital in London. The latter is an infill facility built on the historic St. Thomas' Hospital campus in Central London, near the banks of the Thames.
- *Rehabilitation and elderly care centers*: this category is actually somewhat of a hybrid of two allied types: rehabilitation hospitals and long-term care centers with a significant medical component. All but one provides a mixture of inpatient and outpatient care. The sole non-inpatient facility is the Center for the Intrepid in San Antonio, Texas. However, this facility is located adjacent to an inpatient rehabilitation care facility. Two are in Europe, with one in Japan, one in Brazil, and two in the U.S. All are freestanding facilities.
- *Regional medical campuses*: these seven case studies are all freestanding, comprehensive medical campuses that serve a regional population base. These provide specialized inpatient and outpatient care, and bed capacities vary as well as their overall size. They are located in urban areas or in newer areas within a metropolitan area. In many cases patients and families travel long distances to these care centers. Two are located in

China in the rapidly growing Shanghai metro area, three are in Europe, one is in Canada, and one is located in the U.S.
- *Prognostications*: these unbuilt projects were chosen for their vision, intent, and scope of services, location, materiality, socio-cultural significance, and timeliness. Each is worth the investment to make it become a reality. Two of these case studies address the aftermath of natural and man-made disasters, including acts of terrorism, earthquakes, hurricanes, floods, public health epidemics, tsunamis, fires, industrial accidents, and drought. One is a prototype for a new network of medical centers and research institutes in India. Another is a proposal for a functionally deconstructed hospital in the heart of a European urban center. Collectively, these projects are reflective excursions in sustainable architecture for health.

Some overlap will inevitably exist in any such system of architectural categorization.

At the scale of a campus

A distinction is drawn between campuses that are centralized versus those that are decentralized. Centralized campuses tend to be built over time on dense urban sites, as infill projects that evolve from a single building to perhaps twenty on a single campus. Buildings tend to be nearer in proximity to one another, and most buildings on the campus are mid-rise. Exterior space is at a premium. By contrast, decentralized campuses have a higher percentage of open space, with fewer freestanding buildings of a lower density and height. Distinctions are also drawn between urban, suburban, or rural contexts. This has implications, for example, in whether a new or replacement campus was built on a fringe-condition greenfield site versus an inner urban brownfield site. Greenfield sites are previously unbuilt, whereas greenfield and brownfield sites require remediation prior to redevelopment. A distinction is also drawn between replacement campuses versus newly built campuses.

At the scale of a building

The reuse of historically significant buildings, adaptive reuse efforts, whether the case study is an addition to an existing building, and the role of the immediate site context is examined. A distinction is drawn between low rise and mid-rise structures and any attributes indicative of theraserialization, i.e. the interactive layering/superimposition of exterior and interior space. Therapeutic gardens are cited in terms of their intrinsic design attributes as well as their relationship to adjacent interior spaces. Person-nature connections are noted, particularly windows and views. With respect to wayfinding, spatial configuration is examined in relation to the role of nature, works of art, color, graphics, and daylight as navigational aids.

At the scale of a room

Individual spaces are examined for their habitability, aesthetics, environmental sustainability, materiality, composition, and operational functionality. Emphasis is given to the inpatient room and the PCU context, including amenities for the patient, families/visitors, their influence on patient and family/visitor empowerment, and provisions for caregivers. Natural daylight and ventilation, and the building's footprint are examined relative to building and room orientation, to the exterior domain, and to adjoining structures. Innovative furnishings and equipment items are cited.

In terms of sustainability

It is difficult to precisely quantify a given case study's carbon neutrality quotient, yet it is possible to examine various contributing factors pertaining to maintenance and life-cycle operations, materiality palette, building design, component assembly systems, recycling provisions, and interior amenities across a spectrum of public, semi-private and private spaces. Innovative landscape strategies are cited, including xeriscaping and green roofscapes that are habitable and/or used as rainwater harvesters, gardens, solar collectors, or as places for refuge and/or social interaction. Geothermal heating and cooling systems are cited for their earthen thermal storage capacities, and locally available materials, fabrication methods, and methods of construction are cited. Sustainable site planning strategies, public transportation linkages, amenities for pedestrians and cyclists, and on-site provisions for automobiles are cited.

1   Providence Newberg Medical Center, Newberg, Oregon

ARCHITECT: Mahlum Architects, Seattle, Washington
LANDSCAPE ARCHITECT: Mayer/Reed
CLIENT: Providence Health System
FEATURED MATERIALS: Cast-in-place concrete, exterior masonry, stone cladding, laminated wood beams, flooring and finishes
COMPLETED: 2006
INPATIENT BEDS: 39
SITE/PARKING: 60 acres (19.2 acres to be developed)/429
HOSPITAL SIZE: 180,636SF (square feet) (and 45,000SF medical office building)

Context/site

This was the first LEED Certified (Gold Level) hospital in the United States. It also received a 2007 Environmental Leadership Award from Hospitals for a Healthy Environment (H2E). It is located twenty-five miles southwest of Portland, Oregon in an agricultural region bordering a suburban community. The hospital and adjacent medical office building is organized around two therapeutic (healing) gardens, bisected by a semi-transparent two-level cafe and dining room situated between an administrative and medical support building, and the core hospital building (Figure 8.1.1). The transitional 'bridge' allows for movement to and from the main entrance and parking areas to the hospital itself, and also laterally between its flanking outdoor spaces. Views to the exterior along this main circulation spine look out onto the site's natural landscape and nearby Parrett Mountain. The bridge is on axis with the main public entrance (Figure 8.1.2).

The public entrance is at the center of the administrative/conference and medical office building. Core hospital functions are housed in a second structure to the rear of the site, with two triangular-shaped courtyards at its center. A staff-only parking area is located to the rear (Figure 8.1.3). The campus plan consists of separate yet connected floor plates, thereby allowing for greater perimeter surface area while improving access to natural daylight, ventilation, and views. The client adopted environmental stewardship as a core value in the mission statement and a green campus was identified as a priority early on. Drought-tolerant plant species on the site reduce irrigation demands by 50 percent. In an innovative partnership with Pacific Gas & Electric (PG&E), the medical center's emergency generators are owned and serviced by PG&E, in exchange

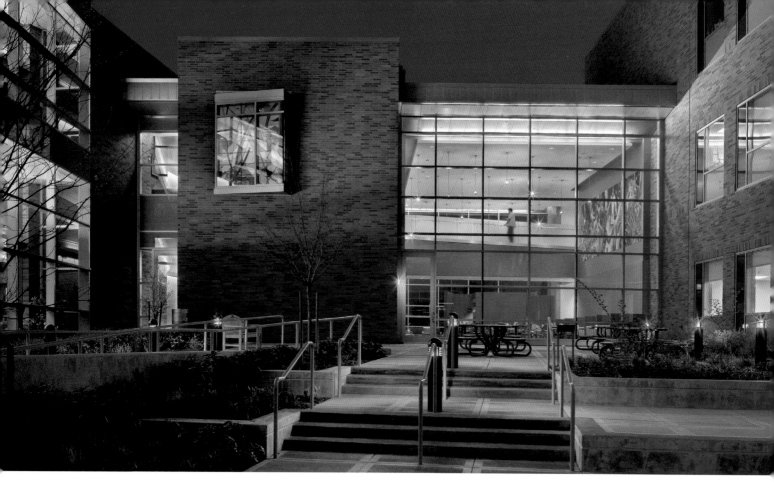

8.1.1 Providence Newberg Medical Center, Newberg, Washington. The hospital and adjacent medical office building features therapeutic gardens

8.1.2 A curved pedestrian path, gardens, and views beyond to nearby Parrett Mountain

for the ability to utilize these systems to generate power for the grid during peak demand periods. This on-demand power system allows the hospital to comply with requirements for e-power while not having to purchase or maintain its own equipment. Additional energy-conserving attributes at the campus level include direct access to public transportation, bicycle racks, mini-auto parking stalls, and showers. Roofs are of high-reflectivity, low-emissivity materials. A network of walking and biking trails was created to promote staff, patient, and visitor access to undeveloped portions of the site, as well as to provide a civic resource for the larger community.

Building/unit

The main level houses general support functions. These departments include the emergency department, cardio respiratory unit, the central laboratory, diagnostic imaging unit, the central pharmacy, surgical suites, and central sterile processing (Figure 8.1.4a-b). The surgical theatres on Level 1 are spacious and adaptable to future needs (Figure 8.1.5). The helipad is located atop the administration/conference end

179

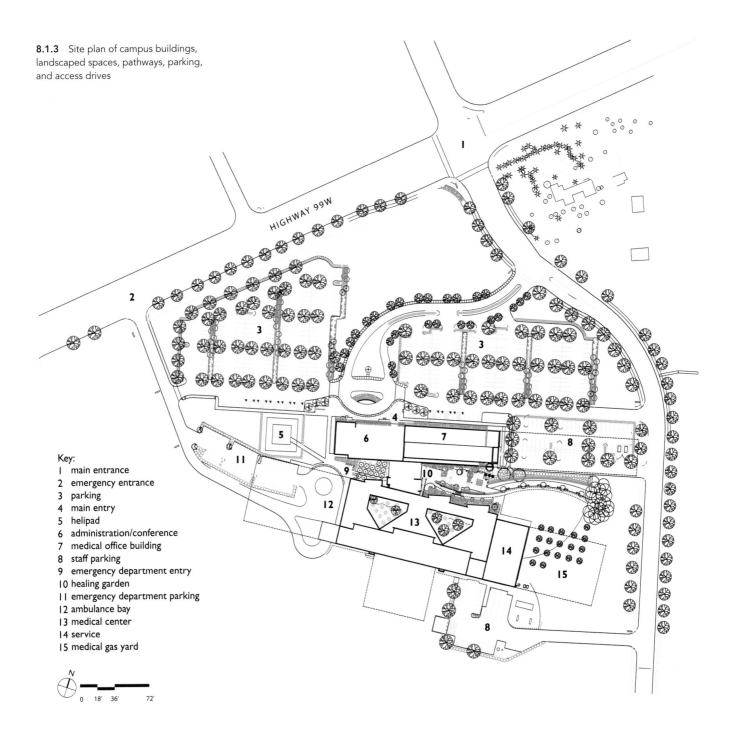

8.1.3 Site plan of campus buildings, landscaped spaces, pathways, parking, and access drives

HIGHWAY 99W

Key:
1 main entrance
2 emergency entrance
3 parking
4 main entry
5 helipad
6 administration/conference
7 medical office building
8 staff parking
9 emergency department entry
10 healing garden
11 emergency department parking
12 ambulance bay
13 medical center
14 service
15 medical gas yard

N
0   18'   36'   72'

of the 'front building'. It also houses the aforementioned medical offices. The second and third levels of this three-level hospital house all-private rooms within two patient care/nursing units (PCUs). Level 2 houses a main waiting area, ICU inpatient rooms, the inpatient rehabilitation unit, a women's birthing center, and in the adjoining building, medical offices and administration functions. The mechanical system uses 100 percent outside air for enhanced infection control; this system operates at 26 percent higher efficiency than required by the Oregon State Energy Code. Water usage is reduced by over 20 percent with efficient low-flow plumbing fixtures and a process-water loop system, thereby conserving potable water.

A two-level glass-enclosed entry and galleria is visually activated with natural daylight. This single point of public entry connects outpatient services located along the main circulation spine with various inpatient units and clinical support functions housed in more private zones within the building envelope. Interior spaces are oriented to receive morning sunlight and to maximize views out to the natural landscape (Figure 8.1.6). Muted earth tones dominate the interiors, combined with residentialist lighting. The inpatient rooms are home-like in appearance, with furnishings able to be rearranged by the patient and/or family members. Large windows in the inpatient rooms afford full views of the site environs. Natural wood and wood

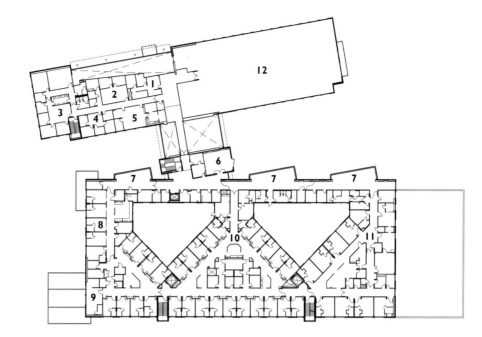

Level 2

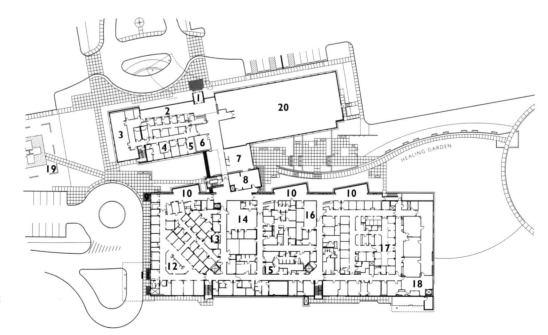

Main Level

8.1.4 The parti' consists of front arrival and backside direct care elements, connected via a circulation artery that houses cafes and vertical circulation. The second level houses administration and medical offices. Support functions are housed on the main level with inpatient units above

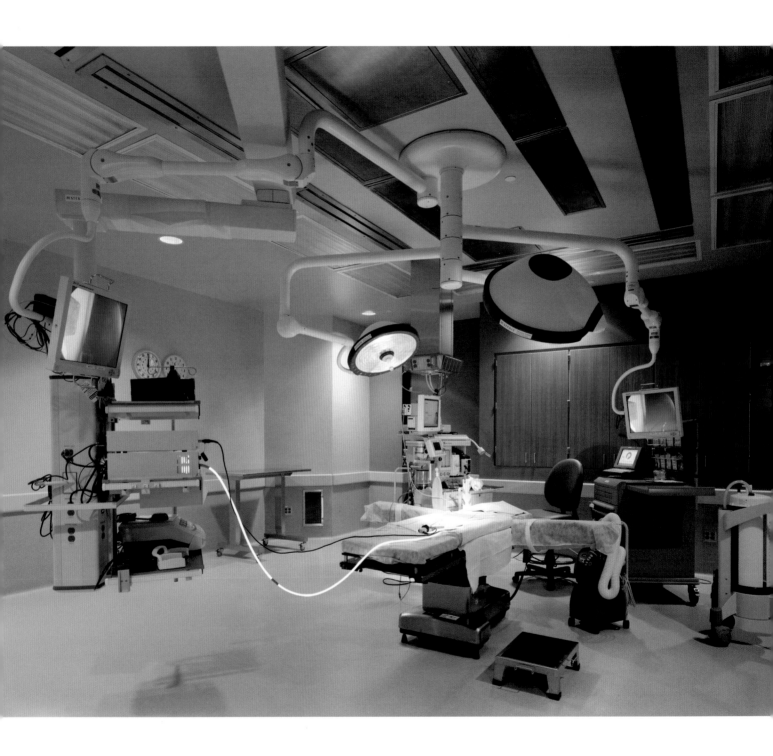

8.1.5 Surgical theater at Providence Newberg Medical Center, adaptable to future medical technologies such as robotic surgical assistive units

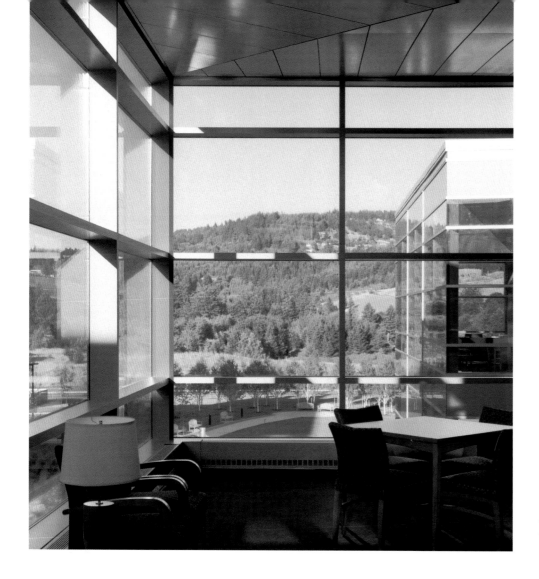

8.1.6 Interior spaces are oriented to receive morning sunlight and to maximize views of the natural landscape

8.1.7 Large windows are provided in patients' rooms

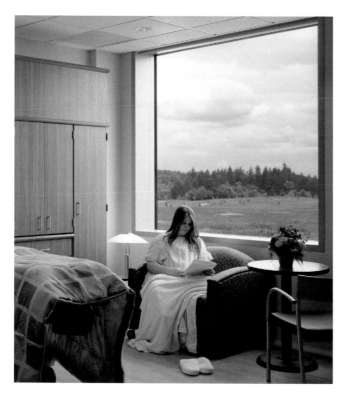

simulated finishes are featured throughout the interior (Figure 8.1.7). Non-toxic, low impact materials were extensively used, with 20 percent of all materials manufactured locally and 50 percent extracted in the local region. Materials were chosen based on life-cycle coats and carbon footprint reductive qualities. Occupancy sensors and daylight controls are installed throughout the campus. Eighty percent of construction waste during construction was either recycled or from salvaged materials. All materials were specified to ensure a high level of indoor air quality by using low-VOC paints, coatings, adhesives, sealants, and carpeting. A post-occupancy evaluation was conducted in 2007. Four main lessons were learned, according to a summary report prepared by the consulting firm *betterbricks. com*. These centered on the need for creative financing strategies in green hospital projects, and the importance of conducting a separate energy charrette so the entire team buys into the project's green goals from the outset.

2 Legacy Salmon Creek Hospital, Vancouver, Washington

ARCHITECT: Zimmer Gunsul Frasca Partnership (ZGF),
    Portland, Oregon
LANDSCAPE ARCHITECT: Walker Macy
CLIENT: Legacy Health System, Portland, Oregon
FEATURED MATERIALS: Steel exterior panel system, masonry,
    travertine stone, water sculpture, laminated wood beams,
    flooring and finishes
COMPLETED: 2005
INPATIENT BEDS: 220
SITE/PARKING: 24 acres/1,464 (7-level garage)
HOSPITAL SIZE: 469,000SF/Pedestrian bridges: 7,000SF
    (Medical Office Building 1: 109,000SF; Medical Office Building
    2: 80,000SF)

Context/site

This medical center was built in Salmon Creek, a growing area in Clark Country, Washington. The site is adjacent to a heavily wooded area. Site planning centered on a clear arrival and entry sequence and a strong visual identity for the medical center. Site amenities include indigenous drought-tolerant landscaping, pervious surface materials, a natural storm-water retention pond, and night-sensitive site lighting. In plan the campus is nearly symmetrical. Two four-level medical office buildings to the right and the parking garage to the left flank the main arrival drive and center court with a bright red logo/sculpture at its center (Figure 8.2.1). The driveways pass beneath a connecting bridge between the medical office building and the garage. Directly ahead are the main hospital and the arrival/departure point. Three interconnected elevated bridges lead to the main entry and atrium of the hospital. The hospital footprint is composed of the curved facade of the linear frontispiece that houses administration, public functions, outpatient diagnostic and treatment services, and general support functions (Figure 8.2.2). Two inpatient housing pavilions are to the rear of the main arrival/support building (Figure 8.2.3). The central courtyard with a fountain, sculpture, plaza area and seating visually connects the various buildings and provides opportunities for social interaction, thereby functioning as the 'front room' of the campus.

Building/unit

The six-level hospital features two L-shaped patient pavilions situated above a two-level base. The main lobby is a two-level atrium with escalators connecting to the network of three connecting bridges (Figure 8.2.4). South-facing outdoor terraces are situated adjacent to the cafeteria, the chapel, and the conference rooms. Each floor houses 64 beds (all private rooms). Shared semi-public space is provided on each floor. The PCUs include a 16-bed ICU, 16 step-down beds and a 15-bed NICU. In each 16-bed PCU the nursing station is situated at the midpoint between two corridors, thereby creating a variant on the classic post-World War II racetrack configuration. The bath/shower room in each inpatient room is on the outboard side, in a back-to-back arrangement. The patient rooms are therefore not single handed, as they are configured in an A/B pattern along the two perimeter corridors in two clusters of eight rooms. Surgery services are clustered together on the second level. There are ten surgical suites, three endoscopy labs and two catheterization labs. Outpatient cancer treatment is provided primarily in one of the medical office buildings (Figure 8.2.5a-b). This 10,000 SF radiation oncology unit is housed on the first level. The waiting areas are colorfully appointed and in one case a bright red structural column becomes its centerpiece, double functioning as an activity area for children.

The chapel is situated at the center of the rear courtyard amid a therapeutic garden (Figure 8.2.6). The connecting corridor is transparent, with full height glass that affords views to the courtyard (Figure 8.2.7). The chapel features walls sheathed in vertical wood slats and the sole window is positioned on an axis with the arrival axis. This element is rotated to give it greater emphasis in the courtyard and to set it off from the patient pavilions to either side. The chapel's arrival axis is defined by the chapel at one endpoint and the ICU waiting room on the other endpoint. This extraction of the chapel from the main hospital block is visually and spatially effective.

The patient housing pavilions are oriented to maximize views to the surrounding natural environs and to Mount Hood, beyond. Natural materials and a warm color palette are featured throughout the pavilions and public areas. Inpatient rooms provide space for overnight accommodations for family members (Figure 8.2.8). Natural daylighting strategies were of priority, particularly in waiting and circulation areas. The inpatient room is large enough to allow for

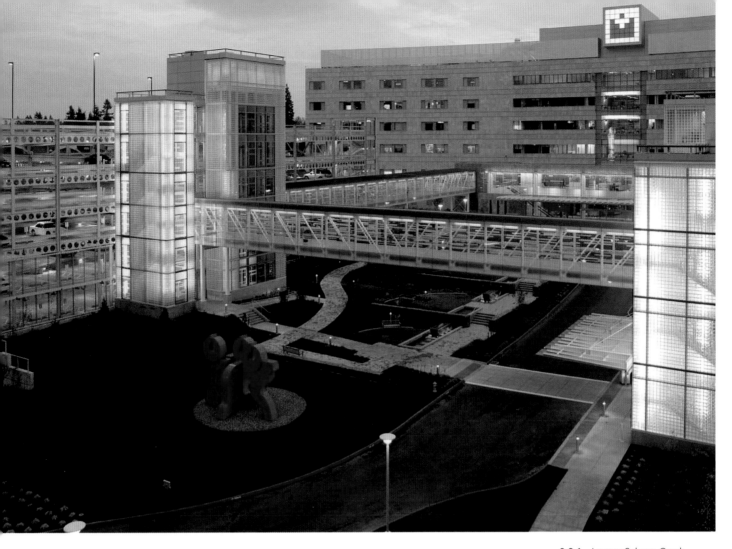

8.2.1 Legacy Salmon Creek Hospital, Vancouver, Washington. The arrival court is flanked by campus buildings, connected to the main hospital via pedestrian bridges

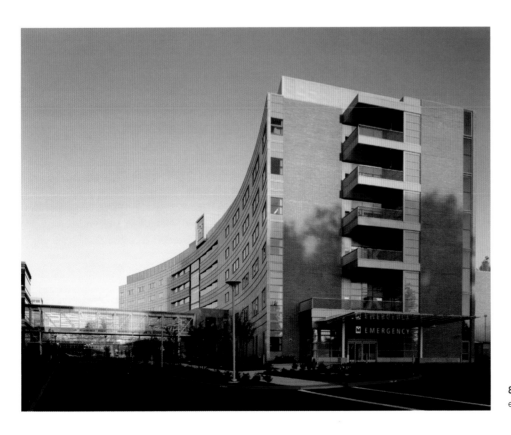

8.2.2 Main arrival drive and emergency department entrance

8.2.3 The campus plan is virtually symmetrical

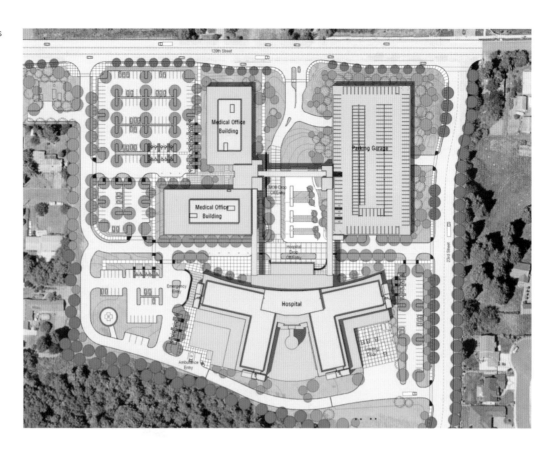

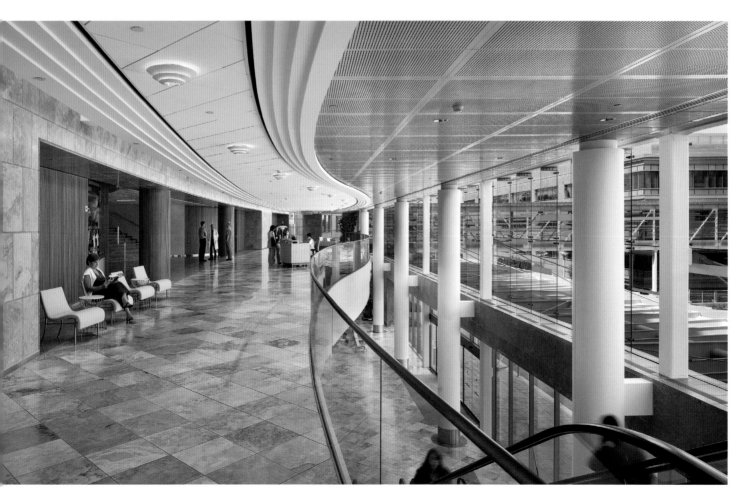

8.2.4 An atrium directly connects to the pedestrian bridges

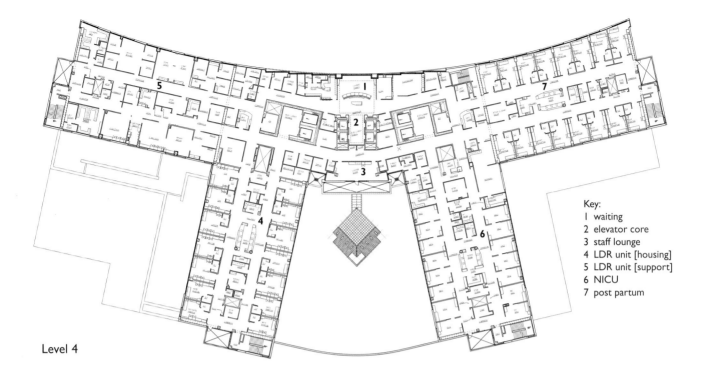

Level 4

Key:
1 waiting
2 elevator core
3 staff lounge
4 LDR unit [housing]
5 LDR unit [support]
6 NICU
7 post partum

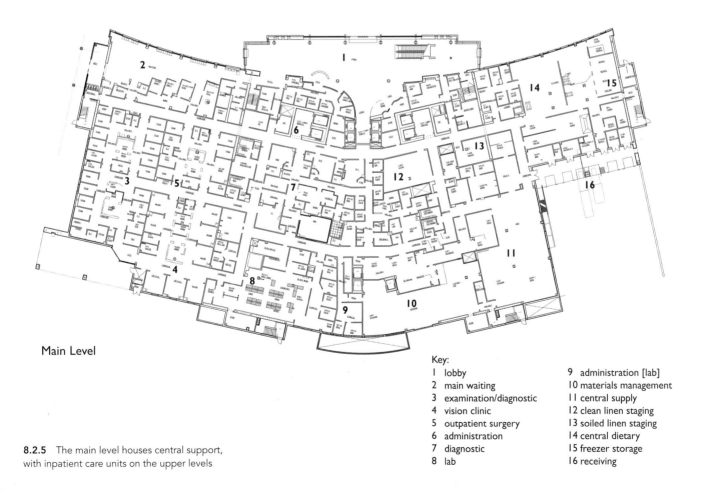

Main Level

Key:
1 lobby
2 main waiting
3 examination/diagnostic
4 vision clinic
5 outpatient surgery
6 administration
7 diagnostic
8 lab
9 administration [lab]
10 materials management
11 central supply
12 clean linen staging
13 soiled linen staging
14 central dietary
15 freezer storage
16 receiving

8.2.5   The main level houses central support, with inpatient care units on the upper levels

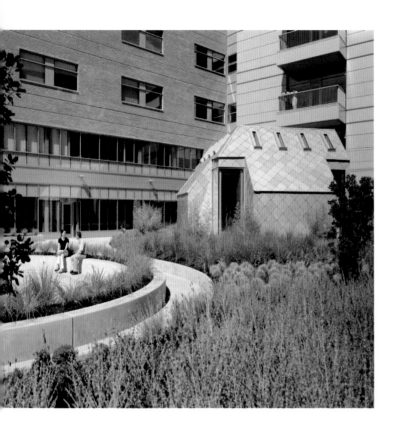

8.2.6 The chapel is semi-autonomous, situated in a therapeutic garden

8.2.7 The chapel affords contact with nature

varied medical and nursing care uses based on the individual needs of each patient. Sustainable design strategies included a rooftop therapeutic (healing) garden, the aforementioned central courtyard, and terraced garden. Three-quarters of all on-site construction waste was recycled during construction, and many building materials were procured locally, including brick masonry, stone, wood, curtain wall assemblies, ceiling panels, and trusses. Legacy Salmon Creek Hospital received an Environmental Leadership Award from Hospitals for a Healthy Environment (H2E).

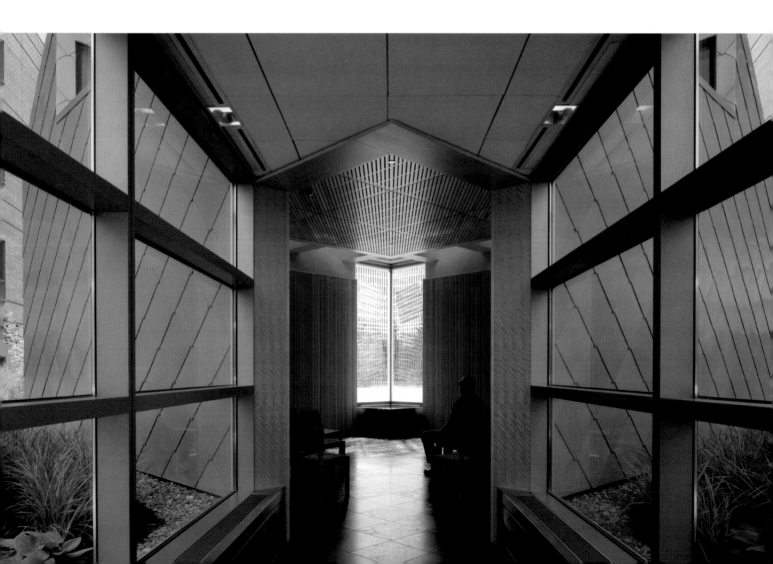

8.2.8 Patient rooms have convertible window seat/beds, and afford views of the adjacent open landscape

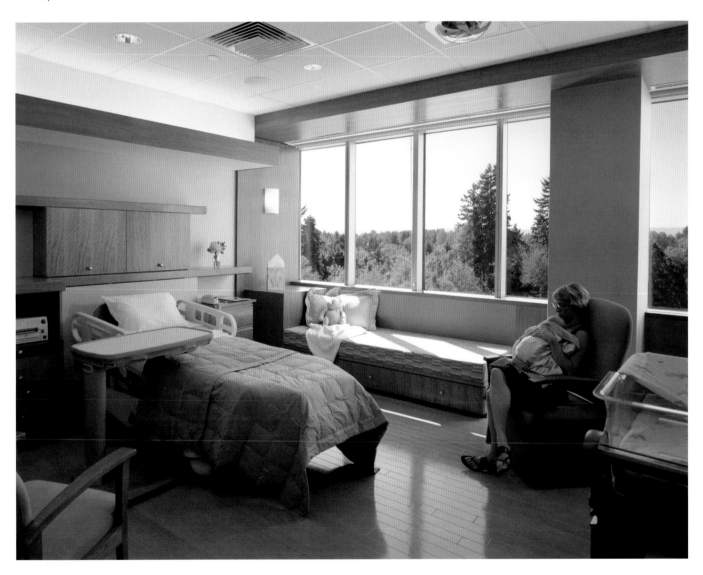

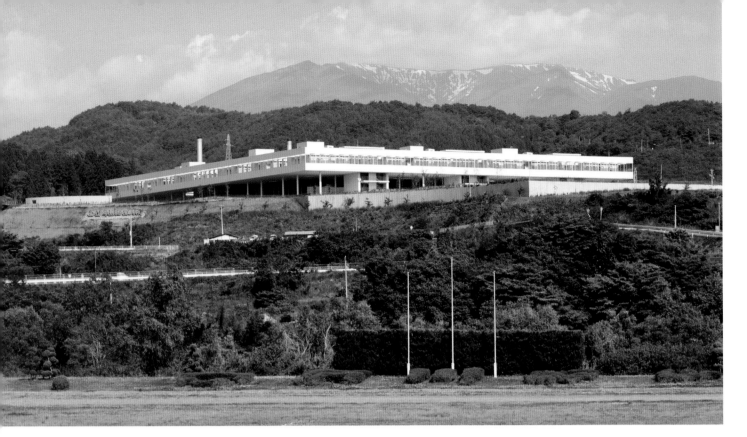

8.3.1 Katta Public General Hospital, Shiroishi, Japan, in relation to its striking site context

8.3.2 The main concourse's transparency contrasts a cantilevered second level, appearing to hover slightly above the natural landscape

3   Katta Public General Hospital, Shiroishi City, Miyagi, Japan

ARCHITECT: Taro Ashihara Architects/Hideto Horike+Associates
PLANNER/LANDSCAPE ARCHITECT: Seiichi Fukukawa/ARK Crew
CLIENT: Shiroishi City, Zao Town, Shichigasyuku Town
    (Miyagi Prefecture)
FEATURED MATERIALS: Steel structural system, glazed exterior walls, stone, aluminum, stainless steel, laminated interior finishes
COMPLETED: 2002
INPATIENT BEDS: 300
SITE/PARKING: 22 acres/276
HOSPITAL SIZE: 132,000SF

Context/site

The Katta Public General Hospital was the result of a Shiroishi-citywide *machizukuri* (participatory planning process). This medical center is a designated disaster response center for the region. The design team developed a strong working relationship with local residents. Katta General was the first healthcare project undertaken by the design team. The traditional design concepts of *shakei* and *kiritori* were employed as a means to maximize, during arrival or departure from the site, occupants' views of the nearby mountains and the pristine aspects of the surrounding landscape (Figure 8.3.1). The hospital achieves both horizontal and vertical theraserialization in its relation to this site context to a degree that is uncommon in large hospitals of its type. The natural properties of the site are therefore reaffirmed in the architectural response.

A low, horizontal profile complements the mountainous context. By 'lifting' the building off the ground, through the use of pilotis' and transparency, a gravity-defying *lightness* is achieved. A seismic foundation isolation system with underground shock-absorbent piers protects the building in the event of an earthquake. The sophistication of this anti-shock system allows for the second and third levels to cantilever outward, appearing to float above the ground plane and also serving as a source of protection from the elements for persons arriving or departing (Figure 8.3.2). In section, the foundation piers are visible as is the relationship to the bridge structure that sits atop this base—the aforementioned element appearing to be held in suspension. The site plan is straightforward: the three-level hospital is directly adjacent to a therapeutic garden, circular in configuration, to one side of the facility, and a staff parking area situated on the other side. A large parking area is to the front and an arrival drive spans the entire length of the front facade (Figure 8.3.3). The hospital is oriented to take maximum advantage of prevailing breezes and sun-path orientation, and a system is provided for capturing and recycling rainwater for use in an on-site irrigation system. A specially designed emergency generator unit allows the entire hospital to remain fully operational in the event of a natural disaster.

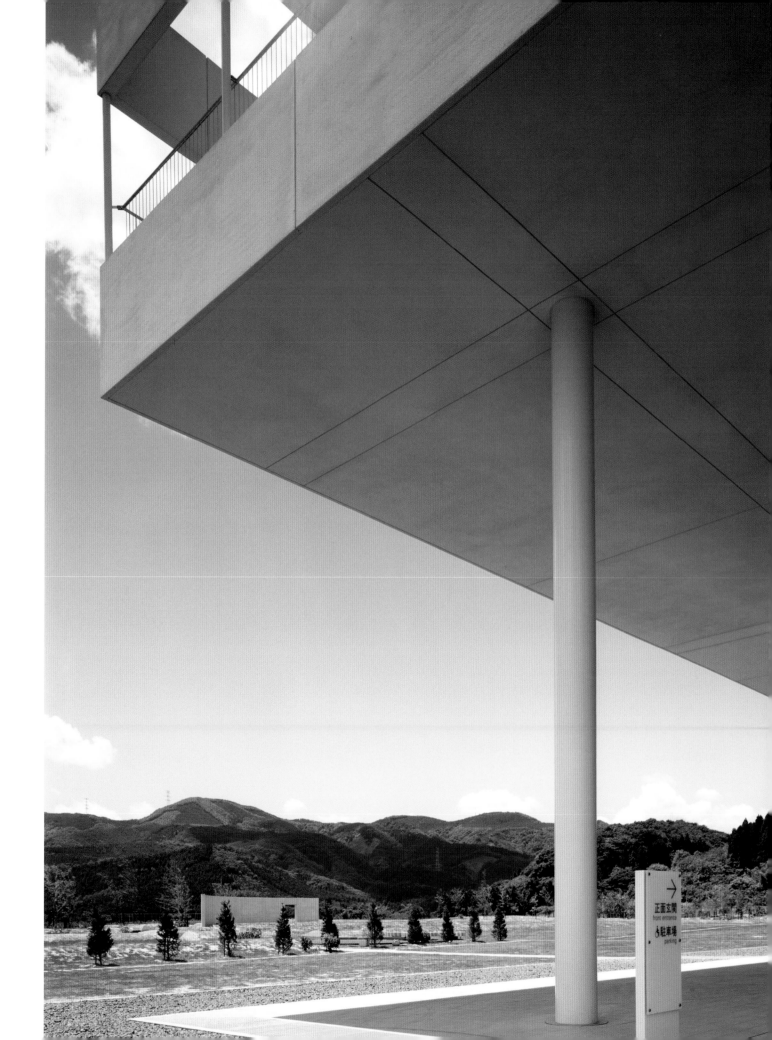

正面玄関
front entrance

駐車場
parking

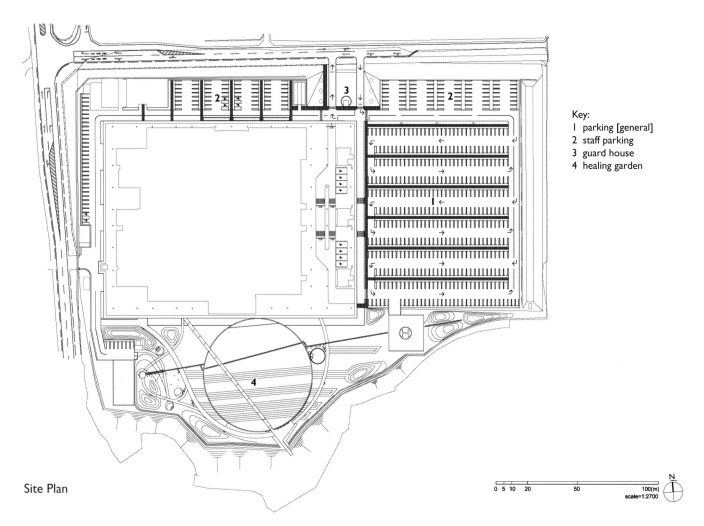

Key:
1 parking [general]
2 staff parking
3 guard house
4 healing garden

Site Plan

0 5 10 20   50   100(m)
                                scale=1:2700

8.3.3 The hospital site plan takes maximum
advantage of prevailing breezes, and sun orientation

Building/unit

The hospital is three levels and rectangular in configuration, measuring
120 meters by 140 meters in plan. Various programmatic elements
are distributed horizontally, including the administration, public
arrival, and diagnostic and treatment functions. The main level
houses the outpatient clinics, emergency department, diagnostic
and treatment services, radiology, medical records, the cafeteria and
kitchen functions, gift shop, waiting areas, and admitting. Level 2
houses the surgical suites, general support, laboratories, and the
central administration. Level 3 houses all inpatient housing (Figure
8.3.4a–b). Natural ventilation and passive solar design techniques are
featured throughout. The building envelope allows for transparency as
well as translucency, depending upon internal functional requirements

of particular units and realms. Patients and visitors enter between a
row of pilotis' into a double-height volume and proceed through a
checkerboard of courtyards and terraces (Figure 8.3.5). Natural light
further accentuates the interiors. Directional graphics are coded in red
throughout, with red crosses and floor graphics to aid in wayfinding
at intersecting corridors. Internal courtyards provide visual continuity
between all three levels while transmitting daylight through skylights
and also on the landscaped roof terrace (Figure 8.3.6). Indigenous
plantings are featured in the courtyards.

A meditation space is housed on the second level beside a rock
garden with traditional wood sculptural elements positioned in a
grid pattern, similar to the grid of cushions in the meditation space

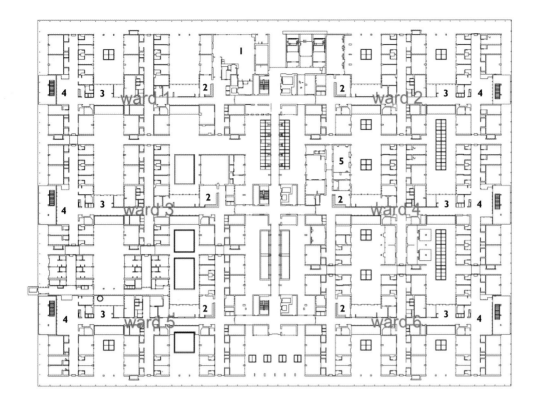

Level 3

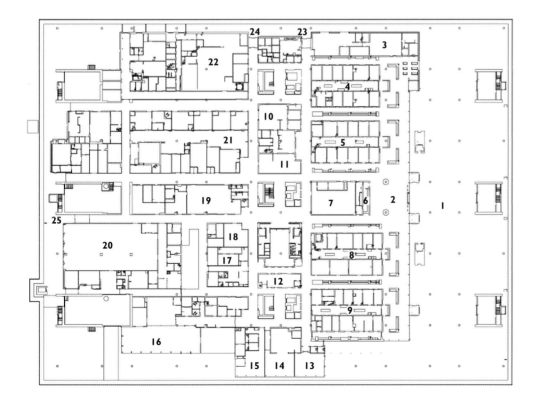

Level 1

8.3.4 Level 1 houses central support and an exterior plaza. Level 2 houses surgical suites, diagnostic and treatment services, and administration. Level 3 houses the inpatient care units

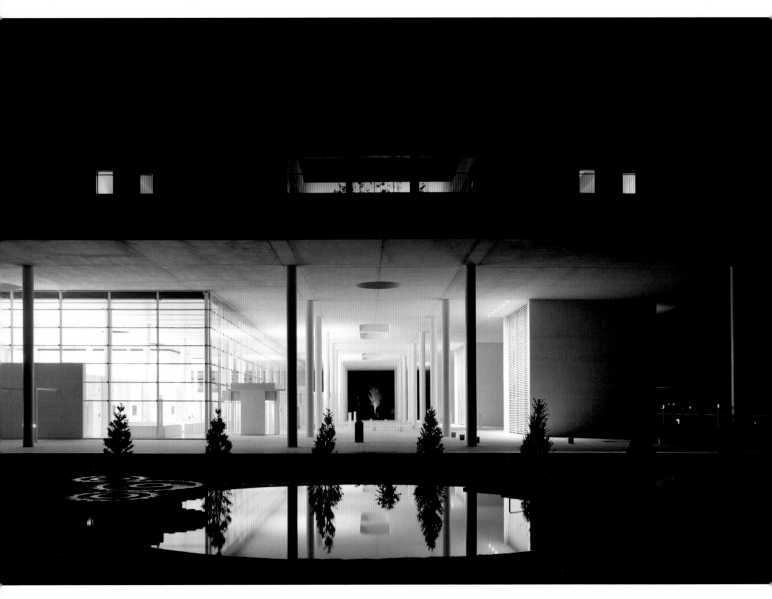

8.3.5 Approach to the main arrival area

8.3.6 Skylights and plantings define the interior atrium that connects all levels. Trees are visible on the roof terrace level.

(Figure 8.3.7). On Level 3, the roof garden and outdoor seating area is provided for inpatients and family members' use for each of the six-inpatient wards. An inviting image is created through the use of wood in the interior spaces as well as wood decking in the adjacent courtyard. This residentially scaled 'outdoor room', one level in height, establishes a horizontal continuum with the interior realm. The architects conceived of these spaces as, in their words, roof garden 'villages' with views (in some cases) projecting outward towards the mountains. From the patient room one has direct access to this semi-private space, with its rock garden, plantings, and trees

(Figure 8.3.8). This space affords respite from the daily stresses of the hospital experience. The laminated wood floors and sliding glass doors in each inpatient room (see Chapter 4) are reminiscent of the *shoji* screens of traditional Japanese dwellings. This project was honored with the Japan Institute of Architecture's Tohuku District Architecture Award, as well as the Japan Institute of Healthcare Architecture Design Award (2003).

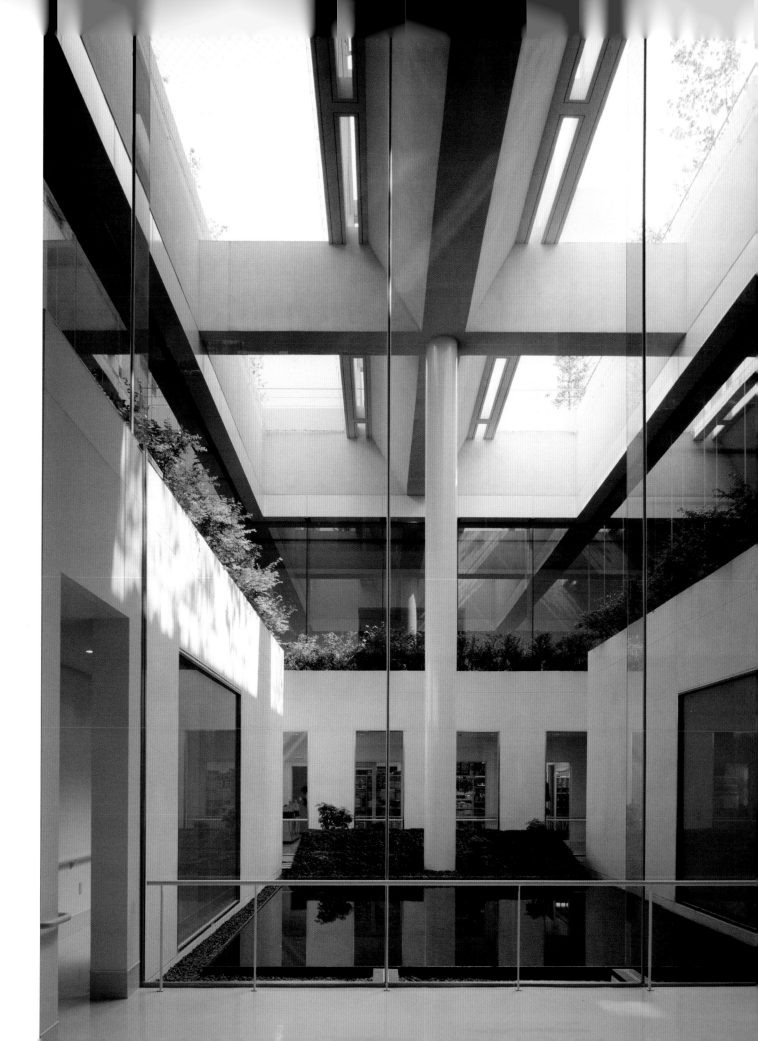

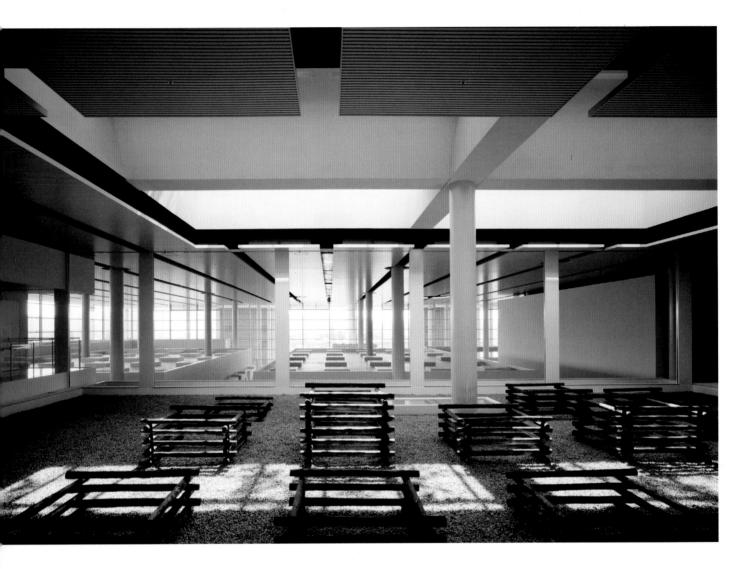

8.3.7 The meditation space is for prayer, and respite

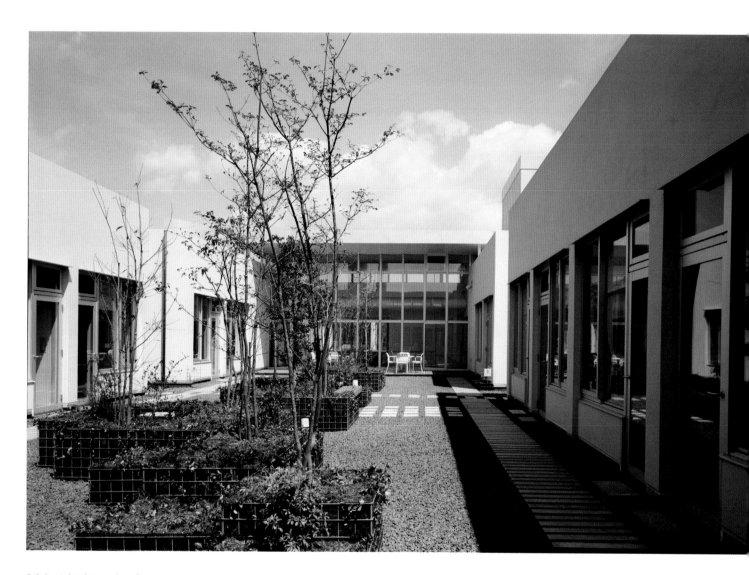

8.3.8 A landscaped roof terrace
is accessed via doors leading
from each inpatient room. It is a
semi-private oasis

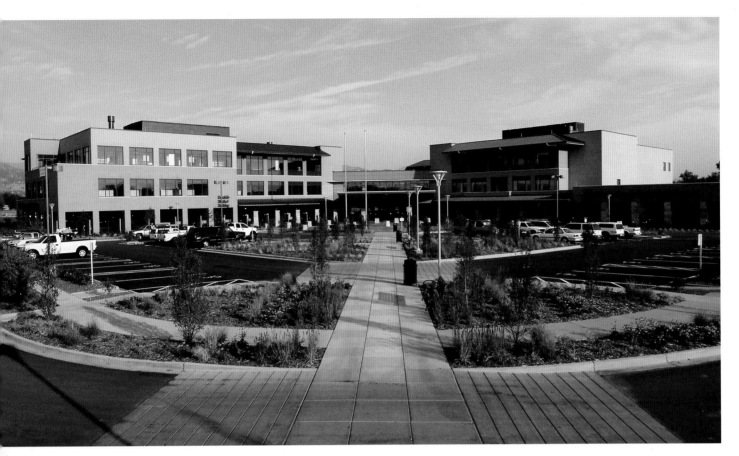

8.4.1 Boulder Community Foothills Hospital, Boulder, Colorado. This was the first LEED certified hospital in the United States. Links to cycling, pedestrian, and public transit encourage transport alternatives to the automobile

4 Boulder Community Foothills Hospital, Boulder, Colorado

ARCHITECT: OZ Architecture, Colorado (Core and Envelope); Boulder Associates, Inc. (Interiors), Boulder

LANDSCAPE ARCHITECT: Civitas

CLIENT: Boulder Community Hospital

FEATURED MATERIALS: Exterior masonry, steel, fieldstone, granite, wood laminate finishes, floors and wall surfaces

COMPLETED: 2003

INPATIENT BEDS: 60

SITE/PARKING: 17 developed acres (49 acre total site)/295

HOSPITAL SIZE: 155,000SF; Outpatient Services: 67,000SF

Context/site

Boulder Community Foothills Hospital was the first LEED certified (Silver Level) hospital in the United States. It was also the recipient of a 2006 Hospitals for a Healthy Environment (H2E) Environmental Leadership Award. The site for this women and children's hospital was an unincorporated parcel the city of Boulder targeted for redevelopment. Over the decades nearby industrial land uses degraded the environmental quality of the site, including a large wetland area and the site of a prairie dog colony. The colony was safely relocated to another site, and the wetlands were remediated.

These site particulars, together with the hospital's commitment to environmental stewardship, resulted in the new hospital as a symbol of sustainable architecture for health. Located on a public transit bus line, a new transit stop was created for the hospital. A car ride-share program was established, bike racks were provided on site, as was a shower/changing facility for cyclists and pedestrian commuters. The site was networked into an existing bike path along Boulder Creek. By encouraging the use of alternate transport modes and through the harvesting of storm-water runoff for on-site uses, the hospital was able to reduce the amount of impermeable surface parking area by 25 percent below the local minimum code requirement for on-site parking. In addition, Grasscrete surface pavers were used to construct the fire lane, precluding the need for a pedestrian sidewalk, and further reducing the amount of unnecessary paved surface area. In a civic gesture, 32 acres of its 49-acre site were returned to the City of Boulder for use as permanent undeveloped green space. Sustainable site planning goals therefore centered on minimal site disturbance, maximum habitat restoration, pervious circulation surfaces, alternate transportation amenities, high reflectance roofs, and xeriscaping with native plant species – thereby saving as much as 40 percent in annual water consumption (Figure 8.4.1).

Building/unit

The formal composition is articulated as three interconnected elements, a main arrival area, and a circular access drive. The arrival canopy is of steel and translucent panels, and it cantilevers forward (Figure 8.4.2). Public areas on all three levels, including the dining room on Level 1, open onto terraces that afford views to the nearby mountains (Figure 8.4.3). The three-level hospital is stepped at intervals thereby relieving the hospital's overall scale and massing. The lower (basement) level houses the central laundry, materials management, mechanical, central laboratory, dietary support, parking for 45 cars, and shell space for future use. The main level (Level 1) houses all the public functions, including reception, admitting, dining/kitchen, emergency department, ICU, women's diagnostic imaging unit, resource center, central pharmacy, conference center, administration, medical records, fitness center, outpatient services, and general support (Figure 8.4.4). The second and third levels house the all-private-room PCUs, a public art gallery, surgical suites, a pediatric unit, chapel, a Boulder Medical Center clinic, and core nursing functions (Figure 8.4.5 and Figure 8.4.6).

The aforementioned dining room on Level 1 opens onto an exterior terrace for outdoor dining. Information desks are decentralized, located at key intervals, often in double height spaces. This strategy enhances the sense of spaciousness and visual connectivity with the site environs, and function as navigational aids (Figure 8.4.7). Waiting areas are located adjacent to clinical departments. Earthen-tone colors and materials are used throughout, and are in harmony with the surrounding indigenous landscape, as is transparency, thereby creating a two-way interactive theraserialization between interior and exterior. A rock sculpture/waterfall is in a large center court adjacent to a therapeutic garden for use by patients, staff, and visitors. Patient rooms overlook the rock waterfall, and it has become a landmark on the campus (Figure 8.4.8). The NICU provides adjoining overnight rooms for family members and the infant stations have lighting options that simulate the circadian rhythms in the mother's womb. A VAV (variable air volume) HVAC system shuts down or activates the heating/cooling capacity on a room-by-room basis, depending on whether the operable windows in the inpatient rooms are open or closed. The facility management team, allowing for readjustment if window use should momentarily cause the system to run inefficiently, monitors this system. The VAV system also manages indoor air quality and humidity levels.

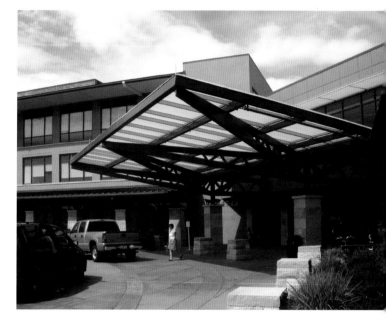

8.4.2 The vehicular canopy is on one end of an arrival axis

8.4.3 A nearby mountain range is visible from a terrace adjacent to the dining room

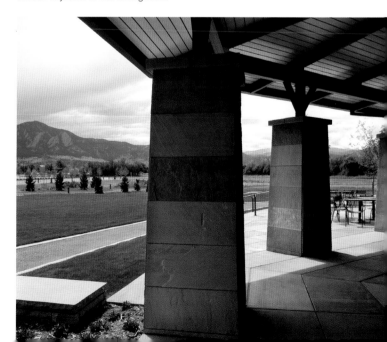

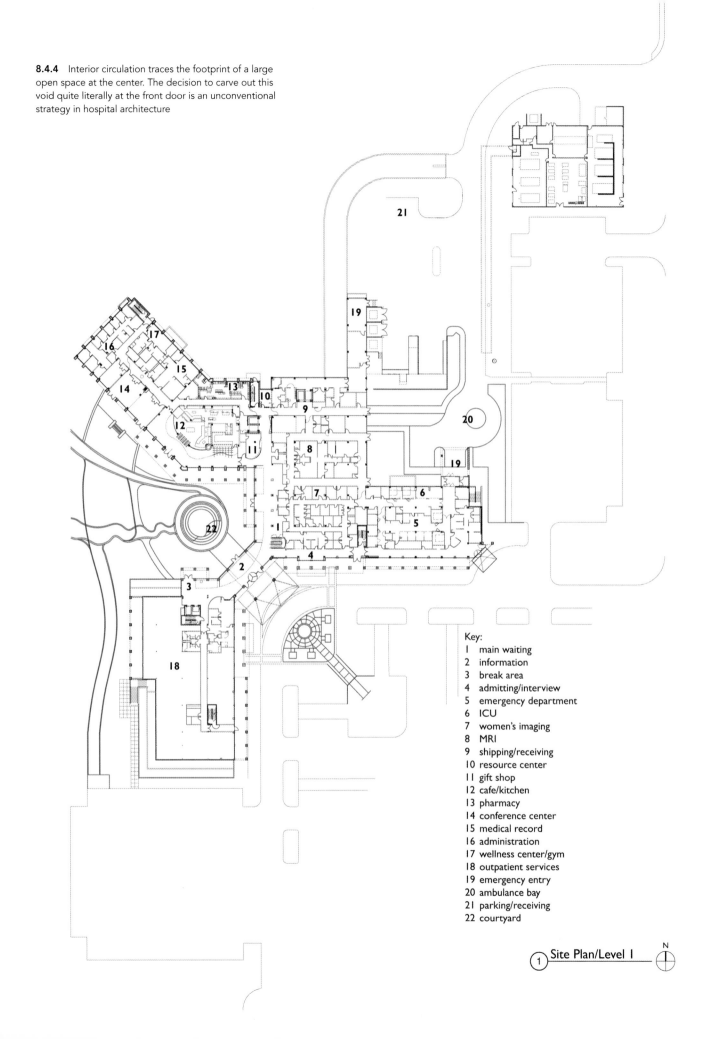

8.4.4 Interior circulation traces the footprint of a large open space at the center. The decision to carve out this void quite literally at the front door is an unconventional strategy in hospital architecture

Key:
1 main waiting
2 information
3 break area
4 admitting/interview
5 emergency department
6 ICU
7 women's imaging
8 MRI
9 shipping/receiving
10 resource center
11 gift shop
12 cafe/kitchen
13 pharmacy
14 conference center
15 medical record
16 administration
17 wellness center/gym
18 outpatient services
19 emergency entry
20 ambulance bay
21 parking/receiving
22 courtyard

(1) Site Plan/Level 1

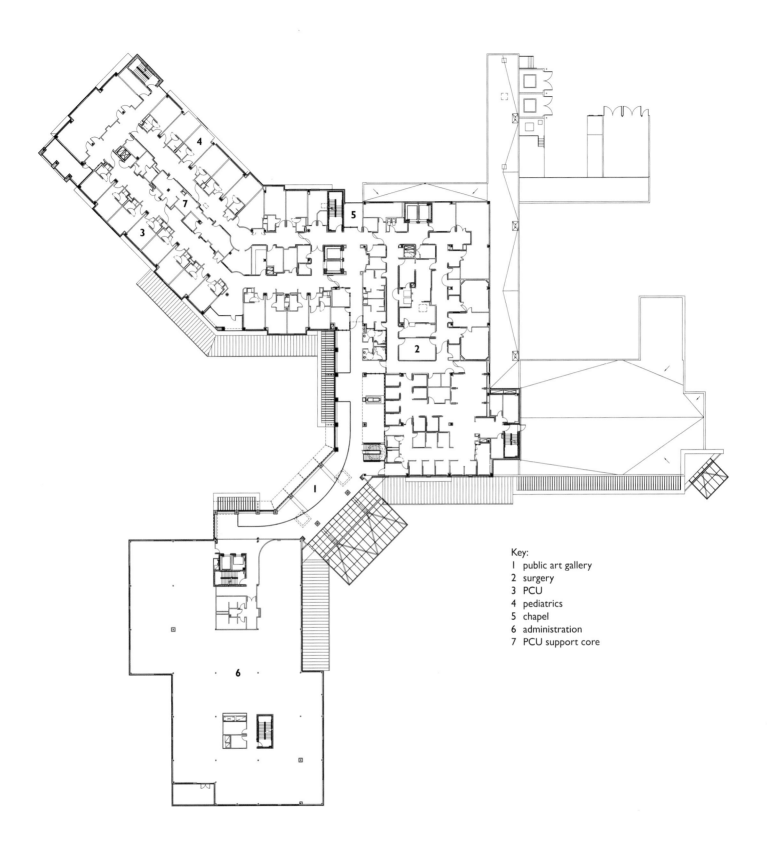

Key:
1 public art gallery
2 surgery
3 PCU
4 pediatrics
5 chapel
6 administration
7 PCU support core

① Level 2

8.4.5 Level 2 houses an art gallery for rotating exhibits of the work of local artists

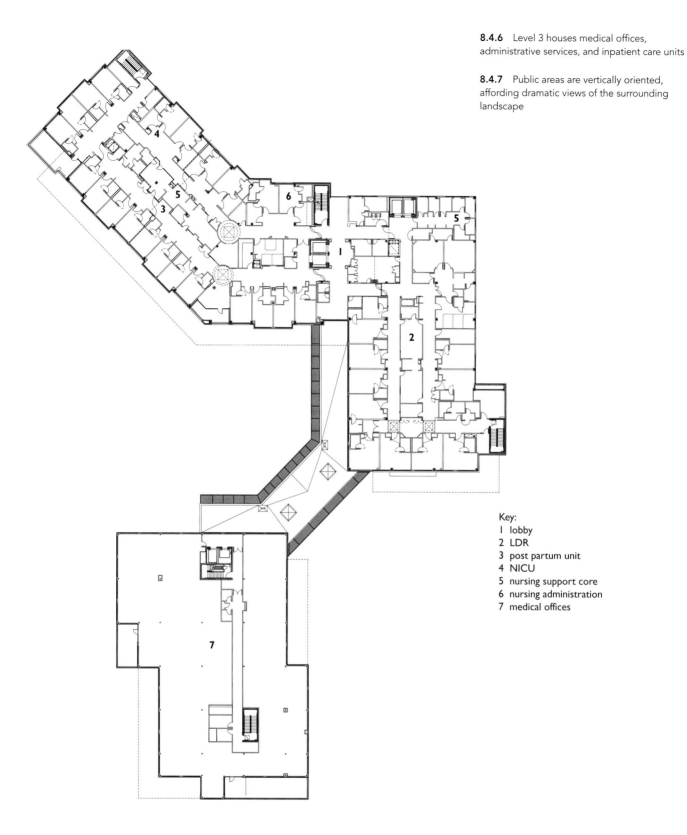

8.4.6 Level 3 houses medical offices, administrative services, and inpatient care units

8.4.7 Public areas are vertically oriented, affording dramatic views of the surrounding landscape

Key:
1 lobby
2 LDR
3 post partum unit
4 NICU
5 nursing support core
6 nursing administration
7 medical offices

1 Level 3

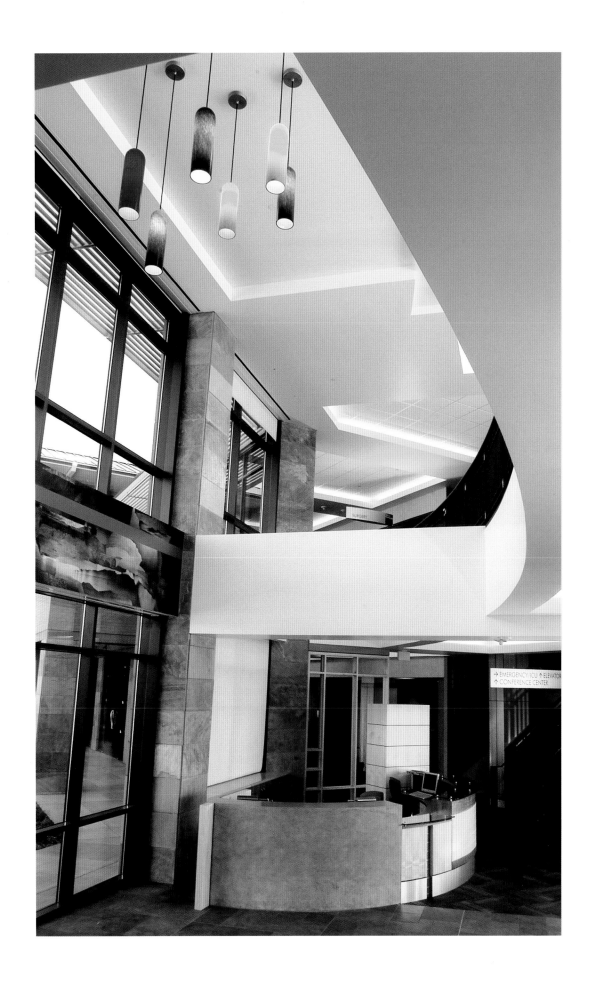

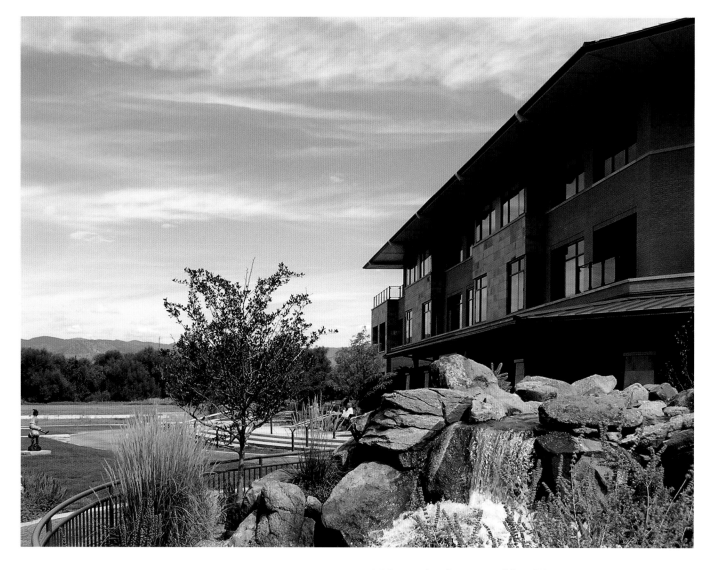

8.4.8 A rock sculpture, waterfall, and therapeutic garden are at the center of the compound. Earthen tones and natural materials predominate

Extended roof overhangs control daylight transmission and were installed only on the south and west sides of the hospital. This provides solar shading, and visually extends the hospital outward into its site. Materials were procured locally including fly ash for cement, bricks, stone, sandstone, and the use of low-emitting VOC paints for interior applications. All art purchases were from artists living and working within the county. This project has been influential in the U.S. and the architects have received many international inquiries because of this hospital's integration of green design principles. Future expansion options allow for a 50 percent increase in inpatient beds and support services on this site without disrupting key view corridors to the site's natural amenities.

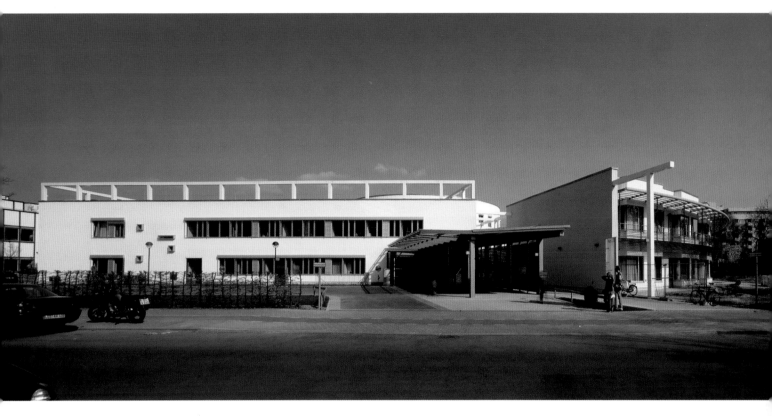

8.5.1 Front elevation of the Vivantes Clinical Center

5   Vivantes Clinical Center, Neukölln, Germany

ARCHITECT/PLANNERS: Schmucker and Partners, Mannheim, Germany
LANDSCAPE ARCHITECT: Same
CLIENT: State of Berlin
FEATURED MATERIALS: Steel, aluminum, cast-in-place concrete, stucco, laminate wood flooring, walls.
COMPLETED: 2005
INPATIENT BEDS: 92 plus 14 (ICU)
SITE/PARKING: 23/258
HOSPITAL SIZE: 132,456SF

Context/site

This hospital was the winning submission in a design competition held in 2000. Unfortunately, it remains rare for a hospital to be the subject of a design competition. It is a dilemma that continues to limit the emergence of new ideas. In nearly every other sphere of architectural practice the design competition is standard protocol as a vehicle to identify new ideas and fresh approaches to specific building types. Competitions have yielded positive outcomes with regard to schools, libraries, university campuses, housing, museums, city halls, performing arts centers, commercial projects, and religious architecture, among the building types advanced through the discourse and precedents set vis-à-vis the design competition format. In the 21st century, the hospital continues to be at a comparative disadvantage in this regard. This addition to an existing hospital houses 92 beds for adults, 14 beds in a children's ICU/NICU, and 7 maternity wards, with 4 equipped with full labor/delivery/recovery amenities. The site planning strategy was to establish a dialogue between two principal elements – a circular element to house inpatient care functions and nursing support, and a second element to house diagnostic and treatment services, related support, and the administration.

Building/unit

A three-level rotunda is situated at the midpoint of the arrival axis. This atrium provides spatial orientation, is a navigational aid, and establishes aesthetic unity. This element also houses the administration, reception, and admitting and serves as a symbolic and functional hub. The arrival axis bisects the two main compositional elements of the parti' (Figure 8.5.1). At the opposite end, an arrival canopy allows for pick up/drop off. The scale, composition, and imagery are at once minimalist and human-scaled. The horizontal emphasis of the fenestration in the patient housing areas further accentuates this. A scale model of the hospital illustrates the overall compositional strategy and the interplay between mass, void, and circulation. Circulation elements radiate outward from the central atrium/hub. This space is linked to the inpatient care domain (Figure 8.5.2). On

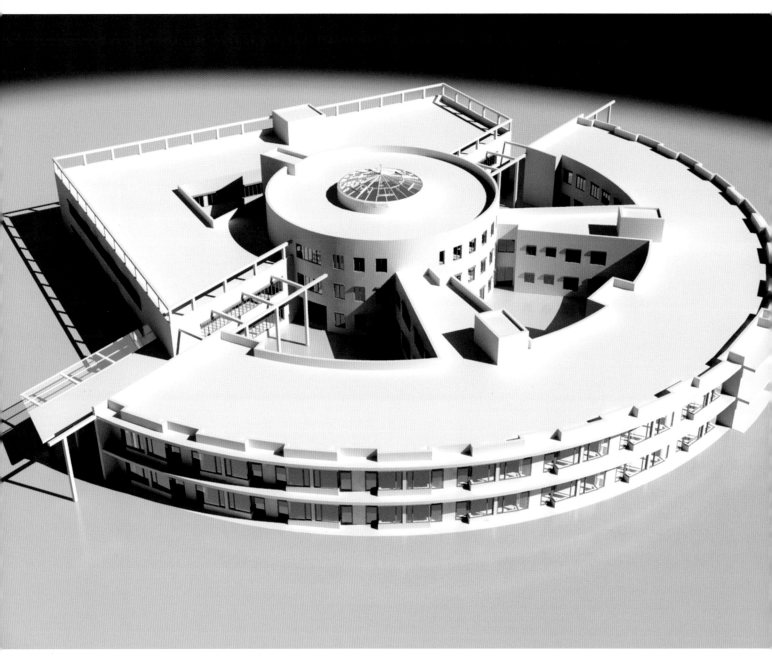

8.5.2 Its parti' is defined by an arrival axis which bisects two compositional elements – a truncated, rotated block, and a semi-circle. Circulation radiates as spokes from a hub, yielding three exterior spaces identical in size and shape

one side of this main circulation axis, its 'spokes' yield a set of three exterior courtyards. On the opposing side, a single outdoor space is created (Figure 8.5.3).

The atrium is a stage for public art exhibitions and a space for special events sponsored by the hospital. It is covered with a glass dome. Interior spaces are white (Figure 8.5.4). Aluminum screens screen the inpatient rooms from excessive solar gain. The screens also provide human scale. A waiting room at the midpoint of the radial element adjoins an exterior walkway. Inpatient rooms open directly to the outdoors on the first and second levels (Figure 8.5.5). The windows in the patient rooms are large and provide full views to the outdoors. The inpatient units provide a mixture of private and semi-private rooms. Overnight accommodations for families appear to be minimal, however.

The radial-shaped structure houses inpatient care units in a fan-like shape reaching outward to the south. All inpatient rooms

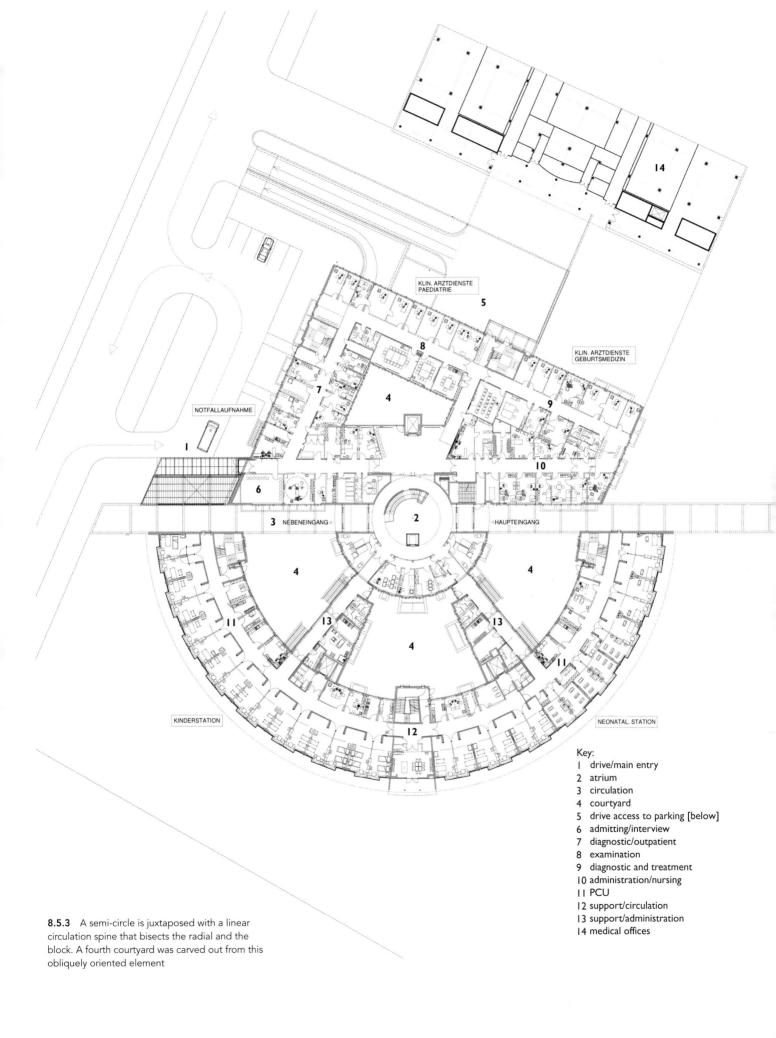

KLIN. ARZTDIENSTE
PAEDIATRIE

5

8

7

4

KLIN. ARZTDIENSTE
GEBURTSMEDIZIN

9

NOTFALLAUFNAHME

1

6

10

3   NEBENEINGANG

2

HAUPTEINGANG

4

4

11

13

13

4

11

KINDERSTATION

12

NEONATAL. STATION

14

Key:
1   drive/main entry
2   atrium
3   circulation
4   courtyard
5   drive access to parking [below]
6   admitting/interview
7   diagnostic/outpatient
8   examination
9   diagnostic and treatment
10 administration/nursing
11 PCU
12 support/circulation
13 support/administration
14 medical offices

8.5.3   A semi-circle is juxtaposed with a linear circulation spine that bisects the radial and the block. A fourth courtyard was carved out from this obliquely oriented element

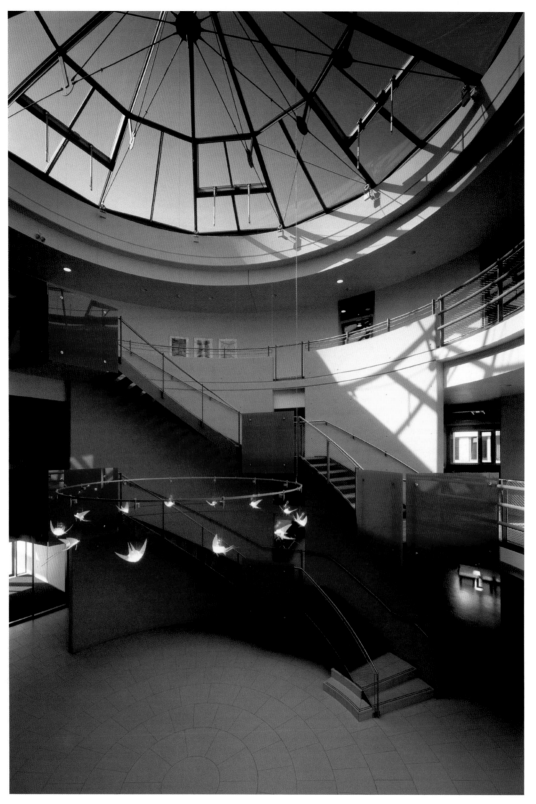

8.5.4 A rotunda, with a large glazed dome, is a stage for public art exhibits and social functions

8.5.5 Rooms on the ground level open directly to patios. Steel sunscreens and rails provide scale and shade. The ambiance is not unlike a hotel or university dormitory

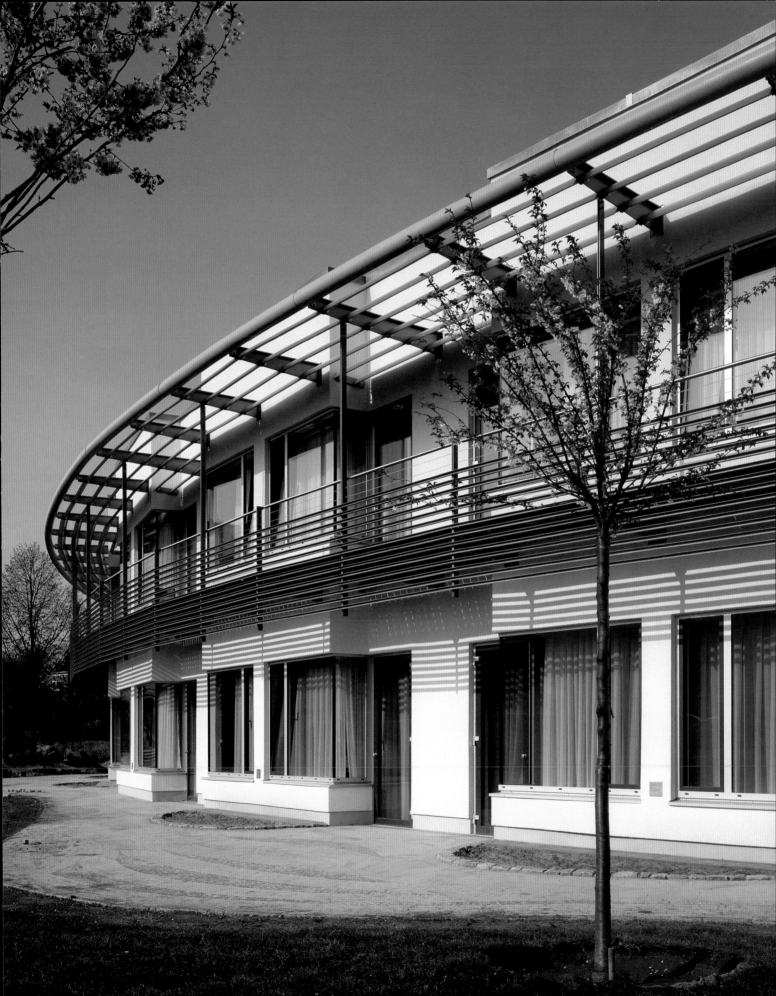

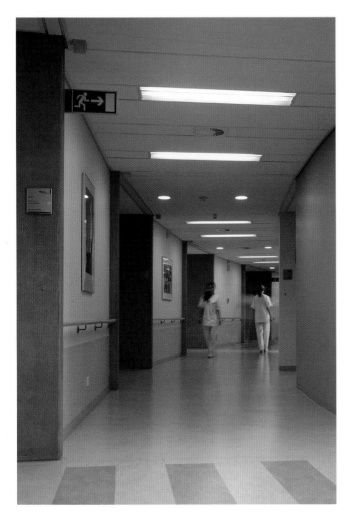

8.5.6 The radiality of the inpatient care units is reflected in the PCU circulation spine

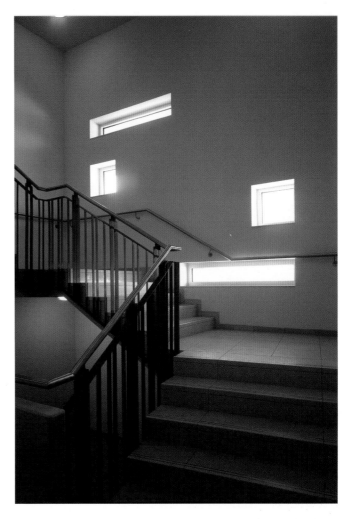

8.5.7 Animated fenestration patterns in the staircases provide light and framed views

overlook a small park. A playground, patio, and seating are provided for patient and family use in this park. A minimal use of color is utilized as an aesthetic feature and navigational aid in the inpatient units. The door to each inpatient room is set back (inset) from the corridor, and all bath/shower rooms are on the inboard side of the radial form (Figure 8.5.6). The pie-shaped courtyards are accessible to patients and their families. Large windows in the atrium rotunda allow views into these spaces, and one courtyard features a staircase element whose windows are abstractly composed (Figure 8.5.7).

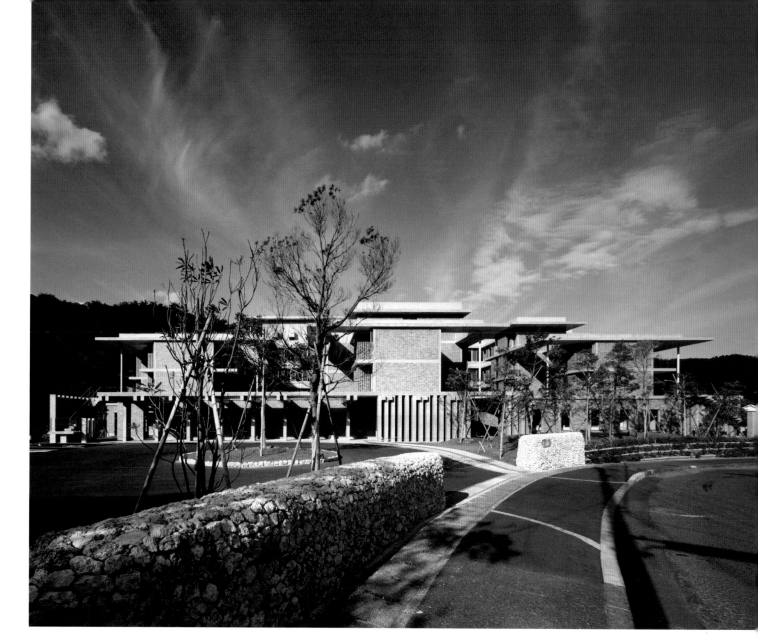

8.6.1 The Jiaikai Amani Hospital reinterprets time-tested Middle Eastern vernacular building traditions dating from the region's earliest hospitals

6 Jiaikai Amani Hospital, United Arab Emirates (UAE)

ARCHITECT: Katsuya Kawashima, Nikken Sekkei, Ltd., Tadao Matsubase, Shimomai Architecture Design Office, Ltd, Tokyo.
LANDSCAPE ARCHITECT: Kimiyasu Tanaka, Nikken Sekkei, Ltd.
CLIENT: United Arab Emirates Ministry of Health
FEATURED MATERIALS: Cast-in-place concrete, exterior and interior masonry, stone pavers, laminate wood finishes and ceilings
COMPLETED: 2003
INPATIENT BEDS: 190
SITE/PARKING: 34 acres/225
HOSPITAL SIZE: 151,542SF

Context/site

This hospital expresses its designers' sensitivity regarding a local vernacular culture, its building traditions, and its architecture. The local architecture and in particular the indigenous single family dwelling provided a point of departure in the site planning and massing of the Amani Hospital. The result speaks to the value of respect for an indigenous vernacular in placemaking in the Middle East. It is a case study on passive solar building design principles. This centered on screening outdoor and interior spaces from the area's intense sunlight. Second, natural ventilation is utilized as a natural cooling device. Third, masonry is used as a visual screen and an air filter. Fourth, the courtyard, a timeless, pervasive ingredient

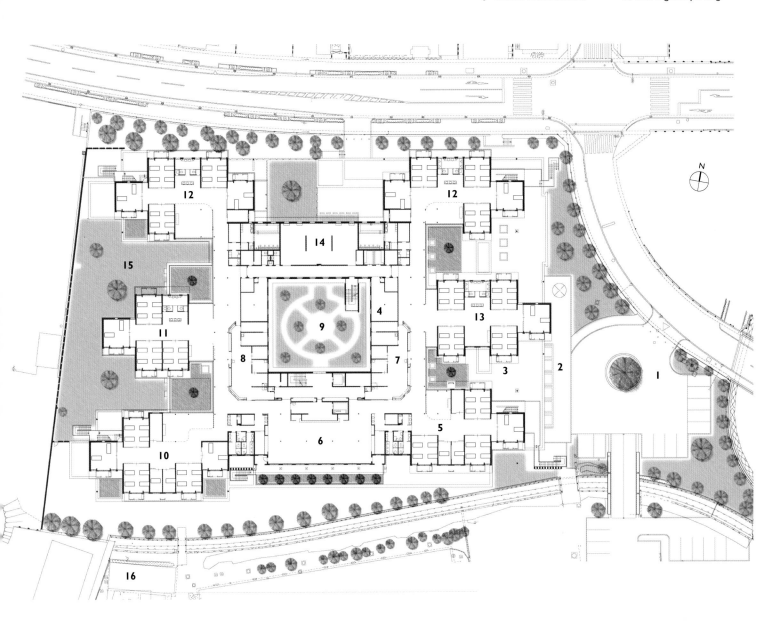

Key:
1	circular entry drive	9	courtyard
2	canopy	10	PCU/nursing support
3	information/admitting	11	pediatric PCU
4	administration	12	PCU/nursing support
5	PCU/nursing support	13	PCU/nursing support
6	dining/kitchen	14	medical records
7	central nurses station	15	gardens
8	central nurses station	16	below grade parking

Plan/Level 2

8.6.2 The parti' is defined by a central court with circulation on all sides. Six inpatient pavilions are articulated by means of landscaped side courts

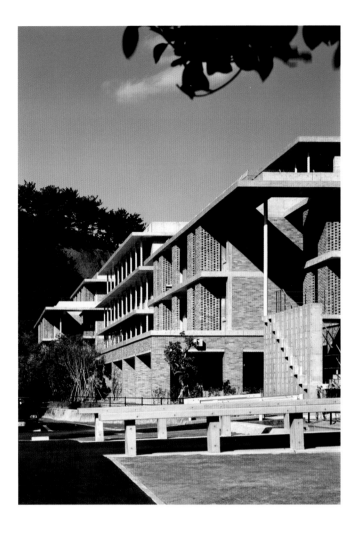

8.6.3 Amani's aesthetic language is defined by extended eaves, structural expressiveness, vertical sunscreen panels, and patterned masonry walls

in the Middle East's indigenous vernacular – including its historic hospitals – facilitates a fluid interactivity between interior and exterior spaces. This indoor–outdoor fluidity has been employed for centuries in Islamic hospitals. Fifth, the judicious use of natural vegetation at Amani – trees, shrubs, vines – is effective in providing visual screening from the harsh elements and as an aesthetic vehicle to bring beauty into the hospital environment (Figure 8.6.1).

Upon first encounter, the Jiaikai Amani Hospital presents an unassuming image. Its stepped massing and pronounced roof overhangs create dramatic shadow lines on its exterior. The graduated massing is achieved through breaking apart its program requirements into a core block, with a main courtyard carved out of its center, surrounding support spaces, and three patient housing wings to one side, and three additional patient housing wings to the other side. A central courtyard functions as the core of the parti'.

8.6.4 Light/dark, mass/void patterns are interwoven throughout, in reference to early hospitals in the region

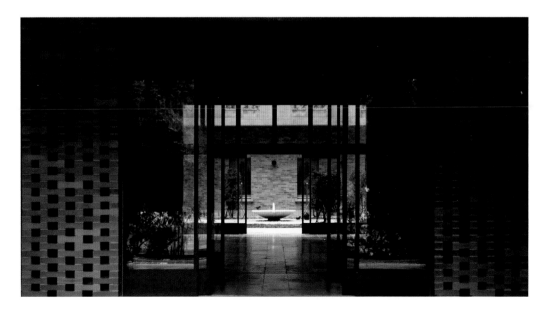

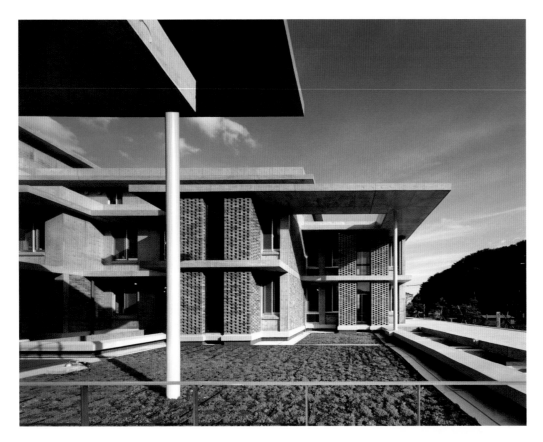

8.6.5 Cantilevered floor plates function as sunscreens, yielding nuanced shadows, textures and modulated effects

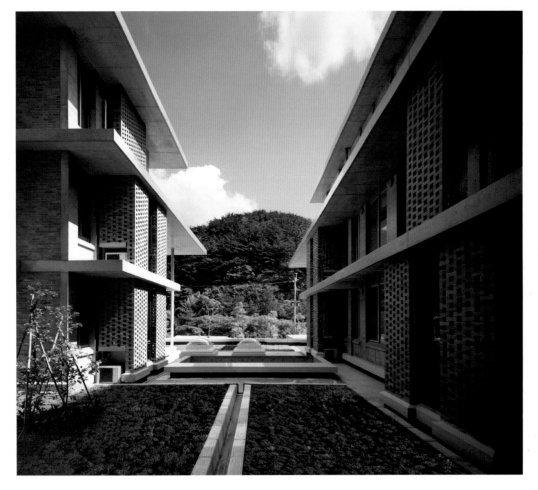

8.6.6 Spatial compression accentuates Amani's materiality, and its relationship to the landscape

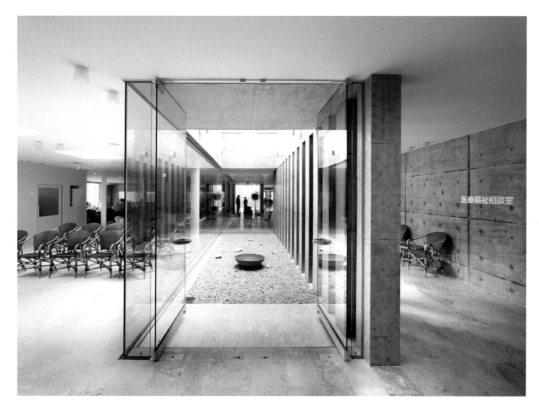

8.6.7 Natural light is judiciously drawn into the building envelope. In this instance, natural light activates a rock garden and waiting area

Building/unit

An access drive leads to a large arrival hall. This space adjoins the reception, admitting and outpatient clinical areas and connects with the large open court. Various departments are deployed around this exterior space. The departments that surround and overlook this open court are housed in a four-level structure. The six surrounding inpatient housing wings are three levels in height. Three of these wings house males only, with the other three housing females. In this manner the hospital is divided, in effect, into two equivalent realms. Key support services are shared, such as the operating theaters, and diagnostic and imaging departments (Figure 8.6.2). The typical PCU houses 16 beds, served by a central nursing station. Each patient room houses 3–4 beds. An allotment of isolation rooms is deployed across the six PCU wings. The floor plates are expressed on the exterior elevations (Figure 8.6.3). As mentioned, the delicately textured brickwork is both ornamental and functional. A tapestry/woven effect is achieved in the openings in these walls, allowing for cool desert-evening natural breezes to flow into the interior. Windows in nearly every part of the hospital are operable. Breezes that pass through and around the masonry 'screens' are filtered to the interior. A light/dark, open/closed dialectic sets a rhythm that further articulates the human scale of the hospital (Figure 8.6.4).

Amani Hospital makes use of a unique solar heat collection system that transforms well water into a coolant, in a variant of a geothermal system. The patient housing wings are shielded from the sun and extreme heat by the aforementioned floor/roof plates that cantilever outward to further accentuate its horizontality (Figure 8.6.5). Narrow footprints of the various wings allow for views to the surrounding natural landscape and allow natural daylight and ventilation to enter (Figure 8.6.6). A waiting room adjacent to the emergency department features an outdoor rock garden. This space also allows filtered daylight to enter the adjacent interiors (Figure 8.6.7). In the nursing dormitory, four nurses share a room; each suite is provided with a study area and bath/shower room. This hospital is noteworthy with regard to its reconsideration of appropriate technology, the virtues of *genius loci*, the value of local vernacular traditions and the rejection of the too often standard practice of superficial importation of Western values and standards to Middle Eastern Architecture.

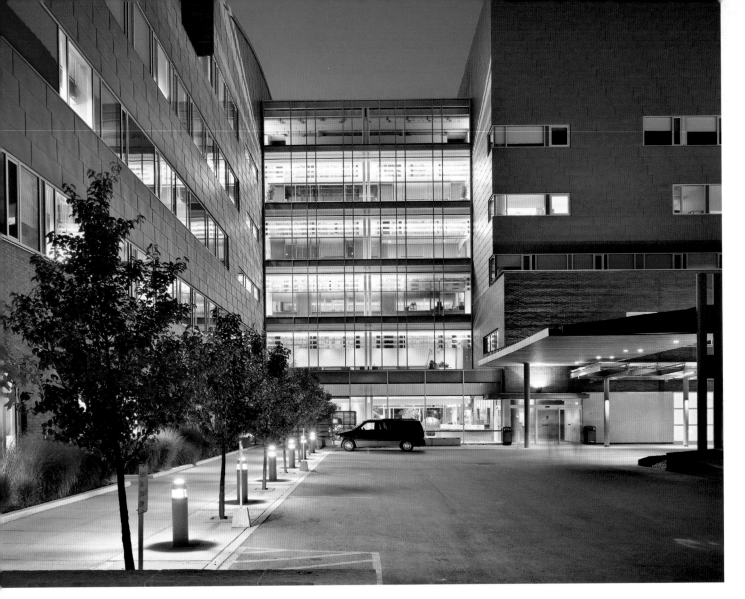

8.7.1 Bloorview Kids Rehab is sited between a residential neighborhood and a wooded ravine. It is Canada's largest and most comprehensive pediatric rehab center

7   Bloorview Kids Rehab, Toronto, Ontario, Canada

ARCHITECT: Montgomery Sisam/Stantec Architecture – Joint Venture, Toronto and Vancouver
LANDSCAPE ARCHITECT: Vertechs Design, Inc.
CLIENT: Bloorview Kids Rehab
FEATURED MATERIALS: Exterior steel cladding, laminate wood, exterior wood decking, limestone, brick masonry, zinc, aluminum
COMPLETED: 2006
INPATIENT BEDS: 75
SITE/PARKING: 12 acres/255
HOSPITAL SIZE: 353,000

Context/site

This pediatric rehabilitation center brings together multiple functions formerly housed at two separate sites. It is Canada's largest and most comprehensive children's inpatient rehabilitation treatment center and its architects strove to create a non-institutional environment. Bloorview houses the following services: a full teaching hospital, a research institute, an all-grades school for inpatients, a family resource center and library, a 24/7 center for rehabilitation treatment, a swimming pool for community-based outreach programs, a therapeutic pool, summer camp, a two-level creative arts studio, cafeteria, therapeutic gardens, play areas, and ravine paths. This facility was built between a midtown residential neighborhood and a wooded ravine that slopes downward to a tributary of the Don River. Outdoor spaces were given careful consideration. A portion of the site bordering the ravine was transferred to the regional conservation authority as a public trail. Indigenous plant species were selected for the exterior landscaped areas. Bloorview Kids features a green roofscape and three accessible roof terraces for inpatient and family use. Roof storm water is captured and stored underground for reuse in on-site irrigation (Figure 8.7.1).

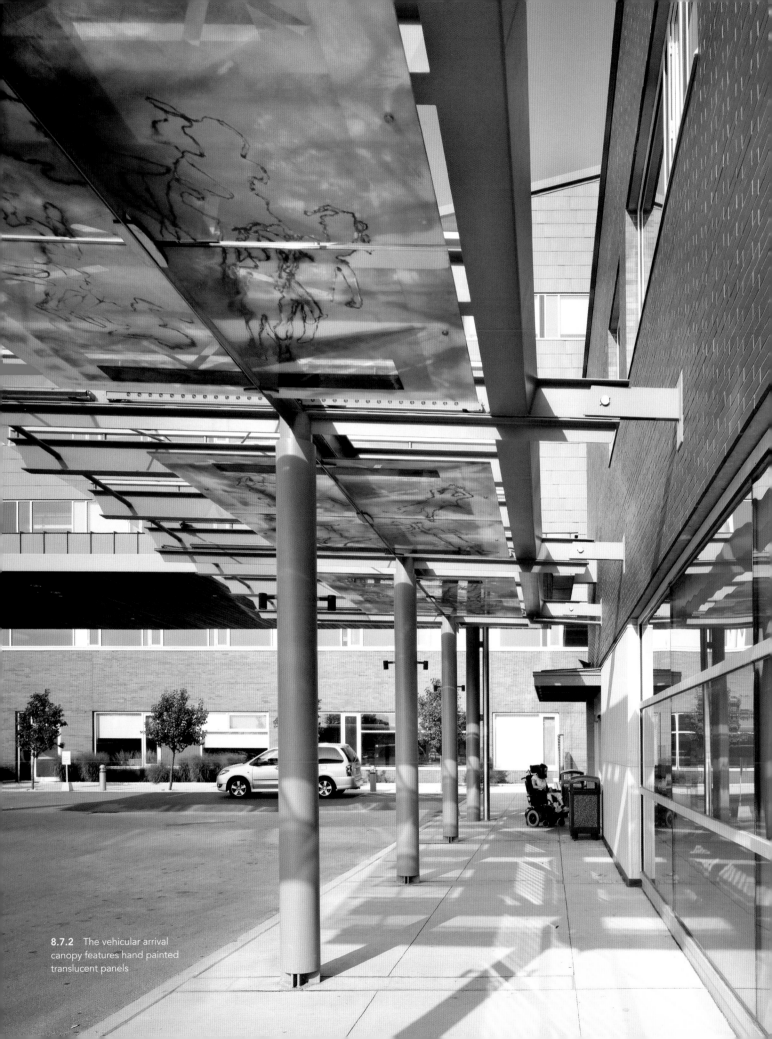

8.7.2 The vehicular arrival canopy features hand painted translucent panels

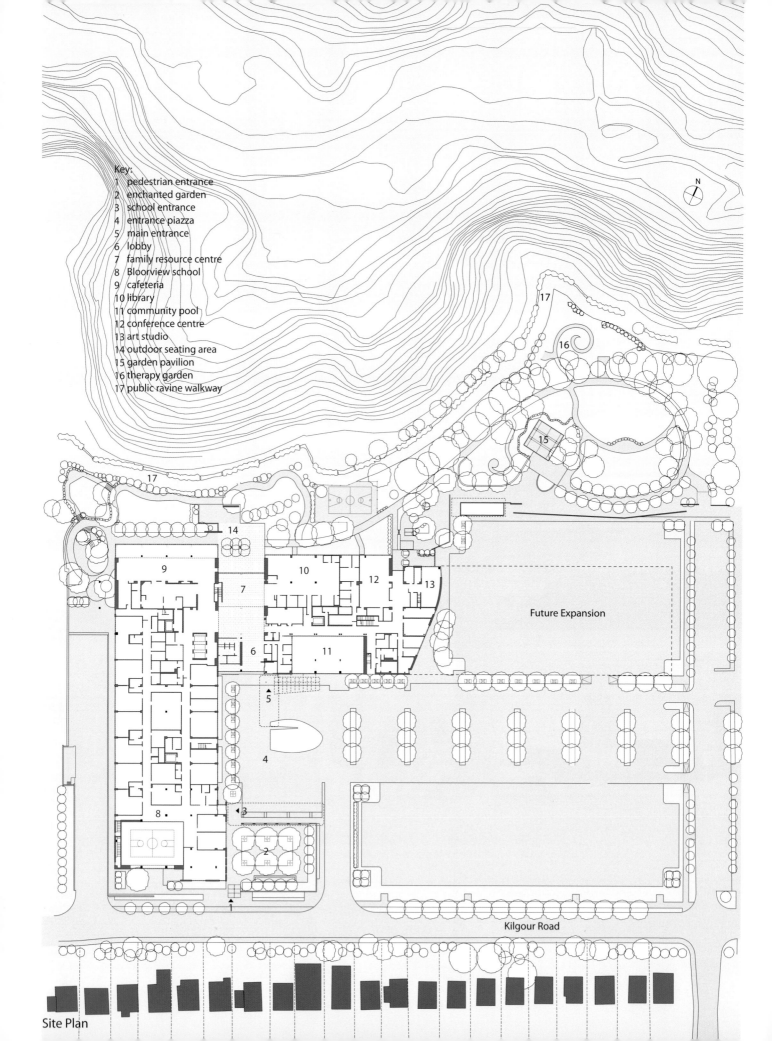

Key:
1 pedestrian entrance
2 enchanted garden
3 school entrance
4 entrance piazza
5 main entrance
6 lobby
7 family resource centre
8 Bloorview school
9 cafeteria
10 library
11 community pool
12 conference centre
13 art studio
14 outdoor seating area
15 garden pavilion
16 therapy garden
17 public ravine walkway

N

17

16

15

17

14

9

7

10

12

13

Future Expansion

6

11

5

4

8

3

2

Kilgour Road

Site Plan

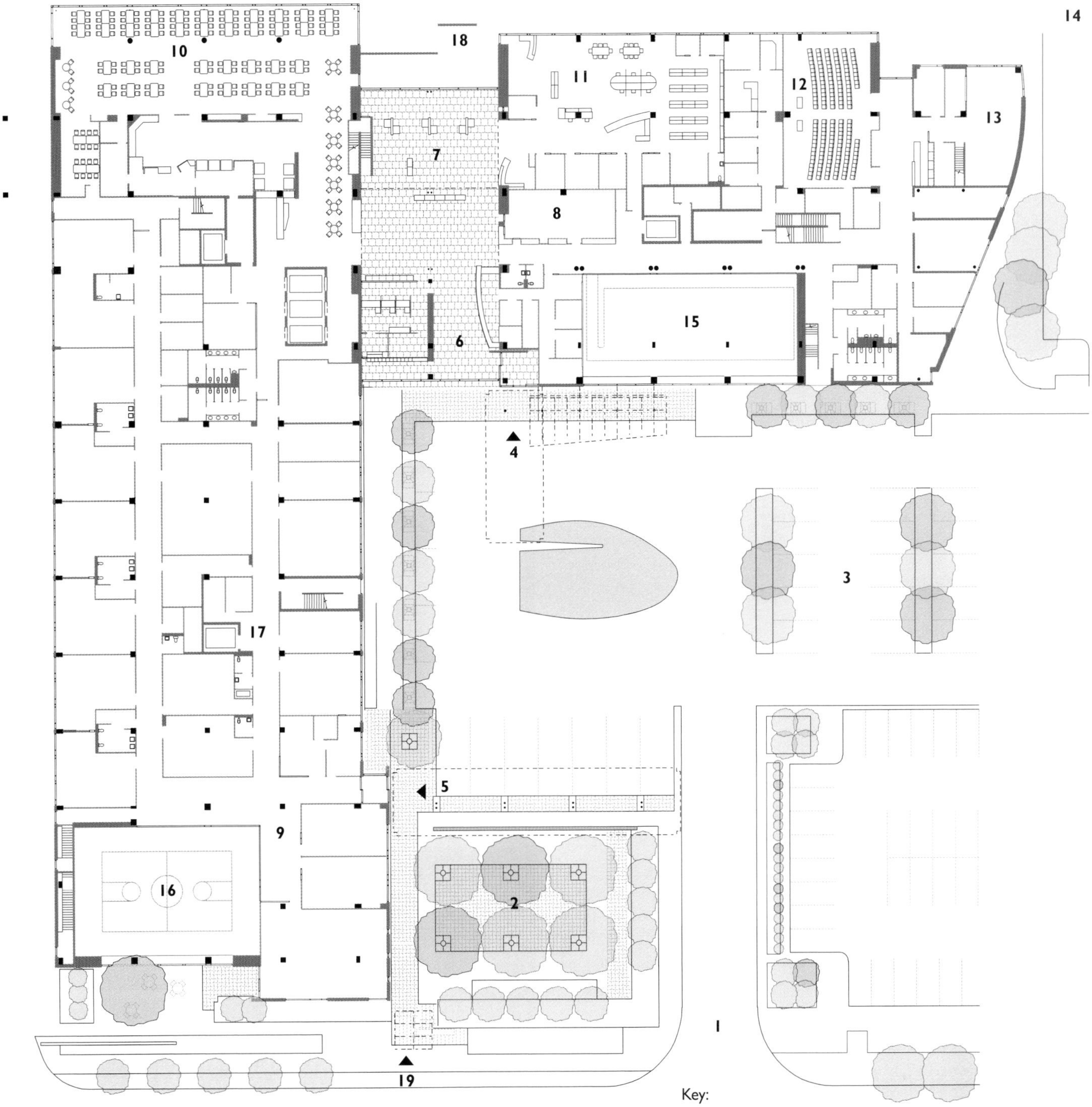

8.7.4 The garden is on axis with the main entrance, visually connected by a row of trees. The main lobby bisects the plan

8.7.3 The L-shaped parti' allows for future expansion. An outdoor pavilion and therapeutic garden are fused with the natural landscape immediately to the north

Key:
1 new public road
2 enchanted garden
3 parking grove
4 main entrance/drop-off
5 school entrance/drop-off
6 lobby
7 resource centre
8 enclosed play area
9 school
10 cafeteria
11 library
12 conference room
13 art studio/greenhouse
14 access to spiral garden
15 open to recreation pool below
16 open to gymnasium below
17 elevators
18 outdoor seating area
19 pedestrian entrance

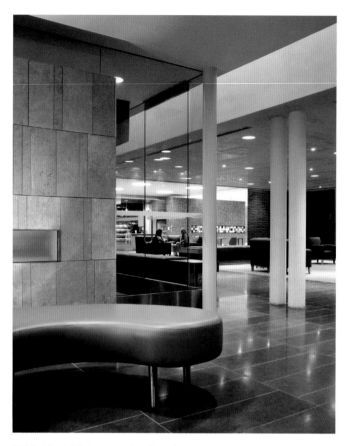

8.7.5 The lobby's textured walls and vibrant colors are reprised throughout

Building/unit

A six-level L-shaped parti' features a sloping, wedge-shaped roof that at once ascends from and extends towards the ravine directly to the north. In silhouette, the sloping roofline mirrors the contours of the site. Setbacks yield habitable roof surfaces. A fully glazed 'bridge' at the center rises upward, reaching all six levels; it affords full views of the surrounding area. A grassy egg shaped mound is situated to the left of the public access drive, across from the arrival canopy and its transparent roof plates. This element is activated with colorful, animated artwork, in stark contrast to the arrival canopies at the entrances to most hospitals (Figure 8.7.2). This landscaped space and the public access drive lead to the main entrance and into a building that at first appears to be randomly composed. The arrival and reception area is unimposing and informal, unlike the formality of the large atriums of many recent urban hospitals; seating in the lobby is configured and painted in a manner reminiscent of caterpillars. Various programmatic components are deployed as follows: ground level – public services, including the school, conference center, cafeteria, and creative arts program; lower level – recreation and therapy pools, gym, video conference room, pharmacy, and staff support; second level – outpatient services; third level – inpatient housing and support services; fourth level – research activities; fifth level – family accommodations and administration (Figure 8.7.3 and Figure 8.7.4).

Sustainable design principles were a priority from the outset and strongly influenced the parti', and the mechanical and electrical systems. The palette of materials, including the materiality of the exterior steel cladding system, were chosen for their energy conservation properties. Windows are operable to facilitate natural ventilation, and the colors throughout the interior are expressed on the facade in horizontal bands. The landscaped roof on the second level provides the adjacent clinic waiting area with views of the surrounding landscape. Photovoltaic panels are housed on the east wing roof. The exterior skin is a case study in recent innovations in window frame, glazing, and weatherproofing technology. All perimeter rooms have operable windows; natural light is transmitted into nearly all spaces occupied by patients.

Wall panels with vibrant colors activate the interior of the ground level and throughout the upper levels of the facility. This is both an aesthetic and navigational aid (Figure 8.7.5). Interiors feature

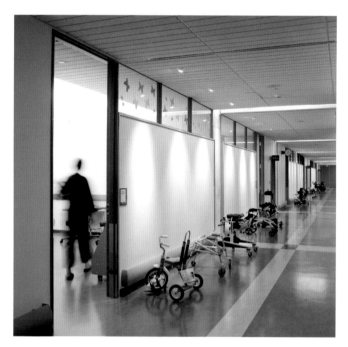

8.7.6 Bikes and mobility assistance devices are parked outside a therapy treatment room. Clerestories draw natural light into the hallway

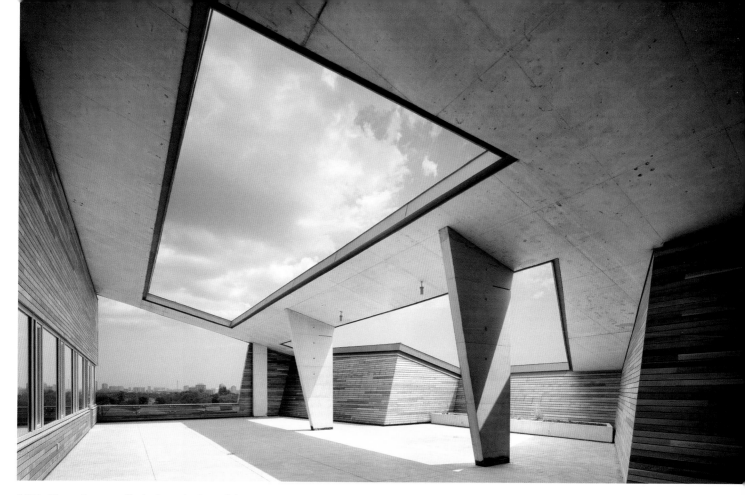

8.7.7 The roof terrace affords dramatic views of the neighborhood and city. Cutouts in the roof transmit light without sacrificing scale or sense of enclosure

natural wood, ornamental glass and ceramic tile. Transparency is employed in the corridor that overlooks the swimming pool, and this simultaneously provides visual access from the library directly across the hall. Corridors are exaggerated in width, allowing young people to test out their mobility skills. Children with wheelchairs, walkers, and tricycles have ample space to turn corners and pass safely. Clerestories transmit light from this circulation space into adjacent rooms (Figure 8.7.6). Artwork produced by 32 Canadian artists is on permanent display throughout the facility. In the Resource Center, a handmade curtain of 5,000 handmade beads and two large wire-sculpted birds provide an uplifting ambiance. The sloping south facade features accessible terraces, including a rooftop terrace with a perforated roof, splayed support columns, and wood-sheathed walls (Figure 8.7.7). The semi-private (4-bed) inpatient rooms feature wood surfaces, wood laminate headwalls, and ample space for family use, i.e. personal storage, social interaction, and overnight stays. Inpatient rooms are interconnected in a suite configuration, with semi-private bath/shower rooms, and with study desks provided across from the patient's bed (Figure 8.7.8).

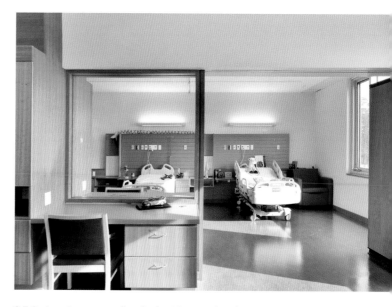

8.7.8 Inpatient rooms allow for furnishings to be placed as per patient and family member preferences. A built-in desk is provided. Note the foldaway wall panels between adjoining semi-private rooms

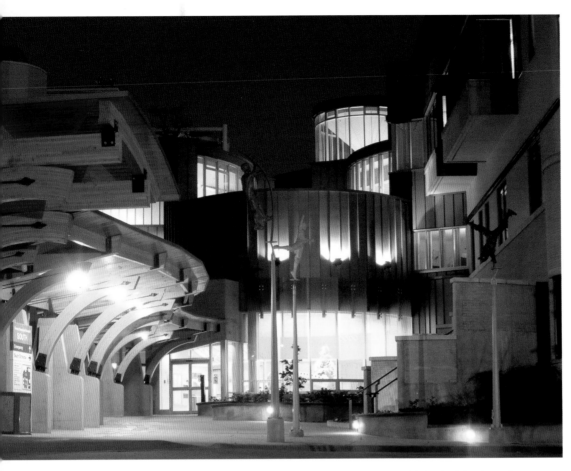

8.8.1 At night, the main entrance at Surrey Memorial is illuminated, underscoring its animated formal language

8 Children's Health Centre at Surrey Memorial Hospital, Surrey, British Columbia, Canada

ARCHITECT: Stantec Architecture, Vancouver
LANDSCAPE ARCHITECT:
CLIENT: Surrey Memorial Hospital/South Fraser Health Region, Surrey
FEATURED MATERIALS: Steel exterior panel system, cast-in-place concrete, bronze, and aluminum
COMPLETED: 2001
INPATIENT BEDS: 95
SITE/PARKING: 28 inpatient beds; 10-OR surgical suite; 36-bed LDRP unit; 84-bed surgical floor
HOSPITAL SIZE: 160,000SF

Context/site

This is a major addition to an existing 400-bed hospital. The fundamental concept was to place the child and adolescent at the center of person-nature transactions at each stage of the healing process. The construction was phased in order for the operations of the adjacent hospital to continue uninterrupted. This major addition houses a children's health center with 28 beds, outpatient clinics, an adolescent psychiatry unit, 10-bed surgical suite, child and maternal care unit including a 36-bed LDR unit and an infant nursery, an 84-bed med/surgical PCU, and related support. Diagnostic imaging and emergency departments were expanded, and a new physical plant and central campus maintenance facility were built in a subsequent phase. An arched, curvilinear arrival canopy, constructed of heavy timber from a local forest, shelters those arriving and departing. This canopy, the access drive, and adjacent landscape space is defined further by a set of rainbow-colored sculptures of children, atop a set of poles, each child engaged in a gravity-defying act (Figure 8.8.1).

Building/unit

This addition is a stage set for various nature-inspired motifs and the color palette invites more nuanced interpretations. The symbolism and geometry of a rainbow was a key form-generative concept in the public areas. The design team reasoned that the rainbow is the single element in nature that provides the most surprise and delight to a young child. For this reason the figurative sculptures at the main

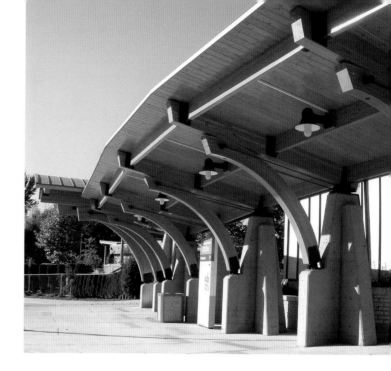

8.8.2 The anthropomorphic arrival canopy's structure is of laminated wood beams, with steel beams rising upward from concrete plinths

8.8.3 From the backside, the canopy's exoskeletal curvature has been described by its architects as a 'sleeping dragon's tail'

8.8.4 A vertically ribbed panel-window system contains operable windows. A horizontal push–pull, not unlike an accordion effect, yields at first what appears to be randomized compression. This yields a series of perforated recesses and projections

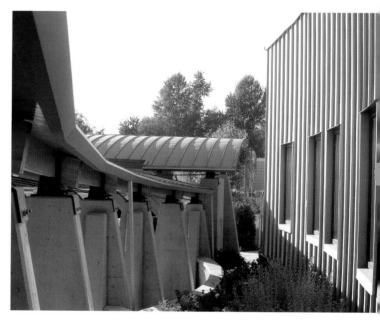

entry are each rendered in a different color of the rainbow – red, green, yellow, orange, purple, blue. The organic geometries of the exterior forecourt establish this theme and it is extended to the interior realm – expressed in plan through concentric rings – not unlike a series of rainbow arcs of varying diameters. The timber beams of the arrival canopy curve outward, which the architects describe as a 'sleeping dragon's tail' (Figure 8.8.2). A garden wall and benches reinforce the playful imagery (Figure 8.8.3). Rainbow colors are depicted in a sequence of sunscreens shielding the atrium lobby from excessive solar gain. Rainbow colors dominate the floor surface at the entrance to the Children's Health Centre. These motifs are expressed on the exterior (Figure 8.8.4). A frog, rendered in bright colors, greets visitors. The lobby's ceiling is rendered in bright hues, with a flock of sparrows etched into the curving 'rainbow beam' that supports the roof. A second flock of birds ascends the main circular staircase to the upper reaches of the space. To the design team, the rainbow symbolizes springtime, renewal, and growth. This composition of concentric arcs and circles are clearly visible from many vantage points, are constructed of steel and glass, and are clad in vertically ribbed steel panels.

The first level of the Children's Health Centre houses a 28-bed pediatric unit and adolescent psychiatry unit, and an ICU and surgical unit (Figure 8.8.5a–b). The reception area is located next to an atrium lobby and contains a play space for young children, overlooking a garden. The adolescent psychiatry unit is provided with its own semi-private courtyard with small alcoves and a basketball hoop in a corner of this space. Outpatients and inpatients share pre-operative and post-operative facilities. An elevator links this unit to the parking garage located in the basement level below. The second and third levels are similar in their overall footprint but not in the details of the floor plans. The second level houses a birthing center, and the third level houses an 84-bed PCU and related family and nursing support. On Level 3, the post-surgical inpatient rooms range in capacity from 1–4 beds.

Rainbow-inspired light tubes help to visually activate the indoor children's play area, and a children's outdoor courtyard celebrates nature, i.e. forests, large boulders that invite climbing, and seating, including a large 'leaf sculpture'. A one-level masonry clad plinth anchors four two-level L-shaped PCU pavilions. The nursing station is located at the apex within each L-shaped PCU. Dayrooms, gardens, and terraces are oriented toward the winter sun. Garden roof balconies provide a place to be outdoors adjacent to the interior spaces.

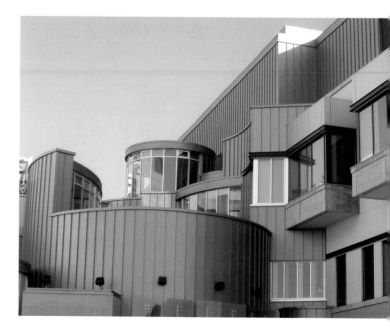

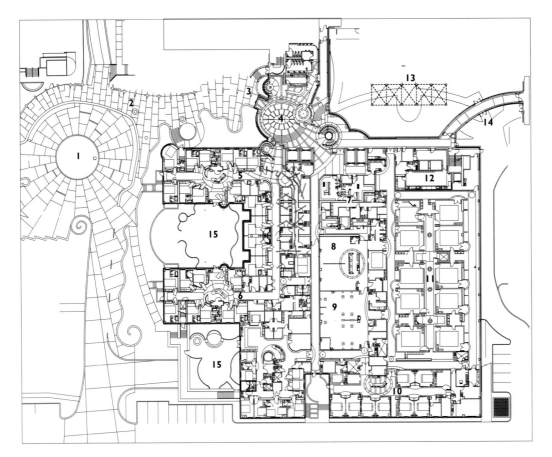

8.8.5 Level 1 houses a 28-bed pediatric and adolescent psychiatry unit, ICU, and surgical units. Level 3 houses four inpatient care units, and nursing support

Site Plan/Level 1

Key:
1 arrival drive
2 trellis/colonnade
3 main entry
4 atrium
5 PCU/nursing
6 PCU/nursing
7 administration
8 admitting
9 PACU
10 ICU
11 surgical suites
12 morgue
13 garden/patio
14 arrival gateway
15 outdoor gardens/ exercise

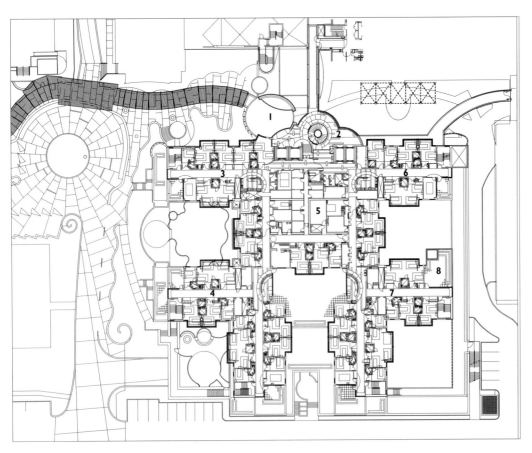

Level 3

Key:
1 atrium
2 circulation
3 PCU/nursing 1
4 PCU/nursing 2
5 support/administration
6 PCU/nursing 3
7 PCU/nursing 4
8 activity

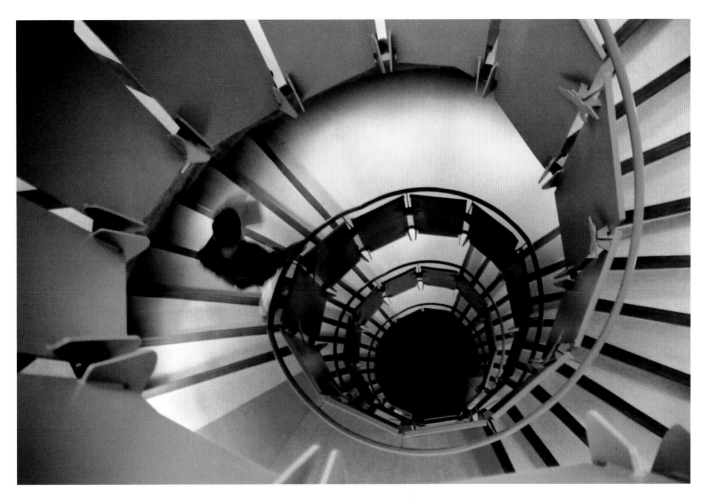

8.8.6 A kaleidoscope staircase is capped with a circular clerestory visible from the exterior main arrival area

8.8.7 Five semi-private courtyards are provided. Inpatient care units feature projecting bay windows, with small patios on the second and third levels. A therapeutic garden is located on the ground level

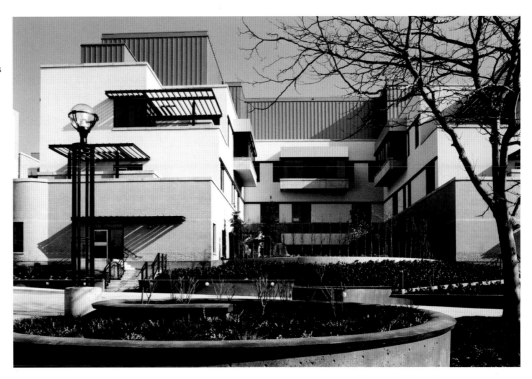

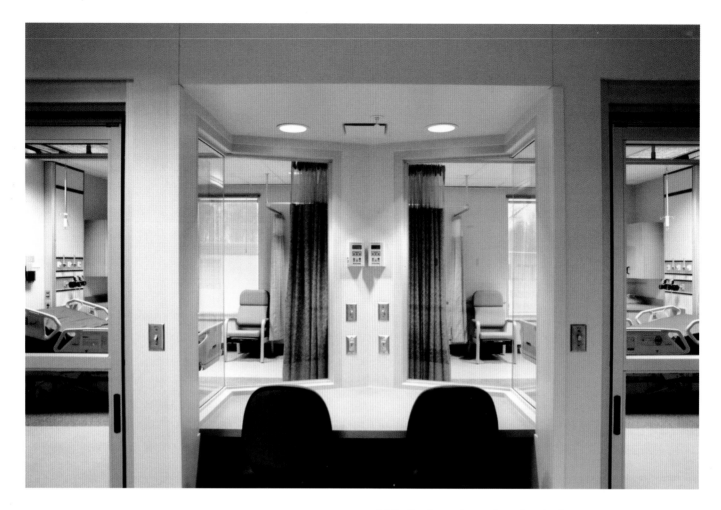

8.8.8 Satelite nursing stations allow simultaneous views into adjoining patient rooms

A kaleidoscope staircase is a principal feature of the main lobby and this has become a memorable feature for patients and families alike, since the facility's opening (Figure 8.8.6). Steel trellises shade semi-private terraces and each is ringed with planters; these spaces are 'carved out' from the ends of each wing. As mentioned, these provide places for social interaction as well as privacy and respite. Every inpatient room features the aforementioned projecting window bays including the 4-bed inpatient rooms. Windows are operable in the inpatient housing units (Figure 8.8.7). Transparency is featured in the nurses' satellite stations next to the inpatient rooms. The bath/ shower room is inboard, on the corridor side of the bedroom. The 4-bed rooms can be partitioned into two 2-bed rooms as patient needs warrant (Figure 8.8.8). This hospital received the 2001 Award of Excellence for Built projects from the AIA Academy of Architecture for Health and *Modern Healthcare* magazine, and a Citation of Merit from *Healthcare Design* magazine.

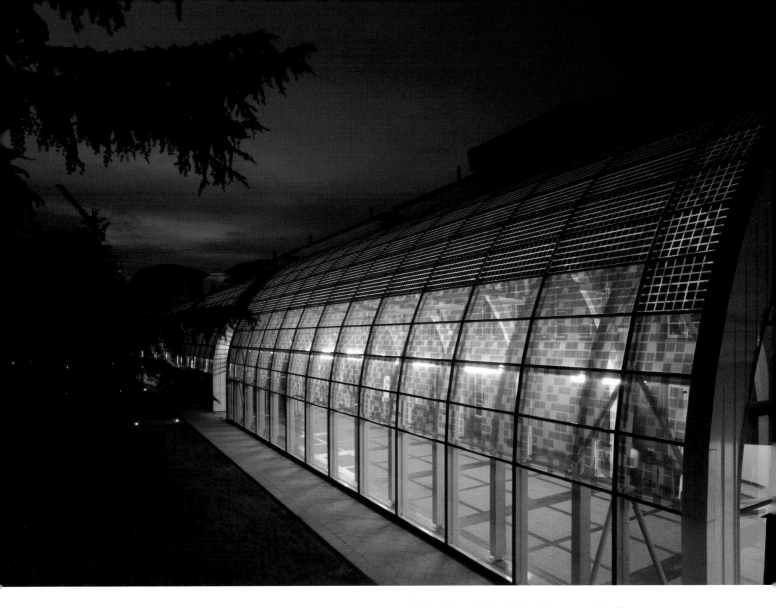

8.9.1 Meyer Children's Hospital was one of the first five demonstration hospitals in the European Union (EU) *Hospitals Demonstration Project*

9 Meyer Children's Hospital (Ospedale Pediatrico Meyer di Firenze), Florence, Italy

ARCHITECT: Anshen + Allen, San Francisco/Centro Studi
    Progettazione Edilizia (CSPE), Florence
LANDSCAPE ARCHITECT: CSPE, Florence
CLIENT: Italian National Health System, Tuscan Region
FEATURED MATERIALS: Structural steel system, laminated wood
    trusses, granite, terrazzo, wood interior finishes
COMPLETED: 2007
INPATIENT BEDS: 152
SITE/PARKING: 17.8 acres/245
HOSPITAL SIZE: 361,667SF

Context/site

Founded in 1884, this hospital was one of the first in Italy devoted exclusively to the care of children and adolescents. The hospital grew in civic importance until it came to be affectionately known locally as the 'Little Hospital'. The original hospital faces Via Luca Giordano. Its fame reached a peak at the conclusion of World War II when tubular meningitis was treated there successfully for the first time in the world. In 1995 the Meyer Hospital, together with the Department of Pediatrics at the University of Florence, became part of the National Health System. An architectural design competition was held. The wining team's scheme is a pediatric hospital that extensively incorporates environmentally sustainable design strategies. This children's replacement hospital, appended to an historic mansion,

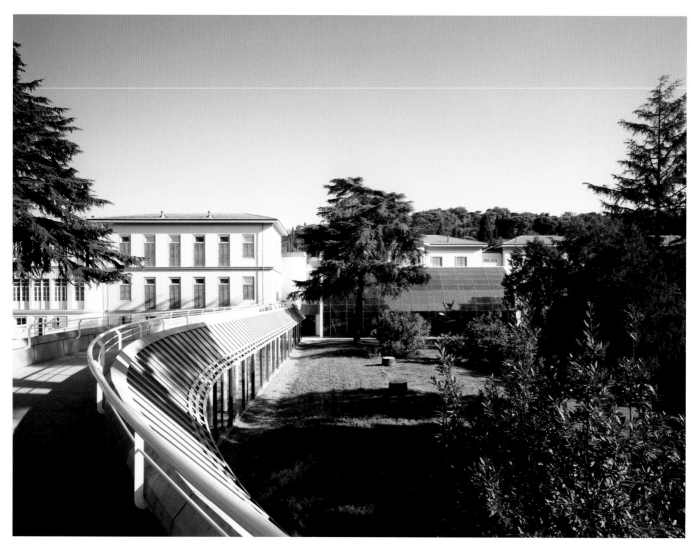

8.9.2 The composition is three levels in height with one level below grade. A glass-sheathed galleria spans its length, and parallels landscaped gardens and an historic villa on the site

features extensive grounds and an extensive roofscape for use by patients, families, and staff. The composition organically slots into its sloping site and therefore minimally disturbs the existing landscape. The hospital is adjacent to a large park. The scheme centers on the transmission of daylight to spaces set deeply into the slope. A goal was to realize a significant reduction in solar heat gain and to provide natural ventilation and natural cooling throughout. The site features old-growth trees, many of which were incorporated into the parti' for passive shading. Natural ventilation is maximized, and the trees and indigenous ground plantings provide a modified microclimate condition near to the building elements and its enclosed circulation arteries. The new hospital has a 53,800 square foot roofscape and a connecting semi-circular rooftop path is directly above an interior corridor on the level below. The Meyer Children's Hospital is perhaps the most ambitious of the five demonstration hospitals in sustainable healthcare architecture built since 2005 within the aegis of the European Union (EU) Hospitals Demonstration Project (Figure 8.9.1).

Building/unit

The facility is four levels in height and these are referred to as Level -1 (basement), Level 0 (main level), Level 1, and Level 2. The building features an energy efficient envelope, including enhanced thermal wall insulation. Occupants are in constant visual contact with the exterior via the radial-shaped circulation arteries. A galleria creates a large central courtyard with the villa at its center, on axis. Vertical circulation nodes connect to a linear circulation spine spanning its full length (Figure 8.9.2). The lower (Level -1) and main level (Level 0) house the administration, general hospital support services, and outpatient clinics, and connect to the main public arrival axis and promenade. Level 1 houses specialized outpatient and inpatient clinics, rehabilitation services, research units, and additional central support. The uppermost level (Level 2) houses inpatient housing, nursing and family support (Figure 8.9.3). The complexity of the site's topography and its intricate interplay with the various *floor trays* is evident throughout the interior.

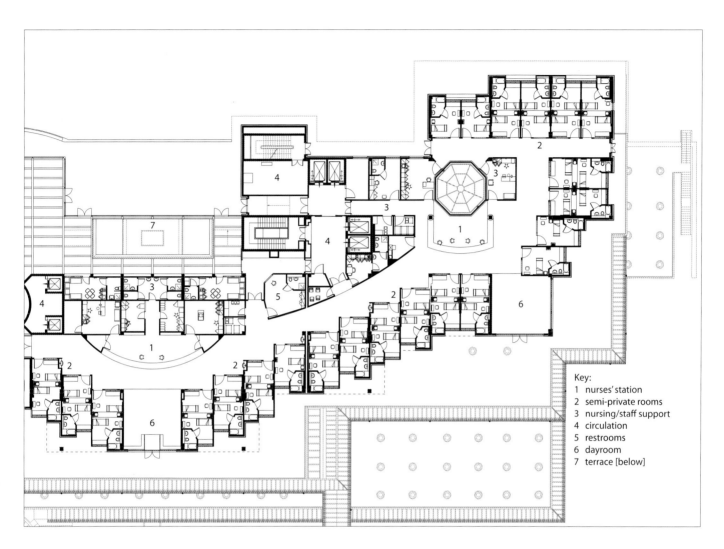

Level 2 PCU [Typical Unit]

Key:
1 nurses' station
2 semi-private rooms
3 nursing/staff support
4 circulation
5 restrooms
6 dayroom
7 terrace [below]

8.9.3 Level 2 inpatient rooms are arrayed in a stepped pattern, opening onto a common terrace. The bath/shower room is on the outboard side. A semi-radial nurses station is at the center, facing a dayroom. A second dayroom is at the end of the unit, slotted between patient rooms

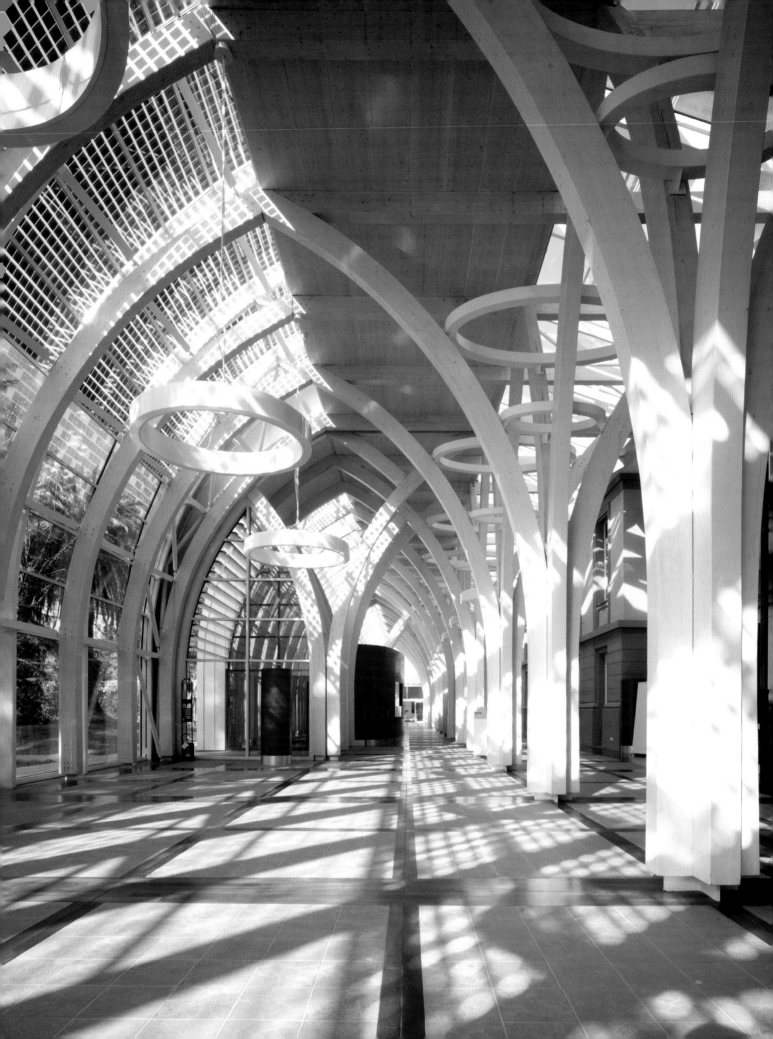

8.9.4 The galleria promenade, with its ribbed, vaulted ceiling, functions as a 'Main Street', providing year-round enclosure and views of the landscaped grounds

The historic buildings on the site were built at varying elevations and the new facility's circulation network carefully negotiated these differences. The central galleria also serves as a social reception area (Figure 8.9.4). At night its glow reaffirms its civic presence. The central information station is housed as a freestanding element within this space, and a commercial arcade is located nearby. This commercial component is featured in numerous recent urban hospitals in Europe (Figure 8.9.5) such as the mall in the main 'city level' of the new public hospital in Groningen, the Netherlands (2000–2004). There, a superblock houses outpatient clinics, health-related commercial shops, restaurants, clothing stores, and cafes (see Chapter 7).

At Meyer Children's Hospital, three skylights and light tubes transmit natural light to the lowest level of the building envelope. These also function as visual landmarks in wayfinding and as colorful sculptures. The three 'sun pipes' were incorporated in a manner whereby each one transmits/injects daylight three floors deep into the building envelope into circulation spaces that would otherwise receive no direct natural daylight – thereby greatly reducing the need for artificial illumination during the day (Figure 8.9.6). The uppermost floor trays feature a glass roof with light filled offices and spaces for research and consultation (Figure 8.9.7). The inpatient housing realm (Level 2) is stepped back, in plan. Most rooms are semi-private (2-bed) while a number of private rooms are provided for patients requiring isolation. Bath/shower rooms are positioned on the outboard side of the inpatient rooms. Unfortunately, this decision cuts off daylight and a significant portion of the direct view to the outside from the patient's bed. However, an unobstructed view is possible from the corridor, into the inpatient rooms. The nursing station is located at the center of each PCU. The stepped pattern of the inpatient rooms yields a sawtooth roof form and its overhangs in turn yield exterior space partially shaded from the elements. This space is for use by patients and their families (Figure 8.9.8).

Meyer Children's Hospital is also innovative in its use of applied photovoltaic technology. A centralized environmental control system monitors and preselects the appropriate ambient temperature and humidity levels. This has resulted in a 35 percent decrease in energy costs. A heat pump (heating and cooling) system is utilized. In addition, the photovoltaic cells are incorporated in the central galleria/solarium. Daylight design strategies provide up to a 36

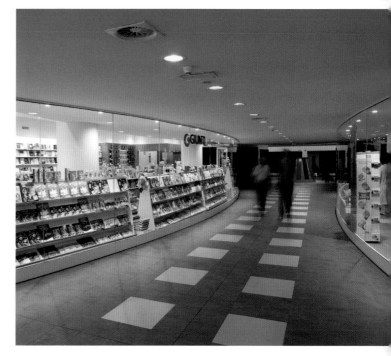

8.9.5 A grocery and a gift shop are located in the galleria promenade

percent life-span cost reduction in lighting energy expenditures compared to conventionally designed hospitals. In terms of the palette of construction materials, low-VOC surface paints were used throughout the interior, as were wood window frames, doors, ceilings and finishes, and copper, in keeping with local vernacular building traditions. Mechanical air conditioning is needed only in certain parts of the hospital. Double-glazed glass was specified throughout many rooms, including skylights, circulation arterial fenestration, and in motorized window screening devices, to control glare and excessive solar gain.

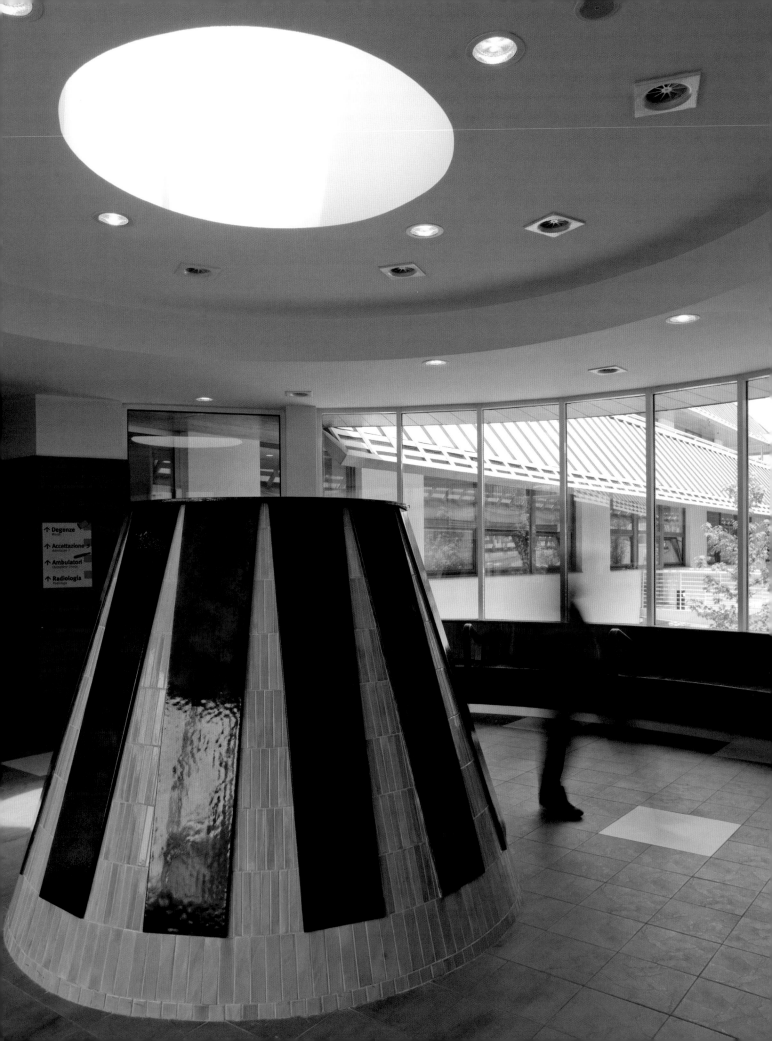

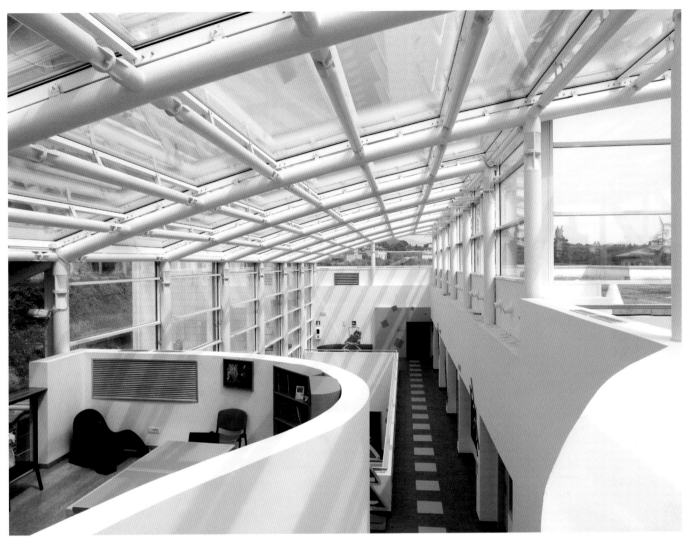

8.9.7 Transparency is emphasized, resulting in a dramatic sense of openness. This administration workspace on an upper level features open plan workstations, a glass roof-wall system, and clerestories

8.9.6 Brightly colored ceramic sculptures are placed at key intervals in the galleria concourse. Each receives daylight via a circular skylight cylinder

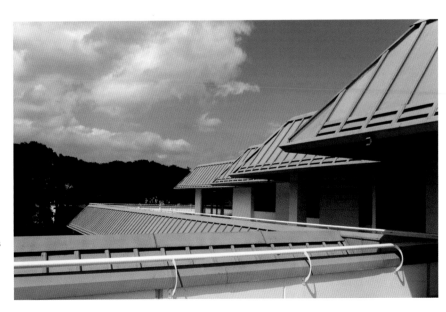

8.9.8 The terrace on the roof allows patients, visitors, and families opportunities to be outdoors while near to their room. Exaggerated roof overhangs provide shade and enclosure

8.10.1 The tower at Dell Children's immediately became an urban landmark when the hospital opened. The campus was built on a brownfield site, formerly a municipal airport

10 Dell Children's Medical Center of Central Texas, Austin, Texas

ARCHITECT/INTERIOR DESIGNER: Karlsberger Architects Planners
    Designers, Columbus, Ohio
LANDSCAPE ARCHITECT: TBG Partners, Austin
CLIENT: Seton Healthcare Network
FEATURED MATERIALS: Reinforced concrete, indigenous sandstone,
    exterior masonry, aluminum, stainless steel, zinc, low-e exterior
    glazing, laminated wood beams and interior panels and finishes
COMPLETED: 2007
INPATIENT BEDS: 169
SITE/PARKING: 32 acres/455
HOSPITAL SIZE: 472,000SF

Context/site

This pediatric hospital is named in honor of The Michael and Susan Dell Foundation, its main benefactor organization. Conceived as a comprehensive children's hospital for Central Texas, it features all private inpatient rooms with family accommodations for use during their child's hospitalization (Figure 8.10.1). The campus was built on the site of the former Robert Mueller Municipal Airport, on a 32-acre parcel that was formerly a 70-acre brownfield site. When Seton Health, the owner, was approached by the City of Austin, the private sector developer leading the master plan process indicated early on that LEED certification was a requirement for every building to be constructed on this 'recycled' site (including all private dwellings to be constructed in the future). The result was the first LEED Platinum Level hospital in the United States. This required innovation from the outset: site planning, landscaping, architecture, interiors, furnishings, and materials, all carefully achieved with sustainability at the forefront of concern.

The planning process involved close collaboration with many local and state regulatory agencies. Without a guiding set of criteria for how to achieve LEED Platinum rating, much extra time and effort was required at every step. A two-day workshop on sustainable design was conducted in Austin with external consultants. The design team and key consultants met on site every four weeks thereafter for the project's duration to assign responsibilities, troubleshoot, and ensure the project was on track in all respects. A LEED point-tracking system was developed to serve as a performance-measuring device. A key 'green' feature is the Combined Heating Power Plant

(CHP) by Austin Energy, the local utility company. Utilizing the most efficient 4.5 megawatt natural gas-fired turbine available, compared to conventional alternatives, the CHP is 75 percent more efficient and generates a far-reduced carbon footprint. The CHP also produces steam as a byproduct, captured as a heating source, and provides chilled water for the hospital through an absorption chiller unit. In addition, power for the CHP is provided by two separate feeds from the local power grid resulting in 100 percent redundancy in power. This therefore eliminates the need for back-up generators and allows the hospital to be fully autonomous in the event of a shutdown of the city's power grid. Natural light and ventilation is transmitted to 80 percent of all interior spaces, as deep as 32 feet into the building envelope. The hospital's two inpatient care pavilions and connecting support spaces feature narrow footprints. Recycled building materials were used whenever feasible, i.e. approximately 47,000 tons of exiting runway asphalt and base material was recycled and re-used on site.

Building/unit

A tower at Dell Children's marks the main entrance and is a local landmark. The hospital is at the center of this new campus, with the CHP and two medical office buildings nearby. The tower is capped with a white Texas 'hat' that to some is more reminiscent of a Catholic nun's head veil and appears as if clipped onto its side. A steel and glass canopy connects to a large atrium. The interior of the atrium features brightly colored panels set in a grid, with residentially scaled siding above. This space houses a gift shop (Figure 8.10.2 and Figure 8.10.3). The gift shop appears to be held in suspension. The space immediately beneath houses the admitting department. The palette of materials featured throughout the facility is highly orchestrated in this space, i.e. Texas field sandstone, natural carpet, polycarbonate wall panels, and wood panels. Daylight filters through the skylights above.

The hospital features six exterior courtyards, two of which are 'enclosed' outdoor courtyards, three levels in height. The panel system, with its tinted glass insets, is reprised here along the courtyard perimeter circulation. This reinforces the theraserialized condition with

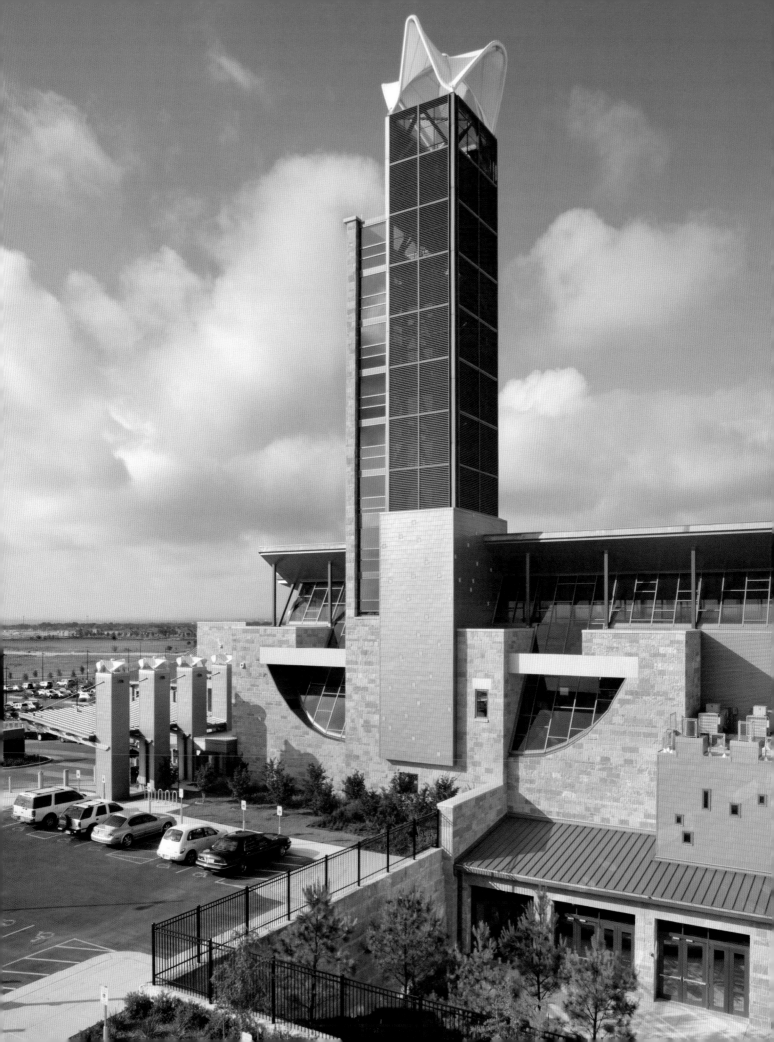

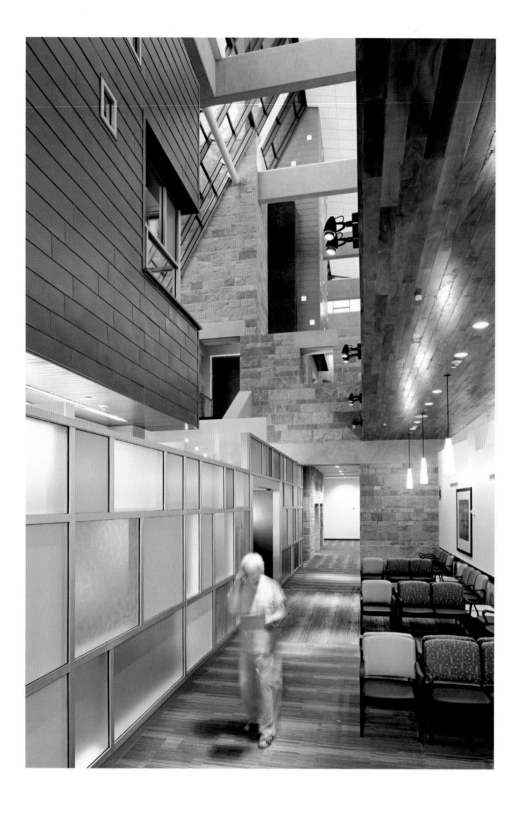

8.10.2 Interior spaces feature Texas limestone and granite, boldly colored polycarbonate panels, and wood. Skylights and clerestories transmit daylight to the interior

8.10.3 In the main atrium, the hospital's gift shop appears as if suspended above an administration area

the adjoining exterior spaces, and also provides a navigational aid. The door to each courtyard is accentuated with irregularly shaped fenestration (Figure 8.10.4). The courtyards are landscaped and include a retention pond, seating, and trellises. The curvature of the inpatient PCU pavilions is accentuated against the rectilinearity of the main element. The arrival axis runs through the hospital, and this creates two asymmetrical zones (Figure 8.10.5 and Figure 8.10.6).

The majority of support functions, diagnostic and treatment areas, and the central administration are housed on Level 1. Inpatient care units are housed on the first, second, and third levels of the pavilions (Figure 8.10.7). The nursing station is at the center of the unit and is also radial, with circular recessed ceilings and cove lighting reinforcing its form, with a sunburst floor tile pattern further reinforcing the overall effect. Staff lounges are located in the corner

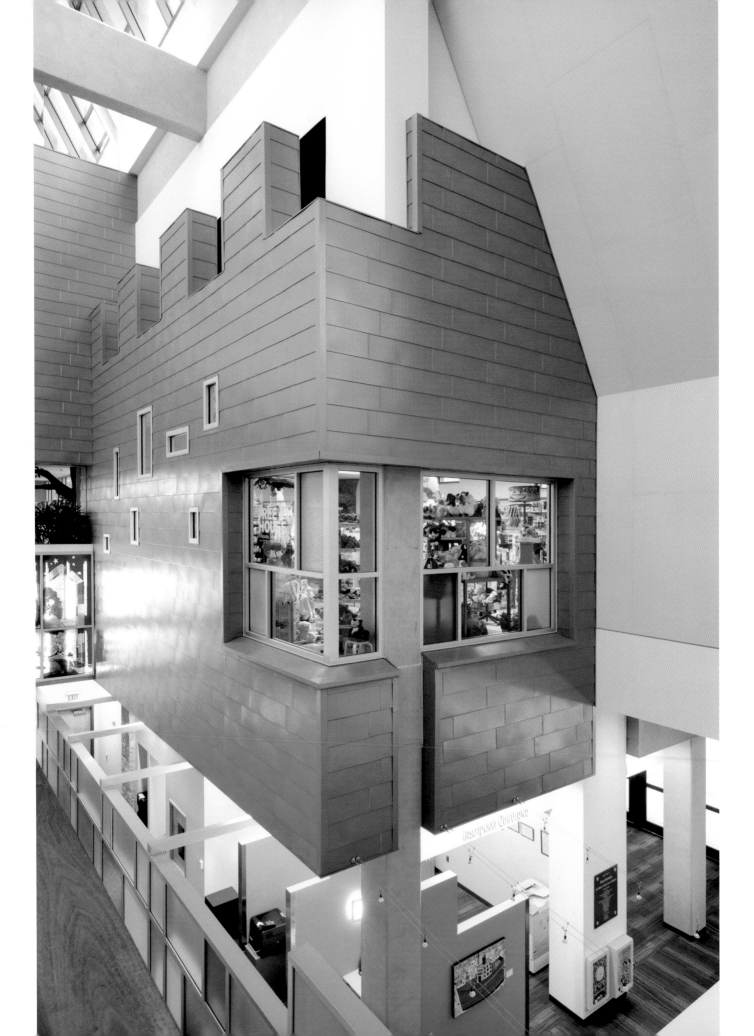

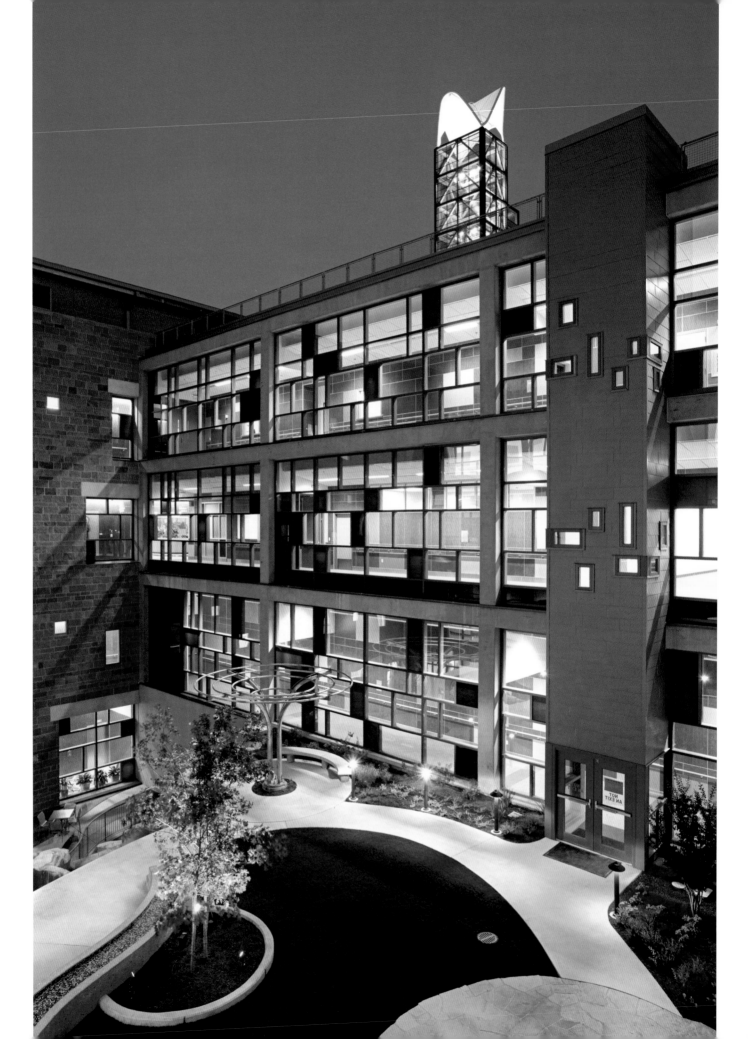

8.10.4 The courtyards reveal a highly articulated fenestration pattern of tinted inset, fixed vision, and operable panels. The tower, illuminated at night, is visible in the background. Landscaped paths are visible in the foreground

8.10.5 Core hospital functions are housed on Level 1. Central support and two ICUs are housed on Level 2. Levels 3 and 4 house radial-shaped inpatient care units and nursing support. The central pharmacy and laboratory are on Level 4

Key:
1 courtyard
2 surgical suites
3 staff parking
4 ICU 1
5 ICU 2
6 support
7 outpatient services
8 imaging
9 administration
10 waiting area

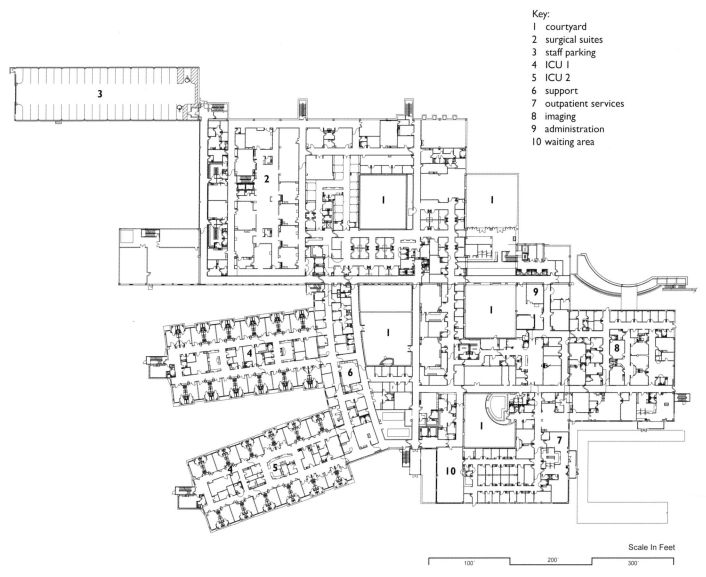

Scale In Feet

100'   200'   300'

Level 2

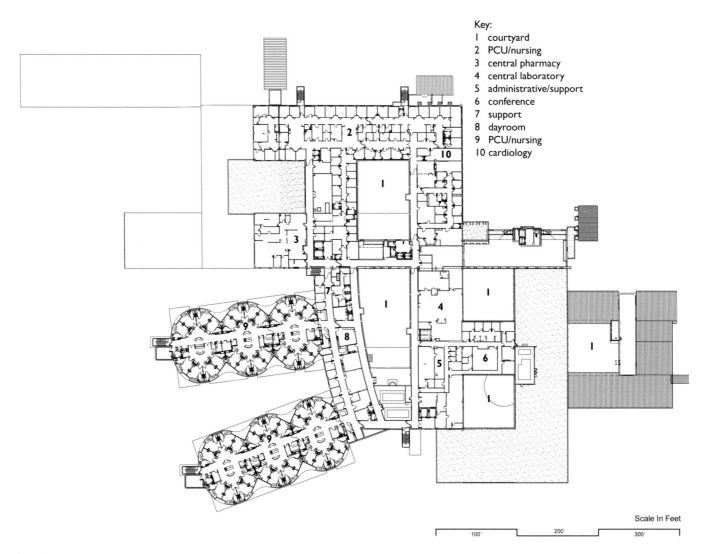

Key:
1 courtyard
2 PCU/nursing
3 central pharmacy
4 central laboratory
5 administrative/support
6 conference
7 support
8 dayroom
9 PCU/nursing
10 cardiology

Scale In Feet

100'   200'   300'

Level 4

8.10.6 Level 2 and Level 3 house semi-radial
inpatient care units, an L-shaped inpatient care
unit, and nursing support

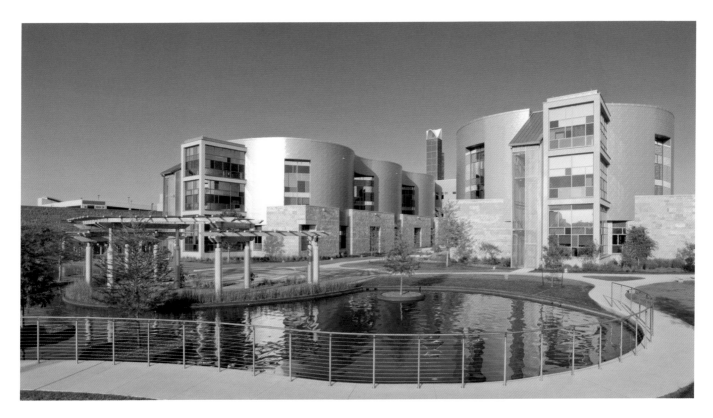

8.10.7 Winding paths correspond to the configuration of a retention pond, with trellises, seating, and gardens. Semi-radial nursing units are expressed on the exterior

of each PCU; these afford full views to the outdoors. The all-private (1-bed) inpatient rooms feature full height windows that are operable, artwork, residential furnishings, a built-in laminate wood veneer desk, and storage closet. The television is perched on a shelf above this desk, and the bath/shower room door is immediately to the left of the desk (Figure 8.10.8).

The building is made of 40 percent fly ash as a substitute for conventional Portland cement, resulting in a reduced carbon footprint. Paints and adhesives with low or no volatile organic content were selected. The flooring is of natural linoleum, and the carpet is 100 percent recycled material (its backing is made of recycled plastic bottles). Dell's innovative HVAC and electrical systems yield significant energy cost savings annually. It is estimated that this translates into enough energy to power 180 private dwellings in the metro Austin area annually. Additional savings were realized by decentralizing the air handling units, using a high-reflectivity roof surface, an under-floor air distribution system, external egress stairways, low-flow plumbing fixtures, motion-detecting light fixtures, heat recovery systems, and the planting of one new tree per every four parking spaces. This reduces the heat island effect during hot Texas summers. Xeriscaping (dry landscape) eliminates the need for conventional irrigation. The sloping roof was designed to house photovoltaic panels, but cost constraints precluded their installation. Locally, Dell Children's promotes its civic role as an environmental steward.

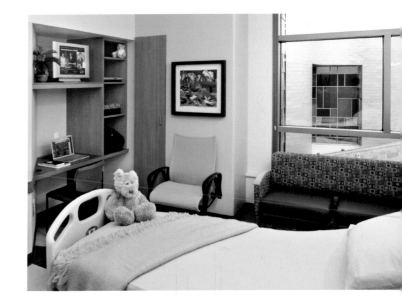

8.10.8 Patient rooms have built-in desks, storage units, multiple lighting options, operable windows, artwork, and adaptable furnishings

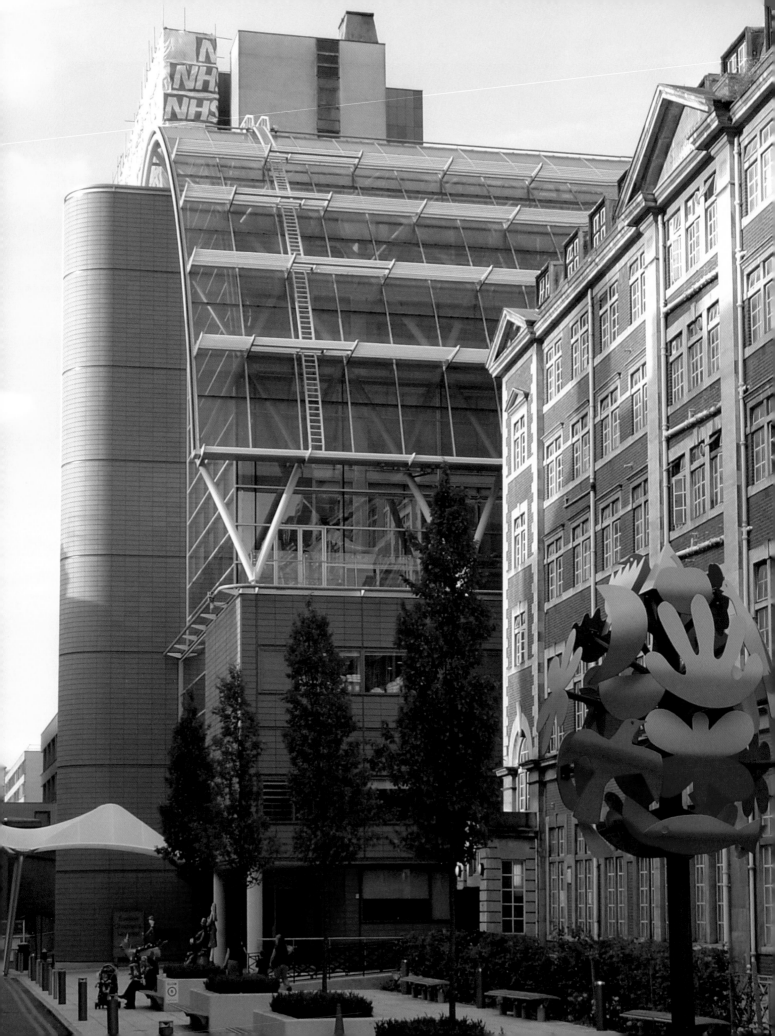

11 Evelina Children's Hospital, London, UK

ARCHITECT: Hopkins Architects, London
LANDSCAPE ARCHITECT: Hopkins Architects, London
CLIENT: Guy's and St. Thomas' National Health Service (NHS) Foundation Trust
FEATURED MATERIALS: Masonry, reinforced concrete, structural steel system, aluminum, low-e glazing systems, wood and laminate interior finishes and surfaces
COMPLETED: 2005
INPATIENT BEDS: 140
SITE/PARKING: 5.5 acres/N/A
HOSPITAL SIZE: 232,400

Context/site

Evelina Children's Hospital is London's first new children's hospital in more than a century. Baron Ferdinand de Rothschild, after the death of his wife Evelina, who died in childbirth, founded the original Evelina Children's in Southwark in 1869. It was merged with the children's hospital at Guy's Hospital in 1948 and it closed its doors in 1973 when inpatients and services were moved to the newly built tower at Guy's Hospital. The new Evelina was built on a narrow, rectangular portion of the historic site of St. Thomas' Hospital (see Chapter 2) and draws together the majority of Guy's and St. Thomas' child and adolescent care programs under one roof. The hospital was made possible by a grant of £50 million from the two hospitals' charities and a £10 million amount provided by the NHS. It serves children in the boroughs of Lambeth and Southwark as well as offering specialist care for children and adolescents from across southeast England and further afield (including internationally). The design process involved patients, their families, and input from staff. Patients did not want a hospital with long dreary corridors, or bedrooms that closed them off from other parts of the hospital or from visual contact with the outdoors. The administration, for its part, did not want merely another 'landmark' building on a landmark site, and stressed it should not look or feel like a hospital at all (Figure 8.11.1).

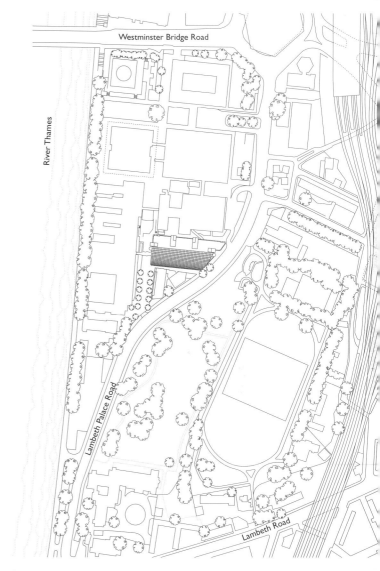

Site Plan

8.11.2 The north side of the hospital faces Lambeth Palace Road. It was decided early on that this roadway would not be the main point of entry

8.11.1 Evelina Children's Hospital makes effective use of its infill site. An arrival plaza contains works of art and invites use by persons from adjacent medical institutions

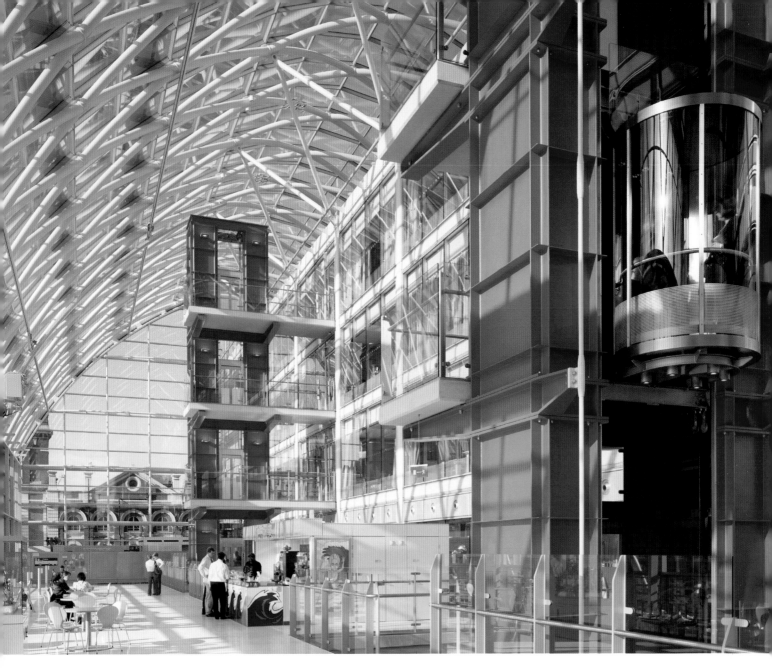

8.11.3 The parti' is defined by an expansive atrium/
conservatory spanning the 100m length of the site,
rising to four levels, above a three level base

Building/unit:

Evelina Children's infill site posed a challenge. The site is hemmed in
by an access drive on the south side nearest to the Thames River; this
drive separates Evelina Children's from St. Thomas' former inpatient
pavilions. Older buildings to either side appear to 'squeeze' the new
hospital and its arrival plaza and drop-off zone, and a fabric-covered
canopy. A colorful sculpture announces the hospital's presence and
serves as a navigational aid. The north elevation faces Lambeth
Palace Road although this is not its entry portal (Figure 8.11.2).
The building's parti' features an expansive atrium/conservatory that
spans the entire 100m length of the site and rises to four levels in

height above a three level base. The inpatient tower and related
functions are housed in a separate seven-level tower, somewhat
compositionally autonomous from the adjacent support base (Figure
8.11.3 and Figure 8.11.4). The south-facing atrium roof transmits
daylight into the interior. The hospital is colorful, with light-filled
spaces and a high level of transparency internally and in terms of
its visual openness when viewed from outside. Brightly colored
sculptures are located in the base, which houses arrival, admitting,
administration and outpatient clinics (Figure 8.11.5).

A wide circulation path connects waiting areas and offices to
either side. The inpatient levels feature a serpentine circulation
path, rejecting outright needlessly long, dark, sterile corridors. This

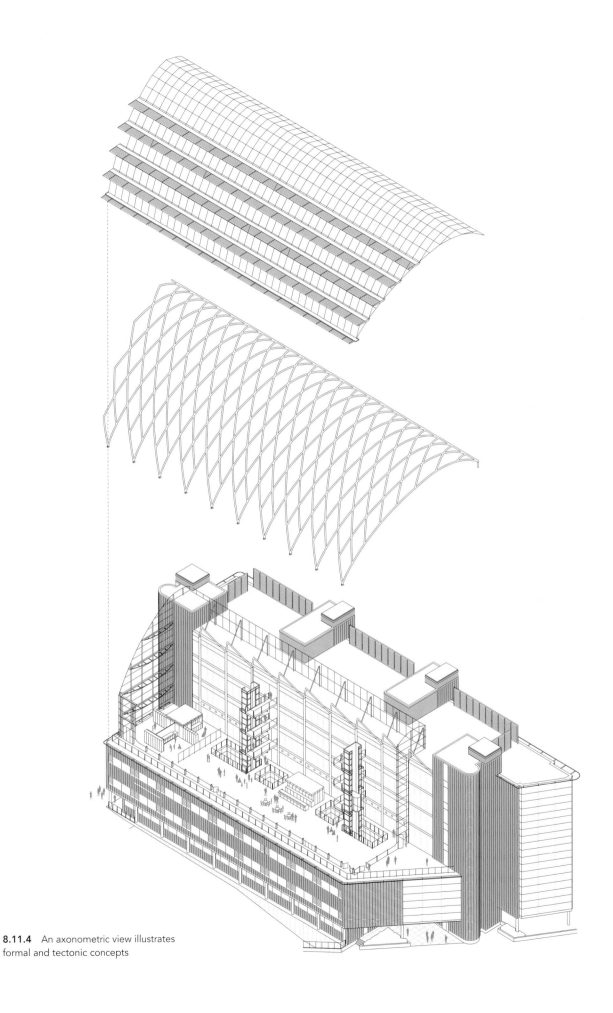

8.11.4 An axonometric view illustrates formal and tectonic concepts

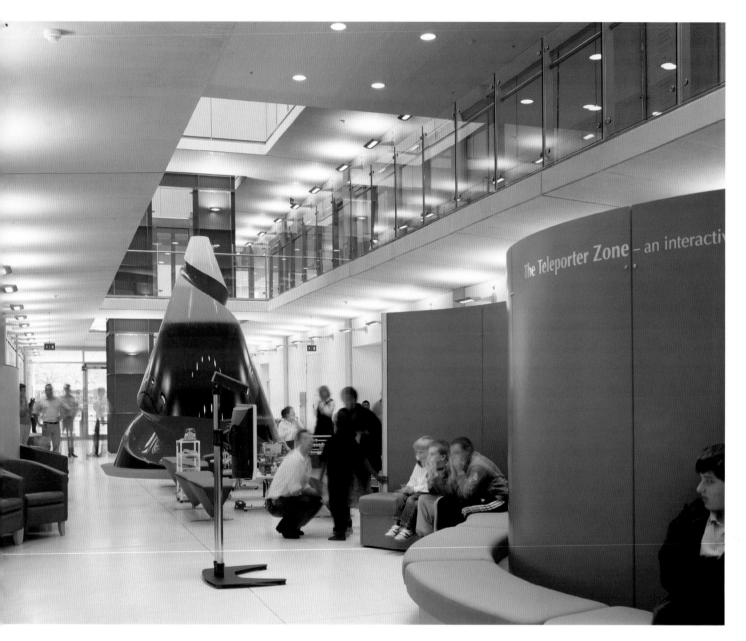

8.11.5 A public concourse houses outpatient clinics, admitting, administration, and waiting spaces, with colorful works of art that invite child's play

path is bisected by inpatient rooms configured as suites of six beds, four beds, and private rooms (Figure 8.11.6). Most patient rooms overlook the large atrium and provide views to the city beyond. The uppermost levels afford spectacular views out to the city.

The elevator lifts are coded in bright red, and are visible from within the large space and from the exterior, transporting occupants up through the four levels of the main atrium/conservatory. A children's activity space is provided on the second level (Figure 8.11.7). Throughout, animated, colorful artwork and sculpture create a welcoming atmosphere. Each floor is coded by means of one of seven elemental symbols drawn from nature – from ocean to beach to savannah and sky. This visual strategy precluded the need for a complex multi-lingual directional signage system (nearly 140 different languages are spoken by local patients and their families). Evelina features diverse play activity areas, as well as a 17-foot high 'helter skelter' structure in the outpatient department waiting room.

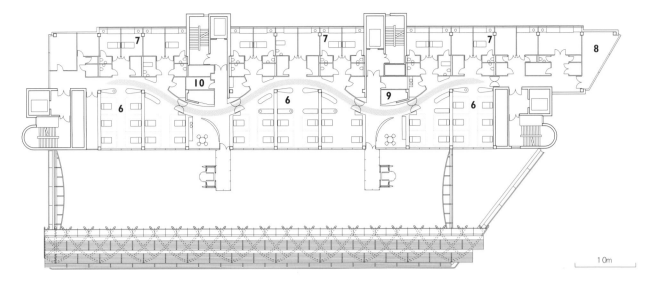

Level 4

10m

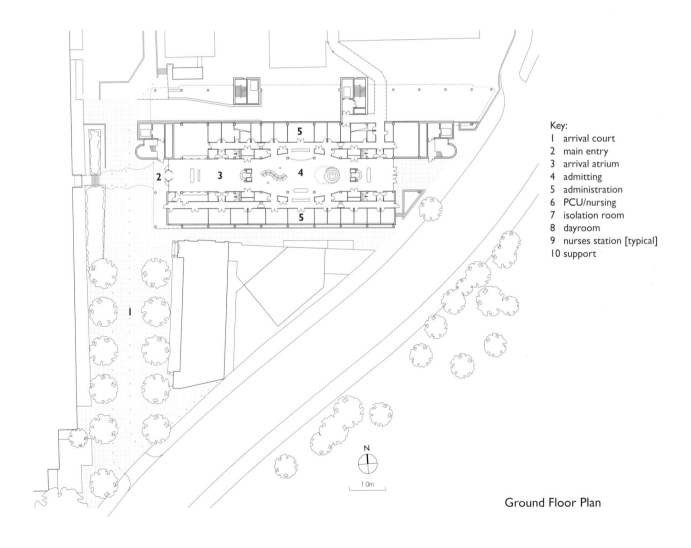

Key:
1 arrival court
2 main entry
3 arrival atrium
4 admitting
5 administration
6 PCU/nursing
7 isolation room
8 dayroom
9 nurses station [typical]
10 support

N

10m

Ground Floor Plan

8.11.6 Circulation spaces are of high priority throughout
Evelina Children's Hospital. The goal was to eschew
the monotonous, drab corridors of the typical machine
megahospital

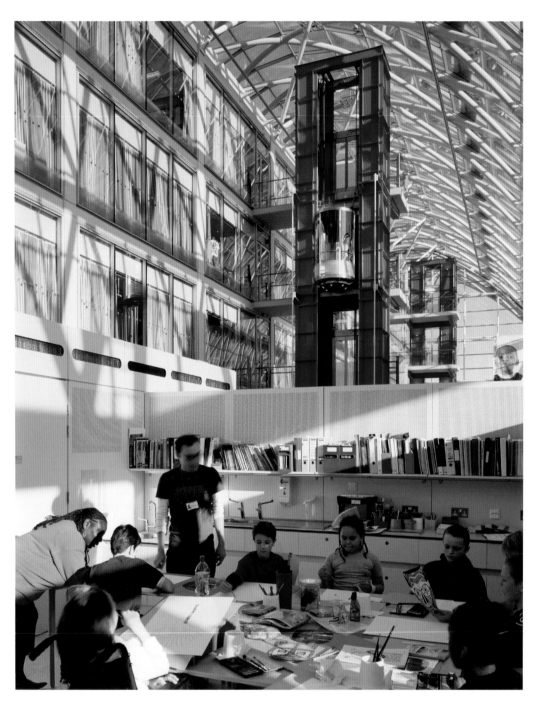

8.11.7 Children's activity areas are loft-like, deployed in trays throughout the atrium/conservatory

Inpatient rooms feature full height windows, wood paneled headwalls, and a personalized TV/media pod at bedside (Figure 8.11.8 and Figure 8.11.9). A nursing station is housed within each 4-bed and 6-bed inpatient suite. A spatial hierarchy was established between the suites, the undulating circulation path, and the private rooms. The floor surfaces are encoded with colorful, animated patterns including a large sphere at the unit entry and at the intersection with the inpatient suites. A semi-private bath/shower room is located across from the bed area. Patients and families are pleased with Evelina, and staff recruitment and retention has not been a problem in this new urban hospital in the heart of London.

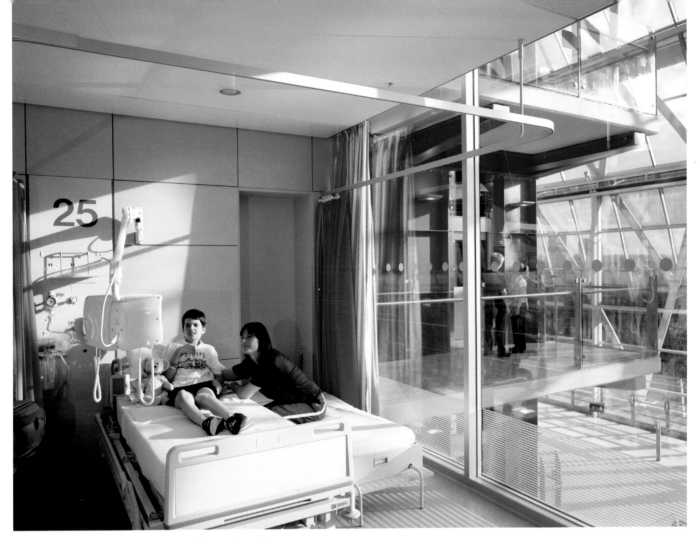

8.11.8 Transparency and anti-institutionalism is achieved. Patients are able to look out into the atrium from their room, or can elect to close the curtains to attain privacy

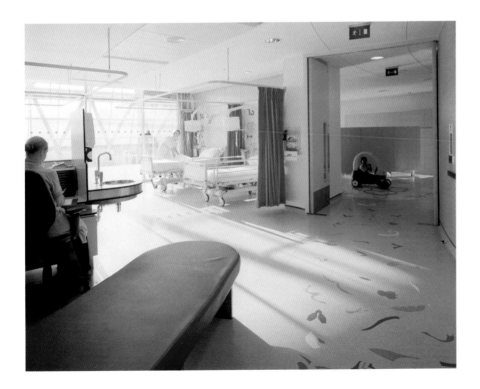

8.11.9 Staff workstations are dispersed throughout the inpatient care units, and colorful flooring and wall surfaces are featured. Natural daylight contributes greatly to a sense of openness

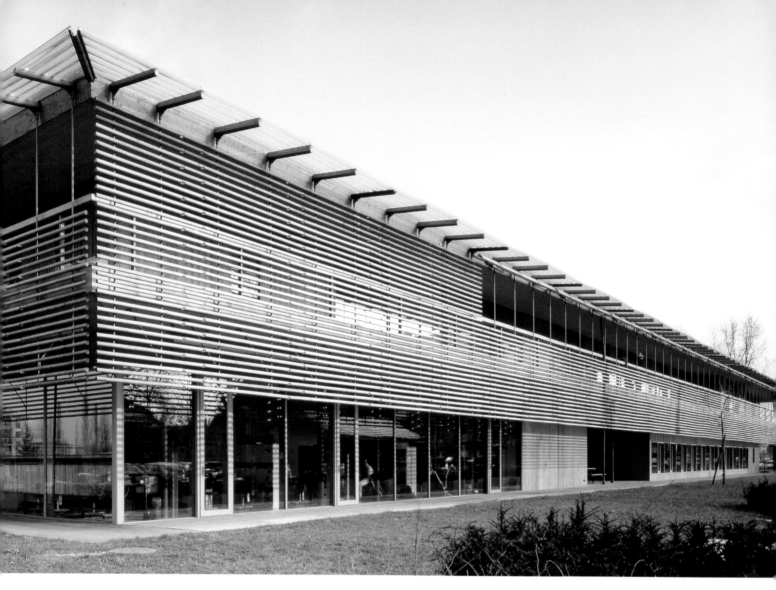

8.12.1 REHAB Basel achieves *lightness of form* by means of its siting, layered exterior sunscreens, roof plates, and a pervasive formal transparency

12 REHAB Basel Centre for Spinal Cord and Brain Injuries, Basel, Switzerland

ARCHITECT: Herzog & de Meuron, Basel, Switzerland
LANDSCAPE ARCHITECT: August Künzel, Binningen, Switzerland
CLIENT: REHAB Basel AG, Switzerland
FEATURED MATERIALS: Wood exterior cladding and decking (untreated oak, larch, ironwood, and waxed pine), steel structural system, masonry, aluminum, low-e glazing, laminated beams, fabric window shades, wood screens, wall panels, sealed oak floors
COMPLETED: 2002
INPATIENT BEDS: 92
SITE/PARKING: 6 acres/200
HOSPITAL SIZE: 246,386SF

Context/site

REHAB Basel is a private treatment center that provides inpatient and outpatient care for persons with spinal cord and brain injuries. It was the winning submission in a design competition held in 1998. In the architects' words,

> The client's express wish, from the beginning, was not to have the new REHAB center look or feel like a hospital. So … what is a hospital? Elevators and corridors, flanked by countless doors leading to patient rooms and examination rooms, a waiting lounge at the end of the hall or next to the elevator. The same pattern repeated on as many floors as permitted by zoning regulations – an economic solution because it is repetitive to the extreme, and requires no modification of staff

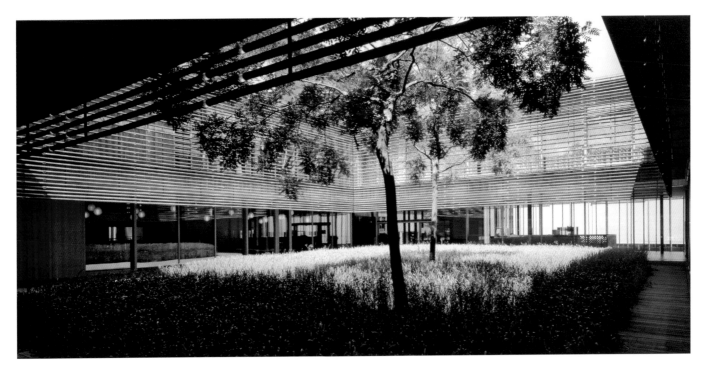

8.12.2 Spaces are hierarchically articulated in an A/B A/B pattern. The main courtyard, shown here, affords respite from a world beyond

behavior. A rehabilitation center is a place where people live for up to 18 months, usually after an accident. It is a place where they learn to cope with their changed lives in order to become as independent as possible again ... Because patients are so restricted, they have to stay ... we have set ourselves the task of designing a multifunctional, diversified building, almost like a small town with streets, plazas, gardens, public facilities, and with more secluded residential quarters where occupants may take different paths to move from A to B ... allowing the patient as much autonomy as possible.

(Architects' brief, 1998)

Its landscape context creates the appearance of timelessness – almost as if it were a reclaimed ruin. It is a low maintenance xeriscape with indigenous grasses, trees, and other species typically found on the open prairie – existing in an urban fringe setting. Oak-fabricated

brisesoleils cover the upper portion of the building, capped with a horizontal overhang/sunscreen (Figure 8.12.1). To the north of the facility a playing field and training course are available for therapeutic exercise activity (Figure 8.12.2).

Building/unit

The REHAB Basel Center is a horizontal building with a ground level and two levels above, and a roofscape with a terrace for patient and family use, conference room, staff exercise room, and overnight sleeping accommodations. All inpatient beds are located on a single level and located around the building perimeter, with ancillary, therapy treatment, and staff functions clustered around five interior courtyards (Figure 8.12.3a–b). This facilitates greater access and fosters an informal, residentialist atmosphere. It is a

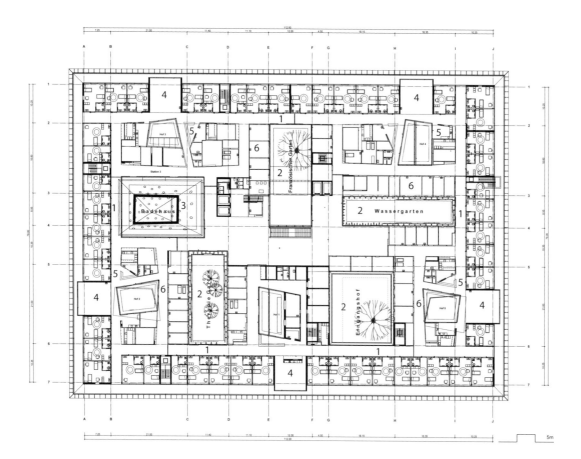

Level 2

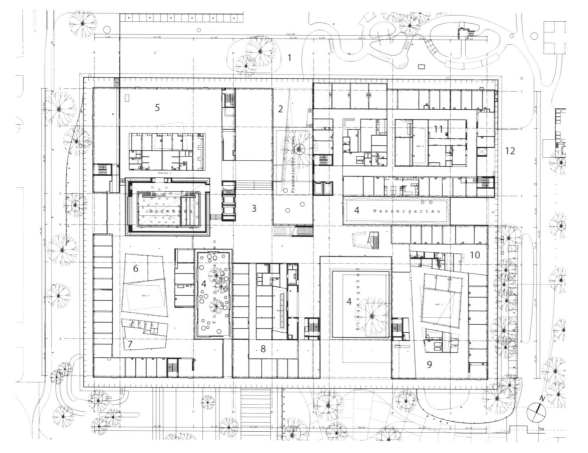

Ground Level

8.12.3 Semi-private inpatient rooms are on the uppermost level at the perimeter of the envelope. Nursing care and therapeutic support is clustered in spaces adjacent to 'interior' courtyards, each of which functions as an outdoor room in its own right

8.12.4 Inpatient rooms feature a circular skylight at the center and a fully glazed perimeter wall. A sliding glass door affords access to a semi-private terrace

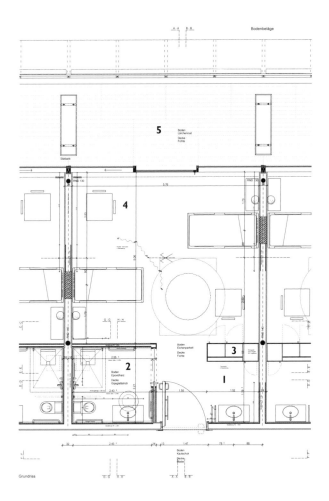

Key:
1   handwash
2   bath/shower
3   storage/supply
4   family area
5   exterior terrace

Typical Patient Room

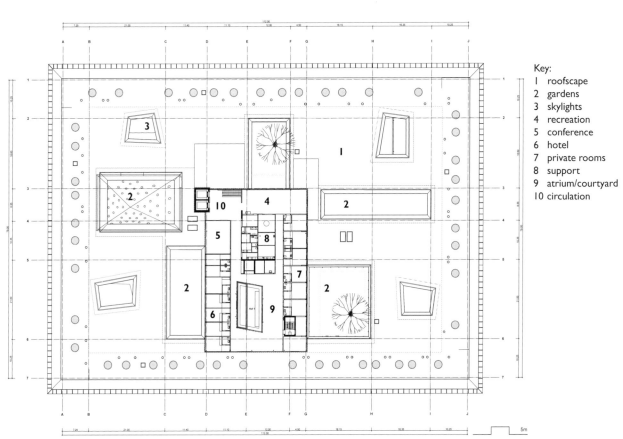

Key:
1   roofscape
2   gardens
3   skylights
4   recreation
5   conference
6   hotel
7   private rooms
8   support
9   atrium/courtyard
10 circulation

5m

Roofscape Level

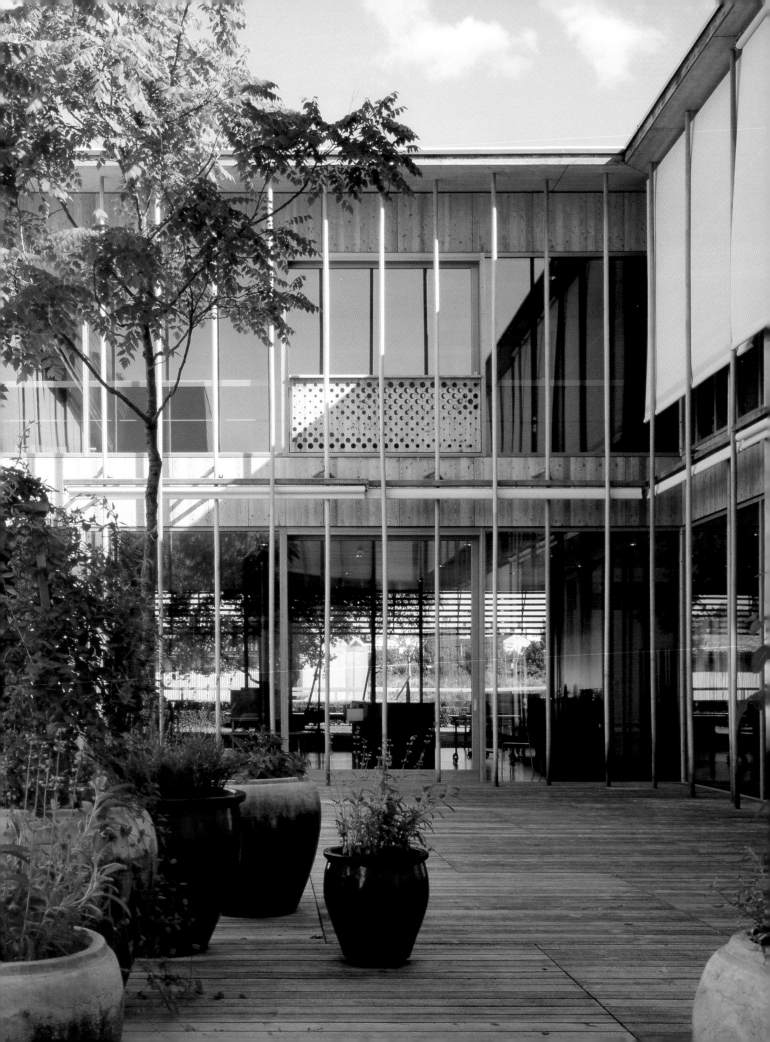

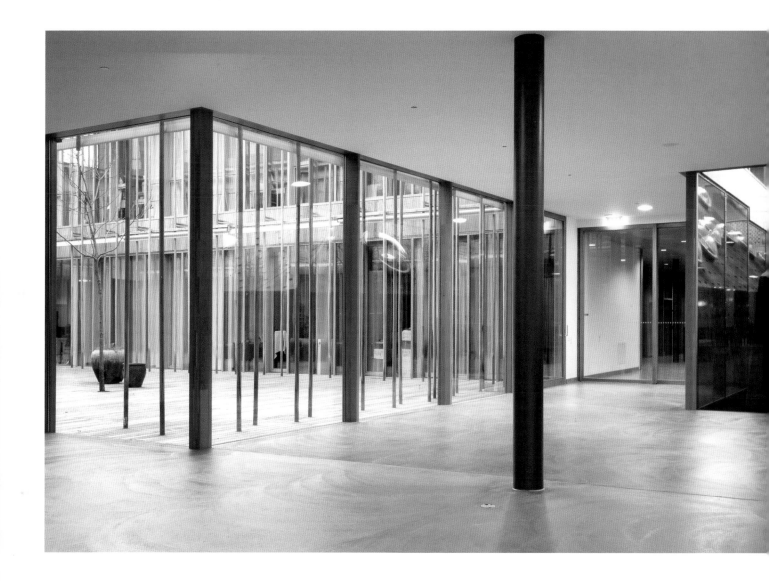

8.12.5 Wood is featured, including courtyards and on the roof terrace. Note the exterior-mounted sunscreens

8.12.6 The intent was for exterior space to be in view from the moment one enters this microcosm of a small village, with its streetscapes and volumes deployed within a single, superordinate structural grid/frame

barrier-free environment from the ground level to the roof – ramps and elevators accommodate horizontal and vertical circulation in a highly visible yet transparent manner – another stark departure from most hospitals (Figure 8.12.4). Connectivity between the interior and exterior realms was a primary design objective. This structure/village is conceived from inside out: instead of an arrangement of discrete departments, the courtyards are positioned informally within a single large rectangular volume. Through a reductive/additive carving out of this volume, courtyards were created which serve as devices for aiding spatial orientation and navigation as much as to draw in natural light and fresh air. Each courtyard corresponds to a particular therapy treatment area (Figure 8.12.5). Transitions between various exterior and interior paces are seamless, organic, and serialized. For this, REHAB Basil is a strong example of *theraserialization* (see Chapter 3 and Chapter 7). Administration and therapy treatment areas are housed on the main level (Figure 8.12.6).

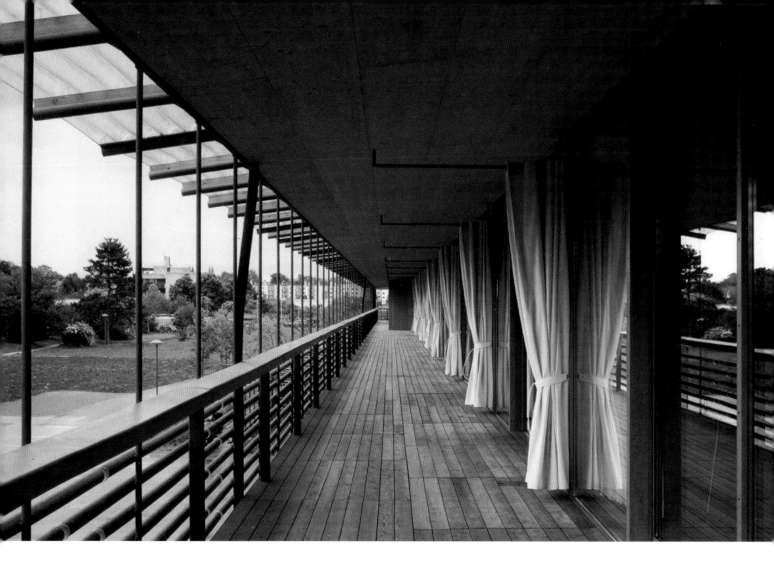

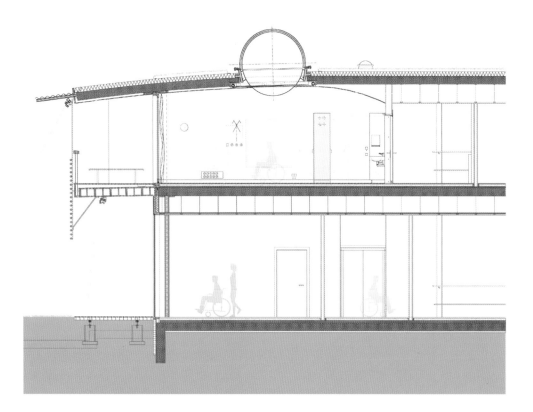

8.12.7 Curtains are provided on the exterior side of the window wall along the length of the terrace, on the inpatient housing level

8.12.8 In section, the spherical sky-dome is shown in relation to the patient room and exterior terrace

8.12.9 A roof terrace provides a conference room, dormitory rooms for overnight visitors, wood decking, and seating, trees, a garden, and expansive views

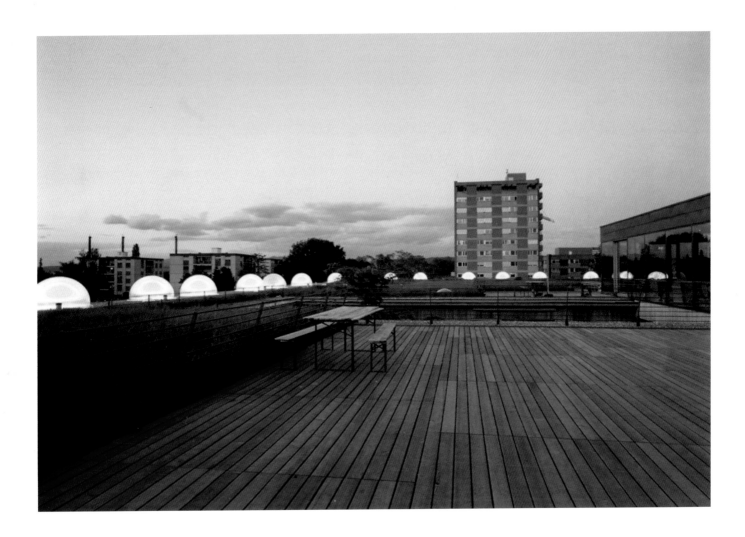

In keeping with the metaphor of the village, streets and plazas were articulated within a single orthogonal volume. One enters the facility through a large central courtyard that doubles as a *landscaped room*. One open space is filled with water, another clad entirely in wood, a bathhouse occupies a third, and so on. Circulation flows through and around a series of mass/void 'events', and large windows afford views of the surrounding landscape. A seamless transition between indoors and outdoors is achieved. In other cases, spaces are inward-oriented: the most extreme example is the bathhouse, located within one open court like 'an erratic block wrapped in black rubber' (Architects' brief). Options exist for personal respite, privacy, and social interaction. Small informal spaces are available for meetings and consultations.

Various species of wood are featured on the facade and in interior spaces. Continuous horizontal wood decking on the building's perimeter provides solar shading. This veranda allows for patients in bed to be wheeled directly outside through large, sliding glass doors. Intricate lattice structures fabricated of wood rods guide fabric screens for visual privacy and thermal comfort. Interestingly (and counter intuitively) these window curtains were installed on the exterior side of the window wall (Figure 8.12.7). A transparent plastic sphere-dome dominates the ceiling of each inpatient room, two meters in diameter: this device eliminates the need for artificial

light sources during the day. This device also affords the patient in a supine position in bed the opportunity to view directly up to the sky (Figure 8.12.8). The skylights supplements daylight entering from the perimeter window wall/door. Windows are operable in the inpatient rooms and elsewhere in the facility. On the roof, the view is of the city and in the other direction outward towards the Alsace Mountains. This roofscape, with its wood deck surface, promotes use by occupants, filters rainwater for reuse on site, and also provides added thermal insulation (Figure 8.12.9). The building features materials applied in their untreated 'natural' state. Passive solar techniques are expressed in wide roof overhangs, the screening system, and shallow floor depths of interior volumes.

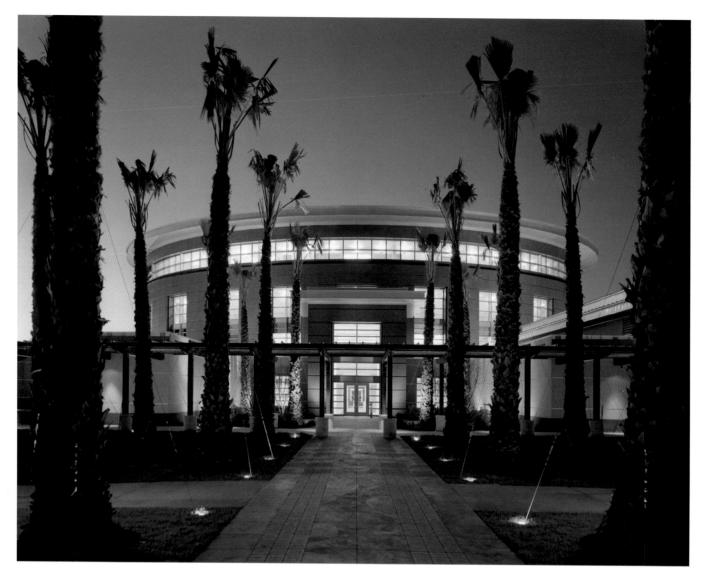

8.13.1 The Center for the Intrepid establishes a striking presence largely due to its elliptical configuration

13 Center for the Intrepid – National Armed Forces Physical Rehabilitation Center, San Antonio, Texas

ARCHITECT: SmithGroup, Washington, D.C.

LANDSCAPE ARCHITECT: SmithGroup

CLIENT: United States Army/National Armed Forces Academy

FEATURED MATERIALS: Structural steel system, reinforced concrete, stainless steel, stone exterior cladding, aluminum, low-e exterior glazing, polylaminate surfaces

COMPLETED: 2007

INPATIENT BEDS: Shared campus with an adjacent 170–bed military rehabilitation hospital

SITE/PARKING: 12 acres/145

HOSPITAL SIZE: 65,000SF

Context/site

Since the Iraq War began in 2002, more than 48,000 U.S. troops have been wounded in the field of combat. To meet an urgent and growing need for the care and rehabilitation of wounded soldiers returning home for treatment, an interdisciplinary team of advanced specialist banded together to construct a state-of-the-art rehabilitation center for armed forces combat veterans. The Center for the Intrepid was designed and built in a period of only eighteen months. Designed as a bold, enduring, national symbol of the sacrifices of Americans who have served in this unpopular war and others, this stone-clad, elliptically configured rehabilitation facility symbolizes the hope that can be instilled in the wounded returning veteran to strive toward a promising future. The Center for the Intrepid was created for individuals returning with severe injuries, such as amputations, burns, and head trauma. The facility provides a range of high-tech therapy

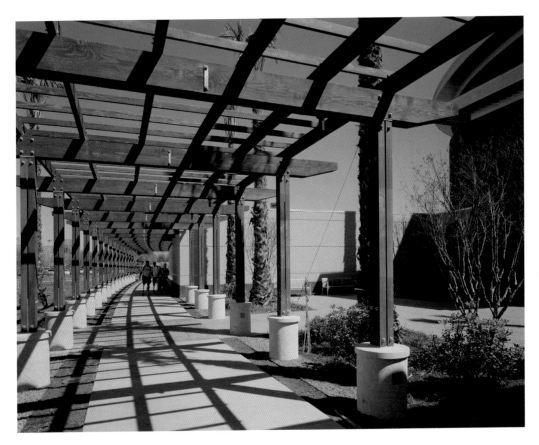

8.13.2 A sidewalk and trellis connects with adjacent buildings on a large military campus

programs based on recent advancements in military medicine. The Center was built on the campus of an existing military hospital in San Antonio. Its elliptical parti' takes on an otherworldly appearance when viewed at certain times of the day and night (Figure 8.13.1).

A thin ribbon of clerestoried windows wraps the facility. The effect is as if the roof hovers atop a platform base structure, especially when viewed at night. The palm trees lining the arrival sequence contribute to its surreal imagery. Near the main entry, a wood trellis structure passes directly in front. This covered walkway will in time be covered in dense vegetation. It is a circulation conduit to nearby buildings on the campus and is used for outdoor physical therapy sessions (Figure 8.13.2).

Building/unit

The four-level Center for the Intrepid houses the most sophisticated amputee rehabilitation technology that exists at this time. Laboratories and therapy treatment spaces are provided for advanced prosthetics, computerized video monitoring for biomechanical research and its application, virtual reality simulators of ADL (Activities of Daily Living) regimens, robotic engineering and nanotechnology applications, and physical movement simulators. The Center for the Intrepid also provides specialized therapy labs for prosthetic fittings and adjustments, consultation and examination rooms, psychotherapy, re-socialization therapy, clinical nutritional therapy, physical and occupational therapy, gait studies, speech therapy, telemedicine, and a physical medicine and rehabilitation research center.

The ground level entrance axis penetrates through the entire parti', allowing direct visual access into adjoining therapy and supports paces.

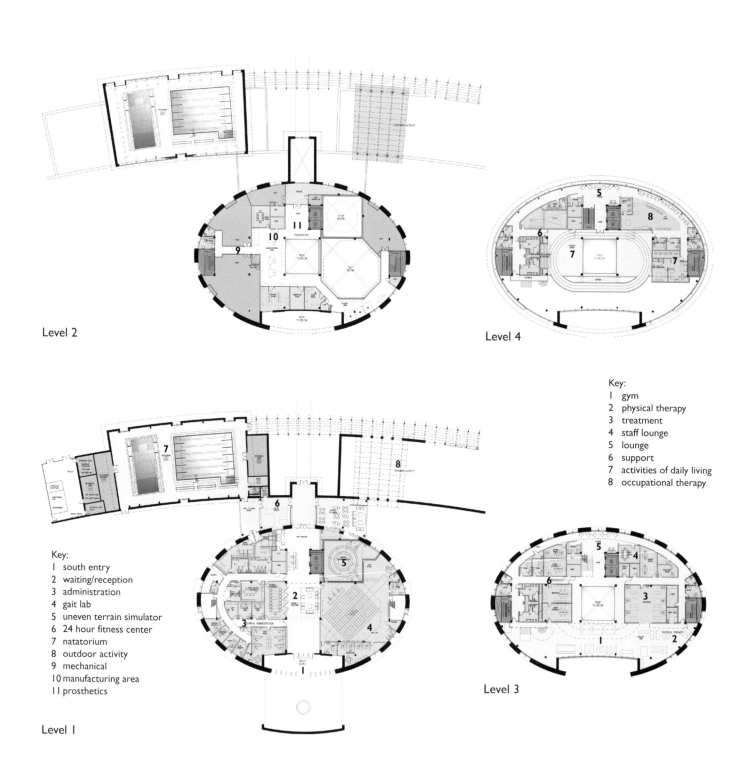

Level 2

Level 4

Level 1

Key:
1 south entry
2 waiting/reception
3 administration
4 gait lab
5 uneven terrain simulator
6 24 hour fitness center
7 natatorium
8 outdoor activity
9 mechanical
10 manufacturing area
11 prosthetics

Key:
1 gym
2 physical therapy
3 treatment
4 staff lounge
5 lounge
6 support
7 activities of daily living
8 occupational therapy

Level 3

8.13.3 High-tech therapy treatment areas are dispersed throughout the four levels of the Center, and include a large pool, gym, jogging track, and multi-terrain simulator

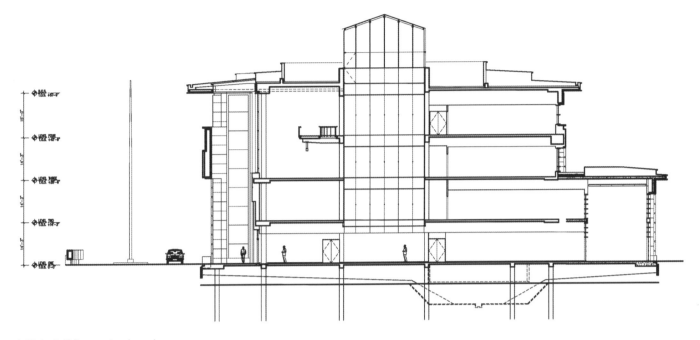

8.13.4 Building section through mid-section of Intrepid's diagnostic and treatment core

8.13.5 Exterior view of immediate campus environs

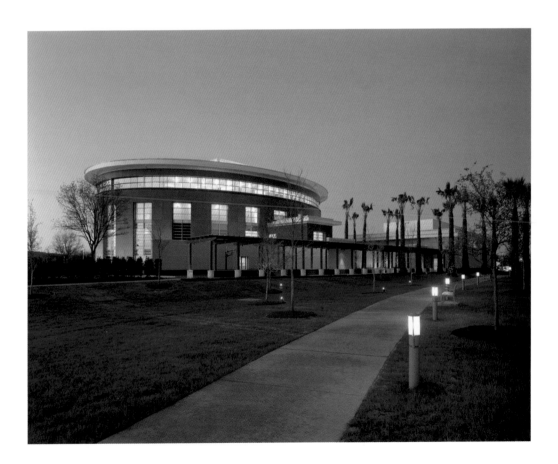

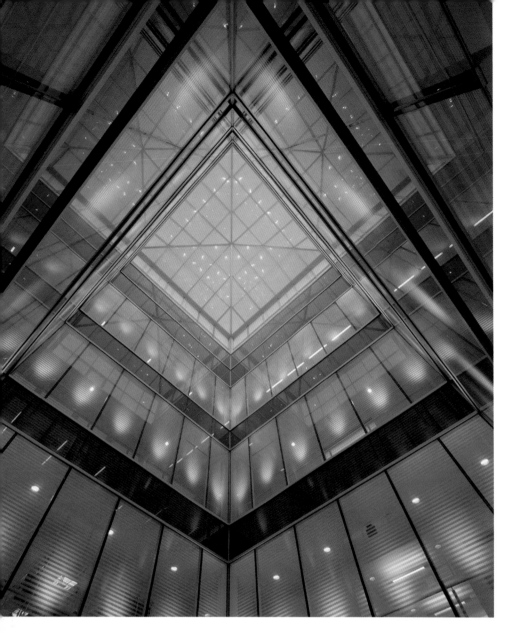

8.13.6 An atrium is the primary organizational element, and is enclosed with a glazed roof

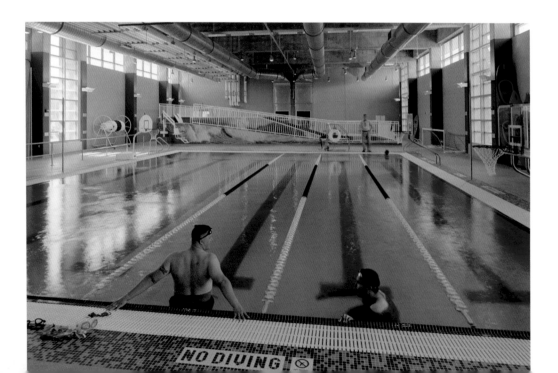

8.13.7 A lap pool and a hydrotherapy unit are located on Level 1

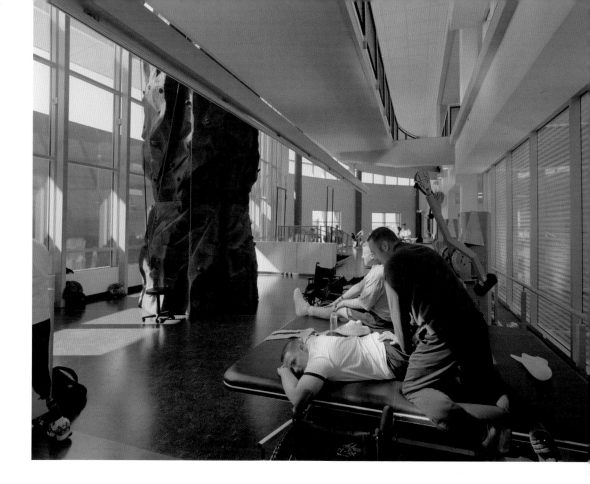

8.13.8 The physical therapy unit contains a climbing wall

A glass-enclosed atrium transmits natural daylight throughout its four levels (Figure 8.13.3a–d). This is a focal point for the entire facility and is a navigational aid. With the atrium as the central organizing element the atrium roof appears to push upward beyond the roof plane. The full height window walls surrounding this space feature a window treatment to control glare and to partially obscure visual access from the atrium (Figure 8.13.4). A second building, connected via the arrival axis, houses a therapy pool, an outdoor activity area, and related support (Figure 8.13.5). The second, third, and fourth levels of the ellipse house labs and treatment units: advanced physical simulators, a running track, climbing wall, uneven terrain and obstacle courses, and specialized equipment for advancing patients' strength, balance, agility, motor-skill therapy, and the virtual reality simulator (Figure 8.13.6 and Figure 8.13.7). The lozenge-shaped running track cantilevers out above a physical therapy space directly below. The largest treatment areas are deployed along the perimeter of the building envelope, notably the main physical therapy gym. There, large expanses of glass afford patients – who often spend their entire day in therapy sessions – fully unobstructed views outdoors to the landscaped grounds of the campus.

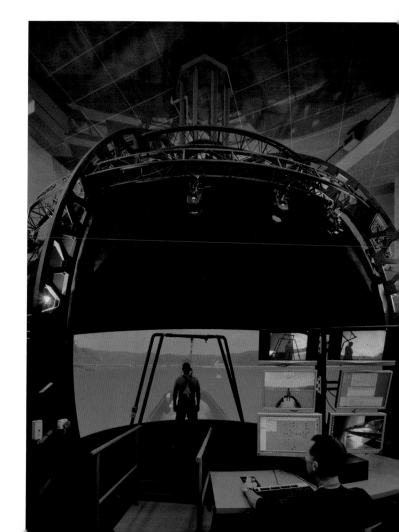

8.13.9 The virtual reality unit simulates activities of daily living

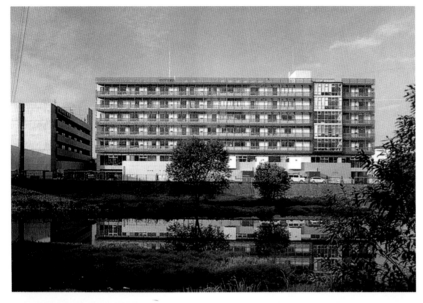

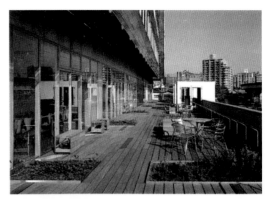

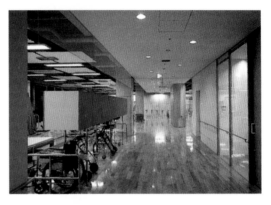

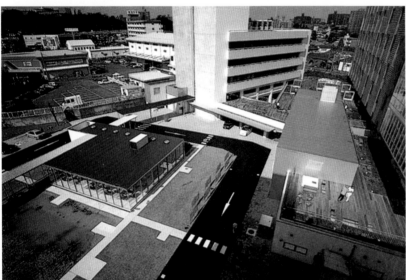

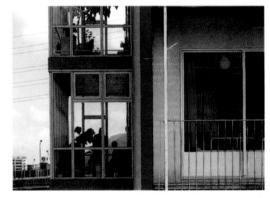

8.14.1a–e The Kokura Public Rehabilitation Hospital is located near the southern Japanese city of Fukuoka

14 Kokura Rehabilitation Hospital, Kokura, Kyushu Prefecture, Japan

ARCHITECT: Yasui Masahiro and Associates, Tokyo
LANDSCAPE ARCHITECT: Yasui Masahiro and Associates
CLIENT: Kokura Rehabilitation Hospital
FEATURED MATERIALS: Exterior steel panels, cast-in-place concrete, low-e exterior glazing, stainless steel, aluminum, stone pavers
COMPLETED: 2001
INPATIENT BEDS: 100
SITE/PARKING: 12 acres/175
HOSPITAL SIZE: 325,000SF

Context/site

This seven-level regional rehabilitation hospital provides comprehensive inpatient and outpatient services to citizens in and near the city of Kokura, in southern Japan. The vocabulary is rationalist, straightforward, and from the exterior appears to be a residential apartment tower. Its deinstitutionalized imagery blends well into its surrounding context of low- to mid-rise residential buildings (Figures 8.14.1a–e). The campus site plan consists of three building elements: a seven-level inpatient tower, a five-level administration and medical office facility, and a one-level dining facility that simultaneously functions as a gateway, located near the public parking area (Figure 8.14.2a–c). A small retention pond provides opportunities for patients and their families to be outdoors.

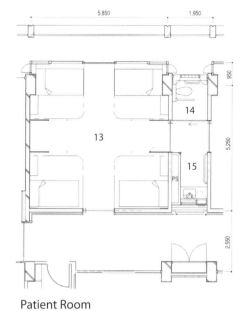

Patient Room

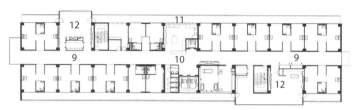

8.14.2a–e The dining facility is a freestanding structure. Administration, admitting, and therapy treatment areas are housed on Level 1. The majority of patient rooms house four beds

Typical Unit

Key:
1 parking
2 cafeteria/terrace
3 main entry
4 atrium/admitting
5 physical therapy 1/support
6 physical therapy 2/support
7 speech/occupational therapy
8 physical therapy 3/support
9 PCU/nursing
10 nurses' station
11 staff support
12 dayroom
13 semi-private room
14 bathroom
15 shower/storage/sink

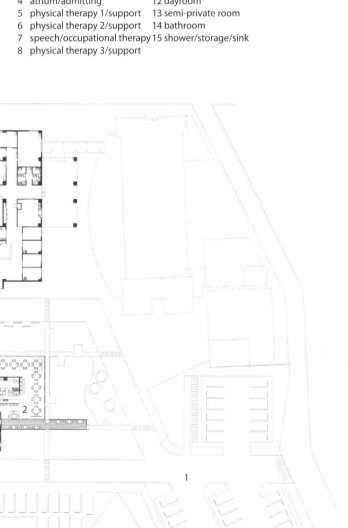

Main Level/Site Plan

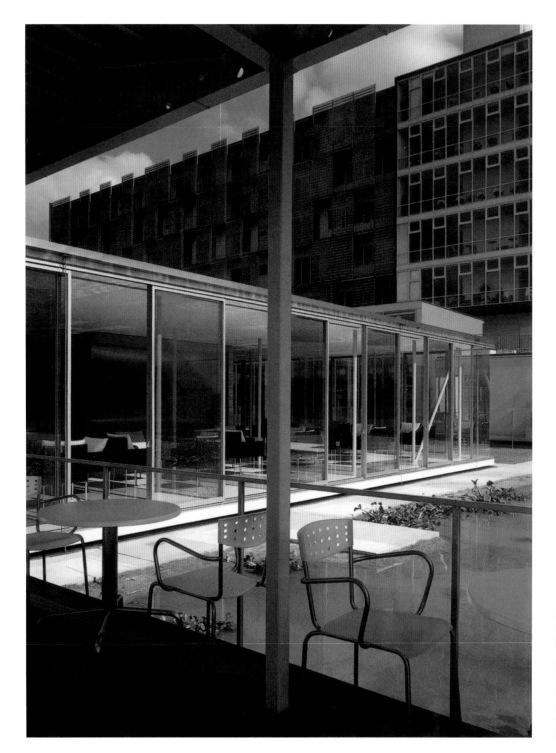

8.14.3 An anti-institutional aesthetic is achieved, with an emphasis on contact with nature

8.14.4 A landscaped courtyard affords opportunities for social interaction, or respite. Note the corrugated steel sunscreens attached to the exterior circulation elements

Building/unit

The main lobby and admitting area features high ceilings that facilitate the transmission of natural light to the interior, and also afford full views to the outdoors. Furnishings and trees create informal places for seating and social interaction. The one-level dining facility features an adjacent outdoor patio and terrace (Figure 8.14.3). The first and second levels provide the support service base. This base contains the core support and administrative areas, medical records, diagnostic, laboratory, pharmacy, central material management, a conference center, research unit, and inpatient and outpatient rehabilitation clinics. A landscaped roof deck is located on the second level. The views from the upper levels overlook a large courtyard. This space has wood decking and light boxes that double function as sculpture while providing shelter. These stainless steel boxes also, and somewhat curiously, establish a human scale (Figure 8.14.4). The entry area to the physical therapy spaces is a two-level volume with narrow light tubes suspended from the ceiling.

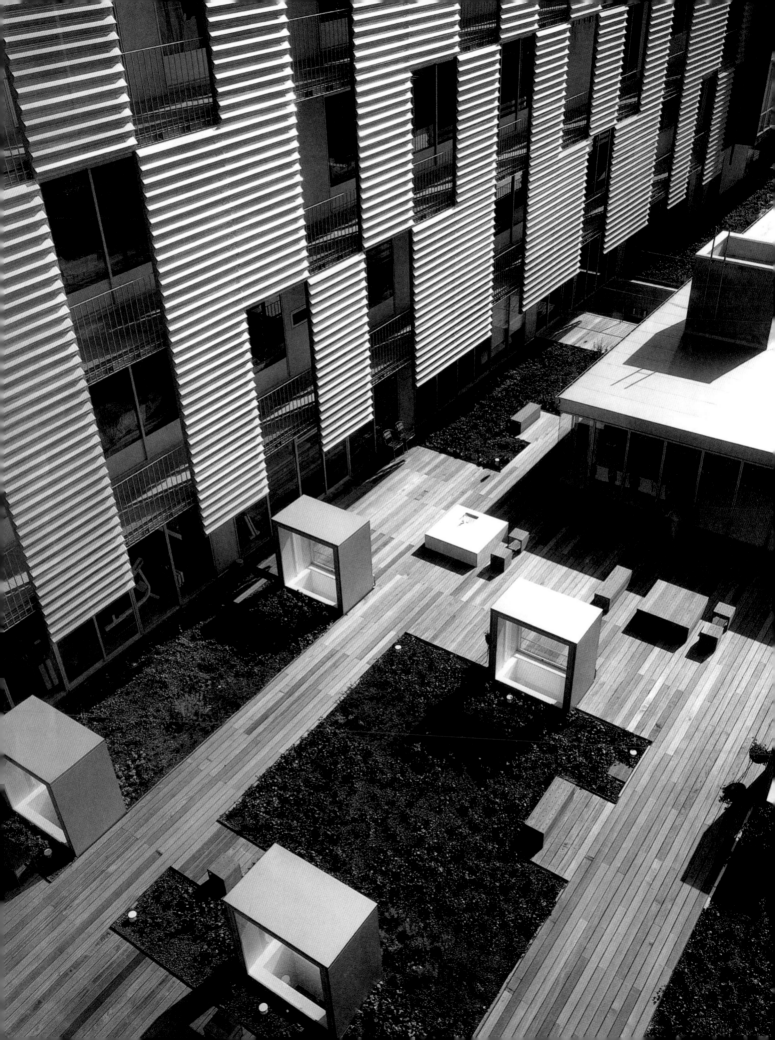

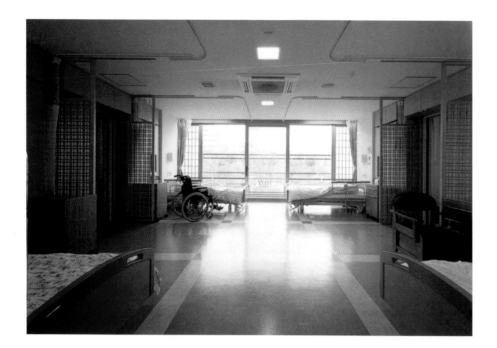

8.14.5 Inpatient rooms have a sliding glass door providing access to a balcony/terrace spanning the full length of the building

8.14.6 Inpatient care units have recessed handwash sinks compartmentalized apart from the water closet. A single communal bathing/hydrotherapy room is provided on each inpatient unit

The semi-private inpatient bedroom suites each house four beds (Figure 8.14.5). Shoji screens and sliding wood doors are featured throughout. Patients can easily move privacy curtains and blinds, and personal privacy is provided without becoming obsessive. The central nursing station and related support functions are located at the midpoint of each inpatient floor. Two dayrooms are provided on each floor, adjacent to vertical circulation. Windows are full height and doors allow for direct access to exterior balconies; these balconies span the full length of the tower. Semi-private bath/shower rooms are positioned on the inboard side of the floor, with a few exceptions (Figure 8.14.6). Perhaps the most innovative aspect of Kokura Rehabilitation is that its entire exterior perimeter circulation and its rooftop are accessible for occupants' use. A perimeter railing made of stainless steel surrounds this expansive deck with a corrugated, perforated steel sunscreen panel system that provides both shade and privacy. At Kokura, as at REBAB Basel, these two innovations – a continuous perimeter veranda that adjoins and extends each inpatient room *into* the outdoors, and a roof that allows patient and family use – are unique among recently built rehabilitation hospitals. The full height glass doors that link bedrooms to the veranda, at REHAB Basel as well as at Kokura, are therapeutic, inviting direct contact with the outdoors while allowing one to remain in the patient housing realm.

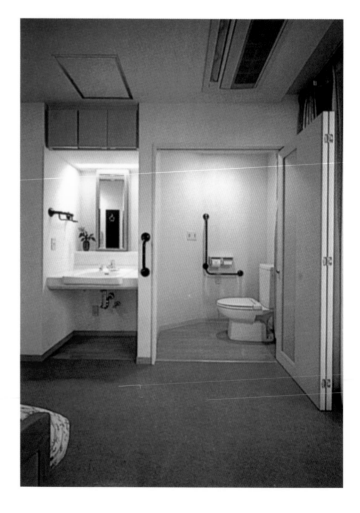

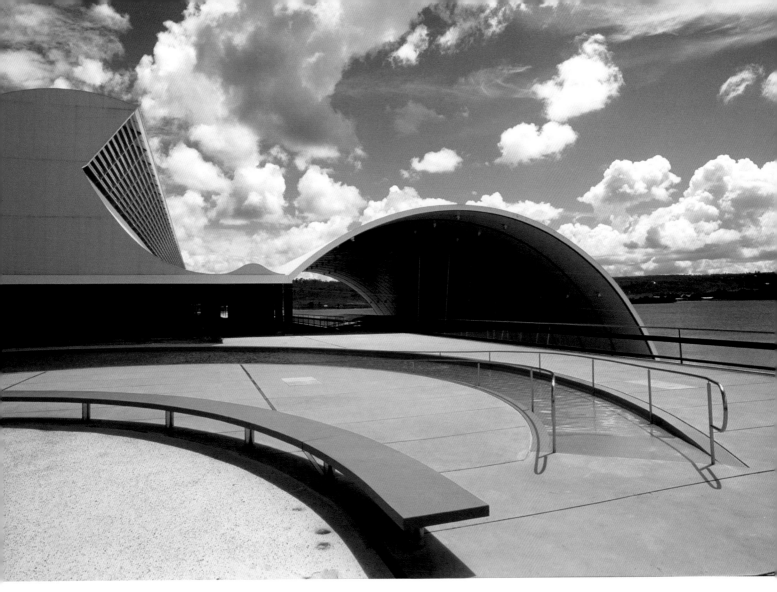

8.15.1 The Sarah Hospital at Brasilia features striking forms adroitly choreographed against a dramatic waterfront setting

15 Sarah Lago Norte Center for the Seriously Handicapped, Brasilia, Brazil

ARCHITECT: João Filgueiras Lima (Lelé), Brasilia
LANDSCAPE ARCHITECT: João Filgueiras Lima (Lelé)
CLIENT: Brazilian Federal Government; Operated by NGO Associacão das Pioneiras Sociais (Social Pioneers Association)
FEATURED MATERIALS: Cast-in-place concrete, wood finishes, ceramic tile, aluminum, copper, granite
COMPLETED: 2002
INPATIENT BEDS: 125
SITE/PARKING: 32 acres/155
HOSPITAL SIZE: 145,600SF

Context/site

The Sarah Lago Norte Center for the Seriously Handicapped is the second Sarah Hospital to be built in the capital city of Brasilia. The site is located in a low-rise urban section of the city approximately 12 kilometers from the center of Brasilia. The waterfront site receives a constant sea breeze from east to west and its topography slopes gently downward toward the water's edge. Its microclimate was ideally suited for the incorporation of natural ventilation throughout the buildings on the campus. These six buildings and the exterior spaces interspersed between exemplify the Sarah Network's core philosophical principles of the promotion of human dignity and individuality, the creation of *genius loci*, and designing for the therapeutic amenity of nature. Collectively, these principles guided an inventive, and frequently highly animated design response to the particulars of its immediate site, and the particulars of a complex functional program brief (Figure 8.15.1).

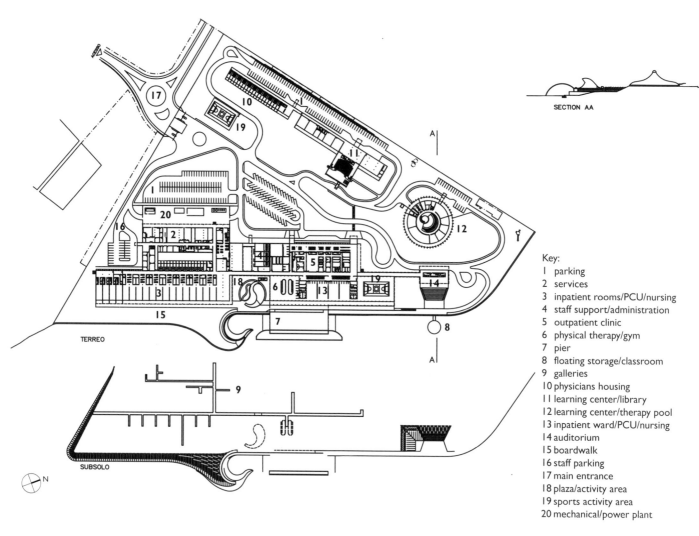

SECTION AA

Key:
1 parking
2 services
3 inpatient rooms/PCU/nursing
4 staff support/administration
5 outpatient clinic
6 physical therapy/gym
7 pier
8 floating storage/classroom
9 galleries
10 physicians housing
11 learning center/library
12 learning center/therapy pool
13 inpatient ward/PCU/nursing
14 auditorium
15 boardwalk
16 staff parking
17 main entrance
18 plaza/activity area
19 sports activity area
20 mechanical/power plant

Site Plan/Level 1

8.15.2 The campus features a boat launch/marina and numerous outdoor therapy areas. The majority of the hospital is one level in height

Building/unit

The formal language of the Sarah Lago Norte campus can perhaps be described as an expressive, late minimalism. Lelé (born 1932) has had a long, distinguished career, earning a reputation as one of Brazil's most revered architects. Unsatisfied with the architectural traditions associated with the neoclassical hospital in Brazil, in the Sarah Network hospitals a reinvention was sought in the relationship between the patient, the indoor realm, and the outdoors. Lelé worked as an assistant to Oscar Niemeyer in the 1950s and 1960s during the construction of Brazil's new-town capital. As a disciple of Niemeyer, his use of reinforced lightweight concrete, interest in rationalization,

and in prefabricated, industrialized building methods sought to extend the formal traditions of the Bauhaus and International Style modernism. At Sarah Norte he rejected the machine-for-healing metaphor that had come to symbolize the modern hospital as a building type in the latter half of the twentieth century. A relatively simple yet animated set of toy-like forms – not unlike colorful children's blocks – resulted in an engaging, human-scaled campus for the manner in which these elements were juxtaposed with one another, and for how they interestingly reinterpreted the functional program brief. From the scale of site to that of individual therapy treatment spaces, this animated expression was transposed from plan to section to elevation and back through color, materials, and a gravity-defying

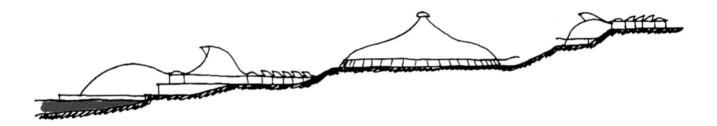

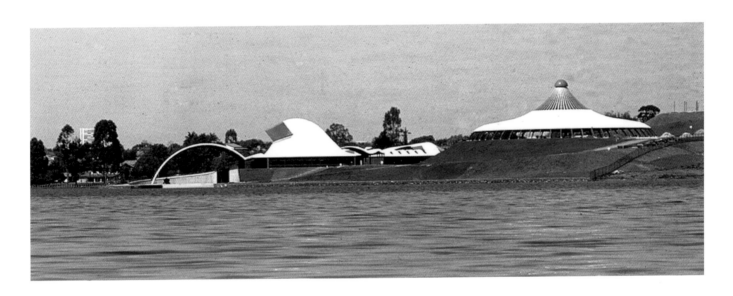

8.15.3 Animated forms are embedded in the hospital's sloped waterfront site

lightness of form (Figure 8.15.2). These qualities characterize Lelé's best work during a fifty-plus year career in Brazil.

Lelé viewed being bedridden indoors for an extended period of time as inhumane. At Sarah Lago Norte the hospitalization experience was therefore reconsidered for the severely injured and disabled by removing formidable physical barriers in favor of an *organic transparency*. The entire campus is on one level, set into its sloping site (Figure 8.15.3). In elevation the buildings take on childlike metaphors – one as a circus tent (the therapeutic pool and learning center) another as a duck (auditorium) and a third as a rainbow arc (the boardwalk pavilion). Theraserialization defines the fluidity of the relationship between interior and exterior realms and

as a continuum of private to semi-private to semi-public zones. The spaces in-between these elements become outdoor 'therapeutic rooms' extending this dialogue between light, organic form, water, and landscape. The large auditorium perhaps most clearly expresses these playful, organic metaphors (Figure 8.15.4).

A dome-shaped activity building houses a learning center, circular pool and an indoor garden (Figure 8.15.5). Circulation spaces are exaggerated in width to simultaneously accommodate multiple wheelchairs and beds. The pool has a ramp, coded in orange, leading into the water (Figure 8.15.6). Not unlike other modernists of his generation, the architect designed the campus' signage and graphics, certain furnishings, outdoor features, and even produced a patient

271

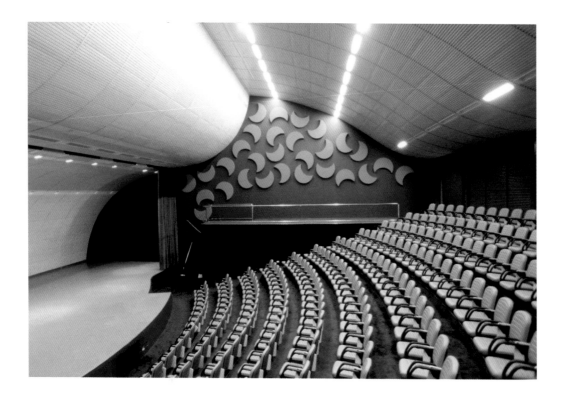

8.15.4 Interiors on the campus are equally expressive, as illustrated in a large auditorium

8.15.5 The hydrotherapy building appears as a colorful wind-up top

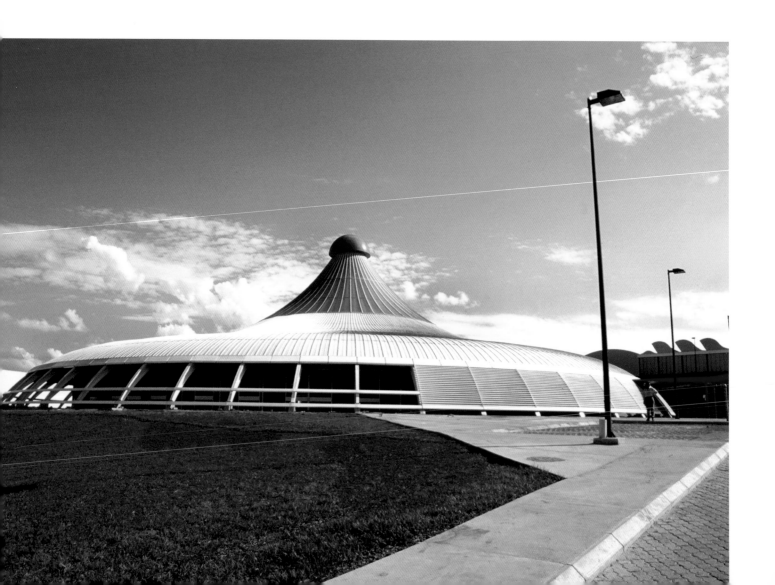

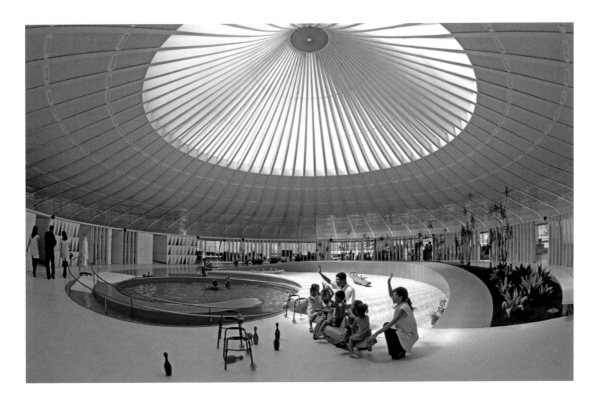

8.15.6 The interior of the hydrotherapy/learning center is equally animated

bed prototype. This bed/stretcher, known as the *camamaca*, is fully ambulatory, able to negotiate physical barriers together with high level of patient comfort. The patient can be easily wheeled from the inpatient unit to adjacent terraces and other exterior spaces on the campus without having to be transferred to a second mobility device (Figure 8.15.7). This device has been particularly successful in enabling patients who otherwise would be restricted indoors to experience the varied benefits of nature. The camamaca has a single steel tubular sphere that arcs above the center of the bed, longitudinally, spanning from toe to head. This allows the patient to pull themself up with the bed's reconfiguration options allowing a fully supine, or an upright chair-like position, enabling him or her to see out towards the open water and the horizon line.

8.15.7 The anthropomorphism of the campus is expressed in a circular canopy, patio, and therapy pool

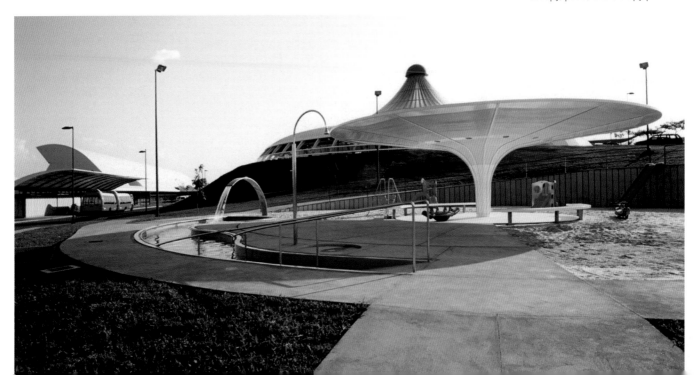

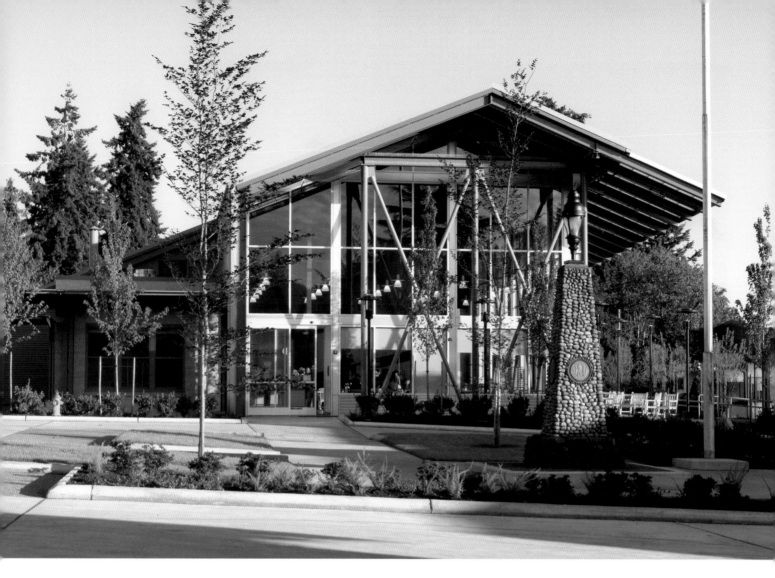

8.16.1 The scale and appearance of the campus at Retsil expresses the region's indigenous vernacular traditions and its seaside setting

16 Washington State Veteran's Center, Retsil, Washington

ARCHITECT: NBBJ, Seattle
LANDSCAPE ARCHITECT: Site Workshop
CLIENT: Washington State Department of Veterans Affairs
FEATURED MATERIALS: Corrugated steel exterior panels, stone, laminate wood beams, bamboo floors, renewable wood wall surfaces and finishes
COMPLETED: 2005
INPATIENT BEDS: 240-bed skilled nursing residential and treatment facility adjacent to 150-bed acute care hospital
SITE/PARKING: 32 acres/225
HOSPITAL SIZE: 160,000SF

Context/site

In the U.S. there are approximately two million veterans of military service aged 85 and older. With the largest veteran population in the nation, the State of Washington faces an increase of 20,000 in its over-age-65 population of veterans, and a tripling of those aged 85 and older, yet its care facilities remained among the oldest in the U.S. In this skilled nursing replacement facility, the campus plan takes advantage of the site's mild microclimate and consistent sea breezes. The campus achieved the second highest sustainability rating (39 points) from the U.S. Green Building Council, at the time (LEED Gold Level). Semi-autonomous wings connect to a central spine, with landscaped courtyards interspersed, collectively referencing timeless healing principles – the therapeutic amenity of view, natural ventilation, daylight, and spending time outdoors – reminiscent of the Nightingale hospitals of the nineteenth and early twentieth centuries. A low-rise silhouette, patios, terraces, and the

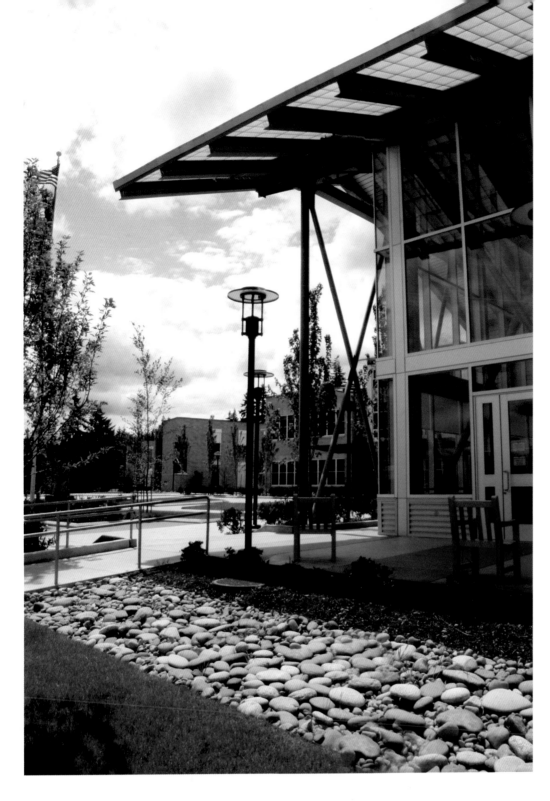

8.16.2 A new campus was built across from the original main campus, which was retained and adapted to ancillary functions

central spine reinforce the effect (Figure 8.16.1). Comparisons may be made in terms of siting and massing with the Slough District General Hospital in the U.K. (1961–1965) by Powell and Moya. At Retsil, key goals were to provide: 1. Non-institutionality and the promotion of occupants' independence, 2. Privacy balanced with opportunities for social interaction, 3. Outdoor spaces universally accessible, protected from the elements, and secure, 4. Interior spaces adaptable to future needs, and 5. On-site support for ancillary medical, dental, counseling, and physical rehabilitation programs.

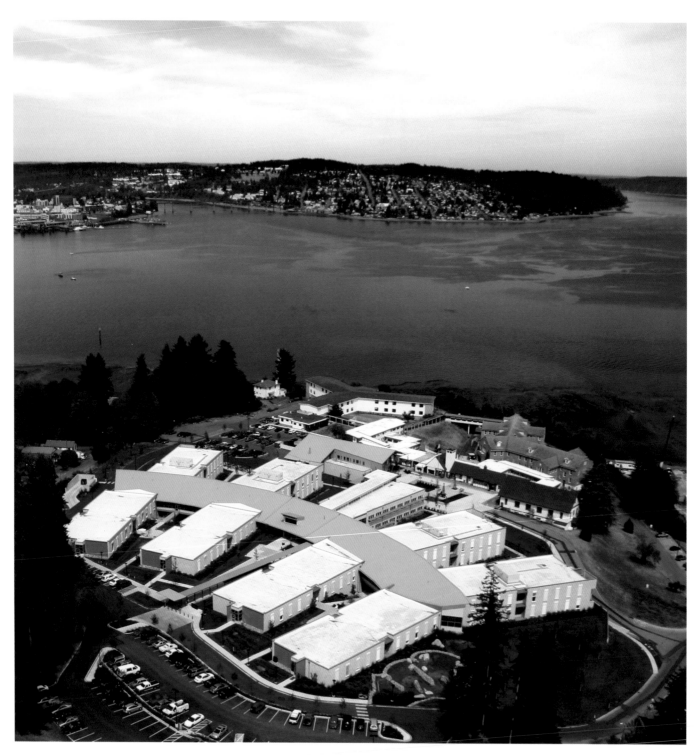

8.16.3 The campus is in some ways reminiscent of nineteenth-century and early-twentieth-century Nightingale hospitals – low-rise, relatively narrow inpatient units, connecting circulation spine, natural daylight and ventilation, and direct access to gardens and green space

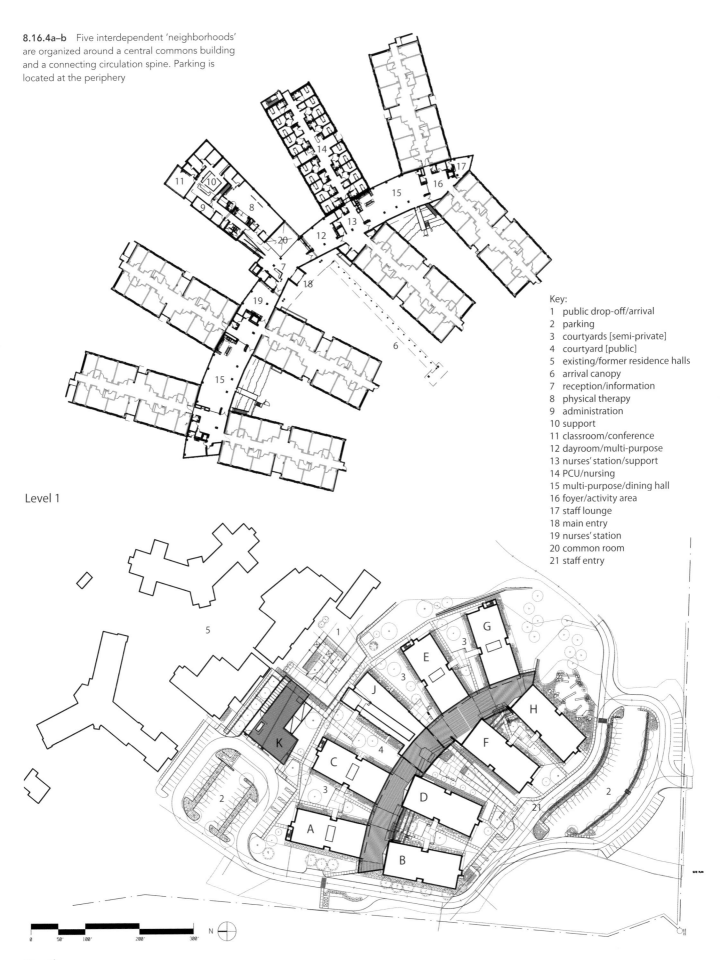

8.16.4a–b Five interdependent 'neighborhoods' are organized around a central commons building and a connecting circulation spine. Parking is located at the periphery

Level 1

Key:
1 public drop-off/arrival
2 parking
3 courtyards [semi-private]
4 courtyard [public]
5 existing/former residence halls
6 arrival canopy
7 reception/information
8 physical therapy
9 administration
10 support
11 classroom/conference
12 dayroom/multi-purpose
13 nurses' station/support
14 PCU/nursing
15 multi-purpose/dining hall
16 foyer/activity area
17 staff lounge
18 main entry
19 nurses' station
20 common room
21 staff entry

0   50'   100'   200'   300'

N

Site Plan

8.16.5 The dining room in the commons building features natural daylight and ventilation, full views, and options to dine outdoors

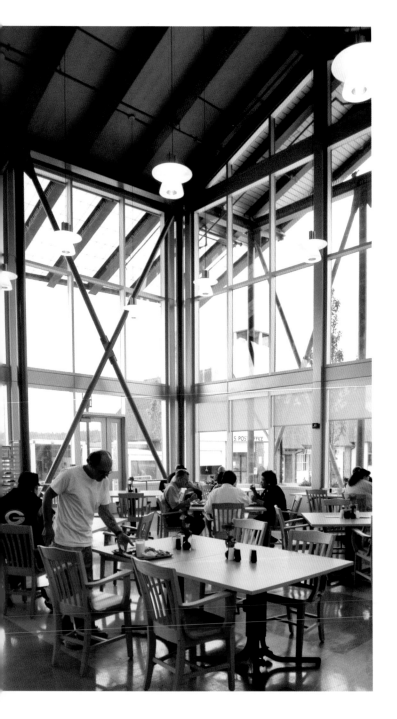

Building/unit

Its residential imagery and openness allows residents an unusually high level of personal choice and autonomy. Residents live in one of five 'neighborhoods' organized around a commons area. Visitors arrive at the main commons building, a structure (Building K) featuring broad overhangs and large expanses of glass. New construction was combined with historic conservation as a means to save funds and also to retain buildings that had outlived their usefulness for patient housing but remained adaptable to new uses. Across the access drive from the commons is the former inpatient care complex, whose buildings were restored and are now used for administration, maintenance, power plant, and campus-wide support services (Figure 8.16.2). The new buildings are partially set into the sloping site to attain consistent grade access with their adjacent outdoor spaces on stepped levels. This allowed for additional thermal insulation without extensive re-grading of the entire site. Every resident has direct access to a therapeutic garden and the new campus is situated next to scenic Sinclair Inlet (Figure 8.16.3).

A curvilinear circulation spine dominates the parti' in plan (Figure 8.16.4a–b). This element links eight 'neighborhoods' – four of which are 'forest' themed (wings B, D, F and H) with the remaining four 'water' themed (wings A, C, E and G). Unit 'J' is situated at the center of an arrival axis that transverses the entire site, linking the main entrance with the staff-visitor parking zone at the opposite end. The exterior spaces situated between the four neighborhoods to either side of this pedestrian street are a mixture of private and semi-private spaces. Each Y-shaped room is bisected by a wall rather than a curtain, yielding two semi-private (2-bed) spaces. A satellite nursing station and handwash sink is provided in an alcove next to each set of semi-private rooms. The nursing units are configured with technical support spaces in close proximity.

The facility's operable windows (totaling 240) required for the hybrid part mechanical/part natural cooling system were custom made to ensure ease of use by the aged. These are lighter in weight and easier to control compared to standard windows. The backup mechanical system filters the indoor air, as needed. Building footprints are narrow to allow for maximum natural light and ventilation. Landscaped spaces function as outdoor rooms, providing opportunities for respite, with provisions for persons with Alzheimer's. The directional wayfinding system is redundant cued – that is, the neighborhood concept is reinforced with letters A, B, C and D and further reinforced with

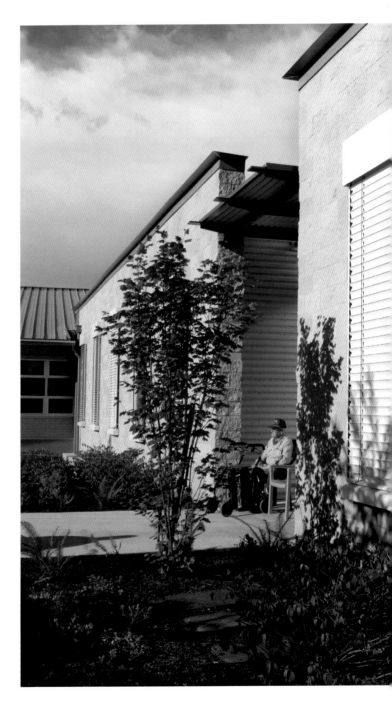

8.16.6 The Nightingale-inspired human scale of the various 'neighborhoods' allow for direct engagement with the landscape

color coding, combined with views to the outdoors at key circulation decision points.

A memory wall, in the commons area near the main entrance, houses a permanent exhibit. It provides spatial orientation and functions as a landmark of sorts, a place where residents meet with visitors and other residents. The exhibit depicts, through large murals and mementos on display, the heroic story of a locally based World War II bomber squadron unit.

The main dining room with its high ceiling and abundant natural light provides access to an adjacent patio (Figure 8.16.5). The low rise silhouette of the campus scale blends into the landscape (Figure 8.16.6). An energy efficient HVAC system is utilized to maximize air exchange and control solar heat gain. This innovative system became the first 'green project' hybrid mechanical/natural HVAC system to receive approval by the Washington State Department of Health. This system allows for future energy savings to be reinvested into the center's day-to-day operations. Additional features include Energy Star compliant appliances, a reflective roof, low VOC points, the use of an indoor air quality plan, renewable hardwood finishes on the interiors, bamboo flooring, a reception desk made of sunflower seeds, and a bio-swale for water runoff. The residential care center at Retsil empowers its residents insofar as ample interior spaces are provided for informal socialization, as well as privacy, combined with direct involvement with the natural environment through the presence of therapeutic gardens and contact with a large, nearby body of water. An innovative site-interior navigational and clustering strategy is combined at Retsil with straightforward, Nightingale-inspired buildings, on a site that possesses many intrinsic therapeutic amenities. This campus is a creative response to a modest construction budget.

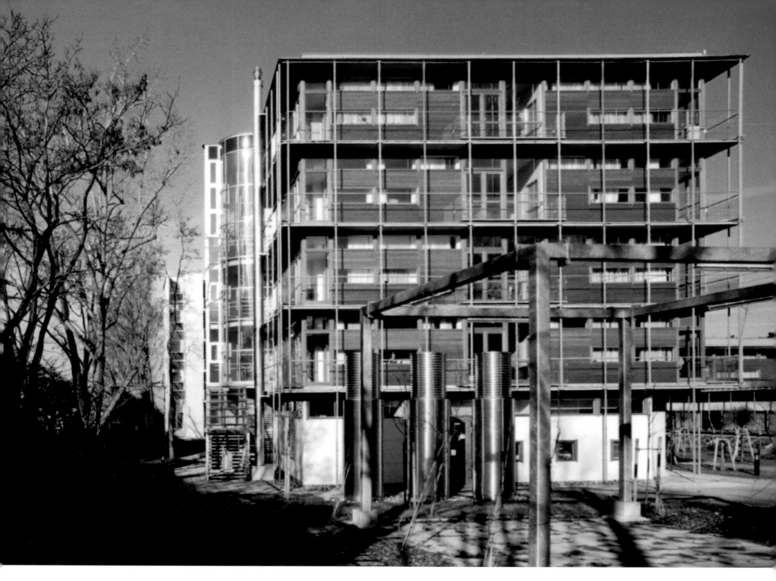

8.17.1 The Favoriten Center was built adjacent to a long-established urban medical center

17 Geriatriezentrum Favoriten (Favoriten Geriatric Center)/ Franz-Josef Hospital, Vienna, Austria

ARCHITECT: Office of Anton Schweighofer, Vienna
LANDSCAPE ARCHITECT: Office of Anton Schweighofer
CLIENT: Wiener Krankenanstaltenverbund (Viennese Hospital Group)
FEATURED MATERIALS: Low-e exterior glass, cast-in-place concrete, aluminum, stainless steel, no synthetic surface finishes, PVC use minimized, i.e. wood window frames in lieu of PVC
COMPLETED: 2003
INPATIENT BEDS: 192-bed skilled nursing residential and treatment facility adjacent to 240-bed acute care hospital
SITE/PARKING: 4.2 acres/105
HOSPITAL SIZE: 183,000SF

Context/site

This facility was the winning entry in a design competition held in 1996. The client stipulated a geriatric hospital to provide a new 'front door' to an existing medical center, as well as options for future expansion, the provision of a below-ground parking deck for 300 cars, and new outdoor landscaped space. It is noteworthy that the winning architectural team (Schweighofer and Associates) had little prior experience in healthcare architecture. Their scheme was selected over designs submitted by many dozens of competing specialist firms whose specialty is healthcare. This is the most recent 24/7 long-term care treatment facility opened by the city-funded Viennese Hospital Group. The facility is part of the campus of the major medical center in Vienna. This organization operates eighteen medical campuses regionally. In the architects' brief accompanying the submittal, the two guiding metaphors were 'hospital as city' and 'housing unit as a tree'. This manifest on the one hand in the

280

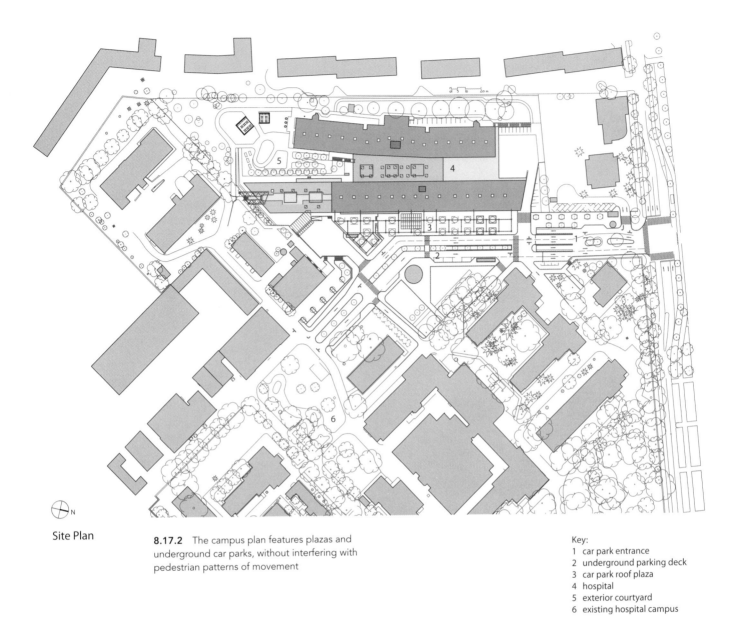

Site Plan

8.17.2 The campus plan features plazas and underground car parks, without interfering with pedestrian patterns of movement

Key:
1 car park entrance
2 underground parking deck
3 car park roof plaza
4 hospital
5 exterior courtyard
6 existing hospital campus

plazas and civic spaces, and on the other in the vertical uplift of the buildings and the balcony/terraces, functioning, in the architect's words, as 'branches of a tree' reaching outward to landscape and sky (Figure 8.17.1).

The new facility houses 192 beds, and fifty 'day patients' divided among eight types of care regimen. The narrow footprint reflected the need to conserve land on this narrow, rectangular site. The main entrance is one level up from the underground parking area. In a break from most hospitals and clinics built in the past decade, this facility does not have its own dedicated public arrival area. The main entrance to the center is on the main level and is accessed via the parking deck or on foot from the neighborhood. The facility's two mid-rise structures sit beside a plaza concourse which doubles as the roof of the parking deck. It was decided at the outset to ascribe high priority to achieving a visual dialogue between the new facility and the

non-healthcare buildings in the surrounding residential neighborhood, rather than attempting to relate to the main hospital (Figure 8.17.2). As a result, particular attention was accorded to relating to the residential scale, materiality, and imagery of the neighborhood and in relating to the scale of the neighborhood's existing open spaces. Patients are therefore able to have direct contact with nature and landscaped areas in this dense urban setting. The main approach to the new hospital is accentuated with a frame of galvanized steel spanning the lower building element and flanked by a row of trees planted on the roofscape of the underground parking deck. In the landscaped area on the south side, a therapeutic garden is provided for patient use, connected by a flight of stairs to a terrace situated between the two main buildings. Residents and families use this space for gardening.

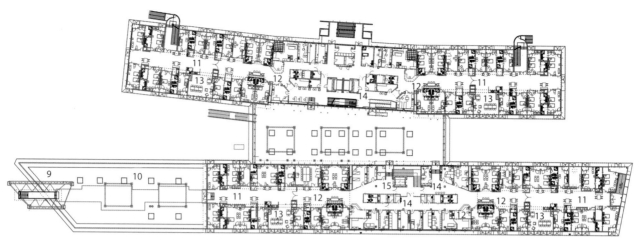

Typical Patient Care Level

Key:
1   car park entrance
2   underground parking deck
3   central materials management
4   laundry/support
5   warehouse
6   materials management
7   shipping/receiving
8   circulation [public]
9   roof access
10 terrace
11 PCU/nursing
12 nurses' station
13 dayroom
14 nursing support
15 circulation [core]

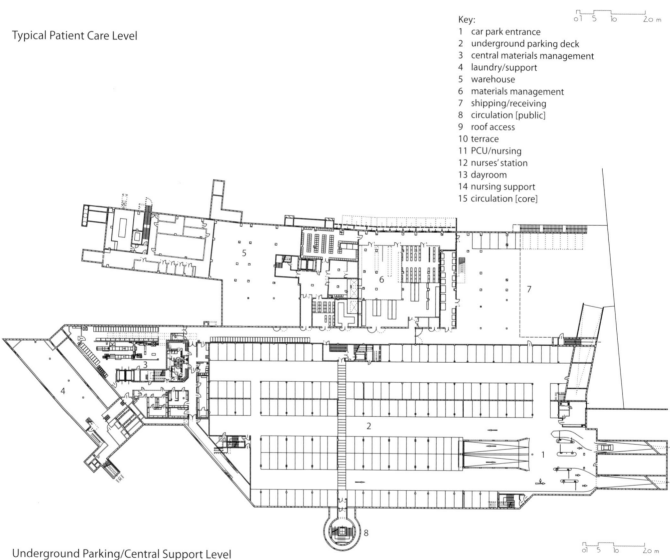

Underground Parking/Central Support Level

8.17.3 Residential care units house semi-private rooms, with dayrooms and the provision of points of access to the outdoors

8.17.4 A large plaza is located above an underground car park

8.17.5a–b Since 2000, the majority of urban European hospitals have been built with underground car parks. By contrast, comparable North American hospital/medical centers in this period were nearly always built with at grade parking lots or above ground car parks. Suffice to say, the latter strategy consumes far more open land

Building/unit

The composition consists of a platform base containing the parking deck and hospital support functions such as central pharmacy, materials management, laundry, and storage space, and two structures housing inpatient units – one five levels, and another three levels in height. The lowest level (also the ground level of the parking deck) provides space for future expansion. The five-level structure houses the inpatient PCUs and nursing support functions (Figure 8.17.3a–b). The plaza above the parking deck provides access to a large, transparent steel grid. This device provides a modicum of human scale and frames a row of trees in a grid containing ground vegetation (Figure 8.17.4). In section, the relationship between the three main compositional elements is illustrated (Figure 8.17.5a–b). The ground level of the residential tower houses the central kitchen/dining, chapel, and the outpatient clinic. Administration, main information desk, admitting, and medical counseling offices are housed on the main level.

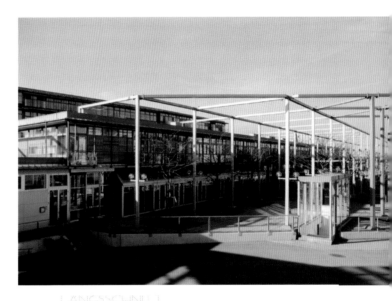

LANGSSCHNITT

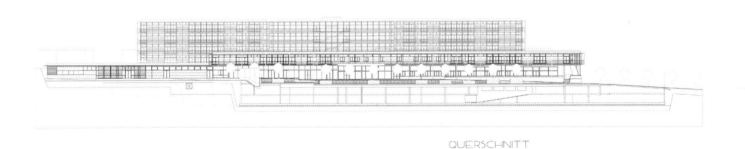

QUERSCHNITT

0 5 10 20 m

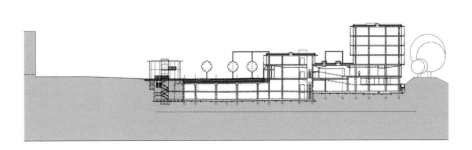

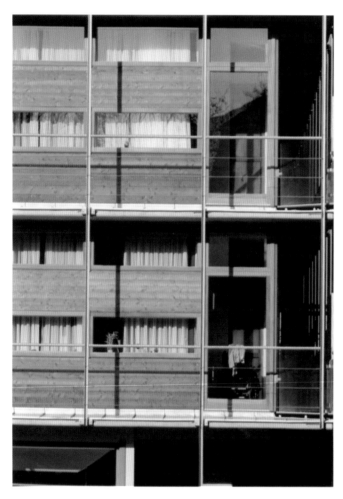

8.17.6 The wood-sheathed exterior trees, with the outer perimeter steel lattice branches reaching outward references a nearby strand (Architects' Brief)

A non-structural grid wraps the outer perimeter of the continuous terrace/balcony on each patient housing level. This device provides natural daylight and views and is made of galvanized steel. Wood cladding, sealed in a natural stain, sheaths the exterior facade. The pair of residential structures house inpatient PCUs and related patient, staff, and family support space.

In the patient housing realm, dayrooms are provided for social interaction, and a mixture of 1-bed, 2-bed and 4-bed rooms. Each PCU has a nursing station, nursing support space, and a dayroom. The narrow footprint of the structures facilitates the transmission of natural light and ventilation. The short corridors have large windows at their endpoints that offer expansive views of Vienna. Each floor has a foyer and winter garden to help establish the hierarchy from public to private zones. The continuous balcony/terrace is directly accessed from each inpatient room, through a vestibule designed to buffer the sleeping area from the cold winter air and to serve as a sunroom at other times of the year. Every resident therefore has a door that opens directly from this vestibule/sunroom to the outdoors. Bedridden patients are able to experience direct contact with the exterior through the large, operable windows. The door, door transom, and windows are made of wood. Curtains buffer sunlight and afford privacy. The perimeter terrace/balcony provides shade and reduces solar heat gain (Figure 8.17.6). The operable windows preclude the need for HVAC during much of the year. The deck is minimally wide enough for a bed or wheelchair (Figure 8.17.7).

All administrative spaces are naturally ventilated: no mechanical HVAC is provided in the administration areas. Corridors are constructed of full height glass walls, achieving visual transparency with the nursing station. This facility, not unlike the Kokura Rehabilitation Hospital in Kokura, Japan, and the REHAB Basel in Basel, provide the occupant with direct access to the outdoors vis-à-vis a balcony/terrace. This passive design strategy simultaneously gives patients control over his or her contact with the outside world. The open grid that wraps the volume gives the composition an air of indeterminacy while at once it represents the overlay of complex urban design and architectural strategies. These express the basic metaphor of the hospital as both city and as tree house. Equal attention is given to the details of the patient care experience in a care setting almost classically organized and proportioned. It is a case study in deinstitutionalized hospital in a dense urban setting.

8.17.7 Residents' rooms in the patient tower open directly to the outdoors. Note the fenestration, and plexiglass panels, and their role in creating transparent connections with landscape

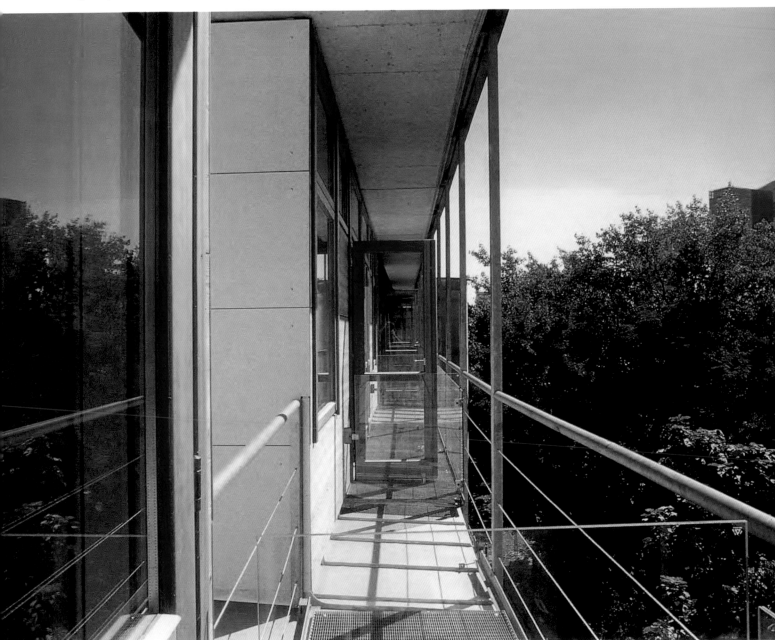

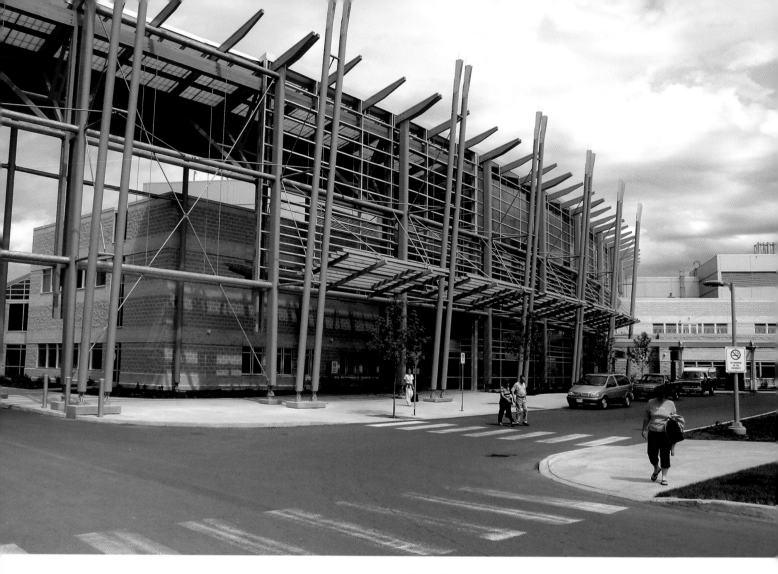

8.18.1 The main concourse at Thunder Bay is arc-shaped, configured for maximum advantage of the sun path and ever-changing rhythms of light and shadows

18 Thunder Bay Regional Hospital, Vancouver, Canada

ARCHITECT: Salter Farrow Pilon Architects, Inc. (successor firms: Farrow Partnership Architects, and Salter Pilon Architects), Vancouver

LANDSCAPE ARCHITECT: Schollen & Co. with Kuch Stephenson Gibson Malo

CLIENT: Thunder Bay Regional Hospital; Cancer Care Ontario; Northwestern Ontario Regional Cancer Centre

FEATURED MATERIALS: Steel, wood, low-e exterior glazing, polylaminate panels, laminated wood surfaces/finishes, native cut Tindal stone

COMPLETED: 2004

INPATIENT BEDS: 375

SITE/PARKING: 60 acres/375

HOSPITAL SIZE: 680,000SF

Context/site

Thunder Bay is a community of 122,000 on Lake Superior in northwestern Ontario. The setting is pristine, affording views of a captivating mountain range in the distance. The community's history is based in timber and in the paper and paper byproducts industries. The terrain is irregular and the campus structures conform to this topography. The medical center's main concourse is arc-shaped, positioned to capture the sun's path and its temporal rhythms throughout the day (Figure 8.18.1). Its orientation allows for maximum daylight penetration into the most public spaces on the campus while affording views of the mountains, from within (Figure 8.18.2). The adjoining structures on the campus are oriented north–south. These consist of the main diagnostic and treatment building, and a series of three enclosed pedestrian bridges that connect to PCUs and to related nursing and family support areas (Figure 8.18.3). The helipad is situated prominently at the far end of the hospital campus. A series of interconnected ponds on the campus divert storm-water runoff and filters it for on-site uses. These ponds are also cold-water fish habitat breeding zones, and 50 percent of the site was set aside as permanent wetlands.

Building/unit

The campus is T-shaped in plan. Central support departments, i.e. laundry, forensics, administration, dietary, and outpatient services, are located behind the concourse, on three levels. Inpatient care units are located to the east of a central circulation spine, originating from the midpoint of the concourse and extending into all three levels of the main hospital. The main concourse is a dramatic, three-level space (Figure 8.18.4). The dining area is on its public arrival level, as is the reception and admitting area. Extensively glazed curves follow the sun's path, facilitating penetration of natural light to the interior and establishing an inviting, welcoming atmosphere. The intent is for this space, in metaphor, to be a path through a forest of trees, with the circulation path symbolizing one's direct connection with nature. This is further accentuated with the laminated wood structural columns and beams.

These elements are highlighted against a neutral background as if for it to recede from the perceptual field, thereby allowing the trees to command complete center stage. This intent is effectively executed. The aesthetic and experiential aim of this 'forested path' is therefore to make its occupants feel as if they are *in* the outdoors, *in* the wilderness. The concourse requires very little fossil fuel-generated energy for its cooling or heating (Figure 8.18.5). On the uppermost level of this arc-shaded element, the 'trees' actually branch outward/upward toward the sky to support the roof (Figure 8.18.6). Balconies overlook the spaces below and afford views to the surrounding landscape. From certain vantage points the concourse appears as if it might be part of a large sports stadium.

The inpatient housing pods are each three levels in height, with additional levels able to be added in the future. Inpatient housing units are organized around the central nursing station (Figure 8.18.7). The pedestrian/service bridge is curved and its glass window wall appears as if *slotted* into the core of the inpatient housing building. This, correspondingly, yields a full height view from the nursing station out to the courtyard. Private and isolation rooms are nearest the nursing station. All other patient rooms on the unit are semi-private. Nine beds are housed on the bridge element, with an additional 21 beds

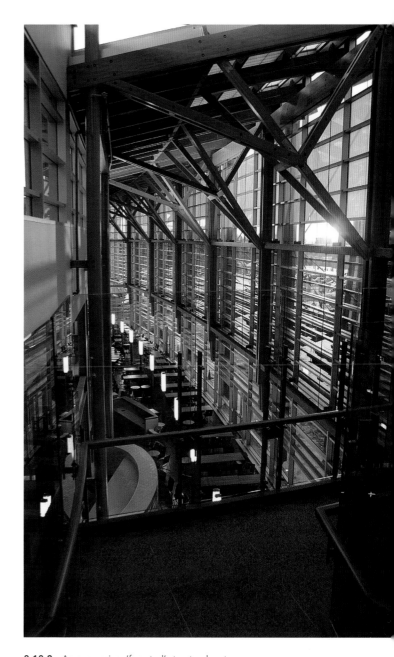

8.18.2 An expressive, 'forested' structural system activates a three-level that affords the dining area expansive views of the surrounding landscape

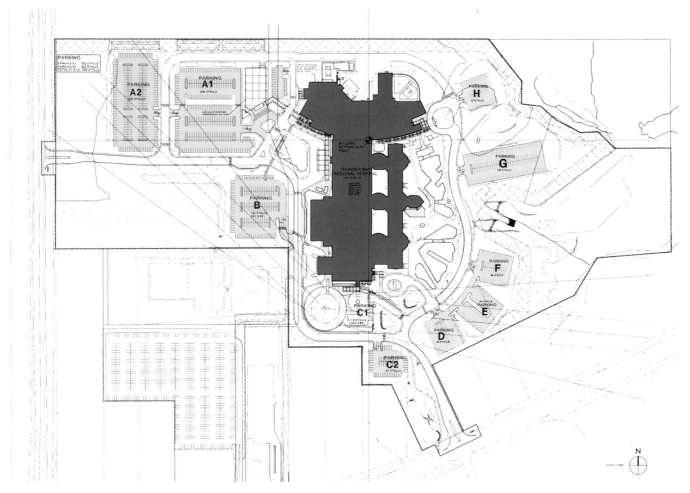

Site Plan

8.18.3 The campus is T-shaped in plan. The semi-radial facade of the concourse building is linked to a diagnostic and treatment building. This, in turn, is linked to the inpatient care realm

8.18.4 The Level 2 plan illustrates the relationship between the emergency department, general diagnostic and treatment realm, and the inpatient realm

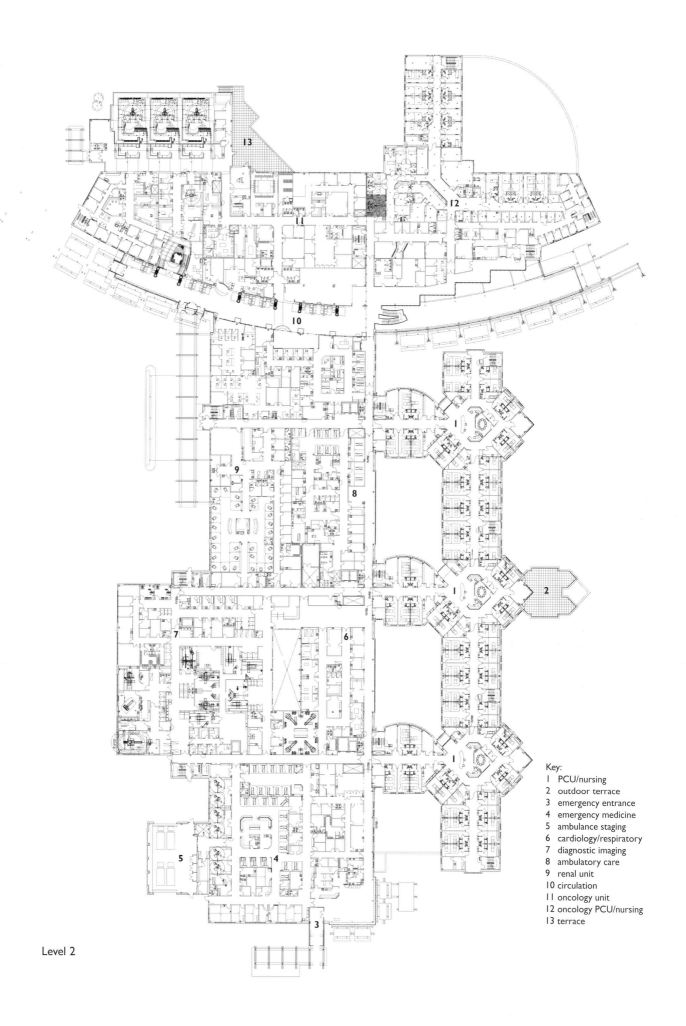

Key:
1 PCU/nursing
2 outdoor terrace
3 emergency entrance
4 emergency medicine
5 ambulance staging
6 cardiology/respiratory
7 diagnostic imaging
8 ambulatory care
9 renal unit
10 circulation
11 oncology unit
12 oncology PCU/nursing
13 terrace

Level 2

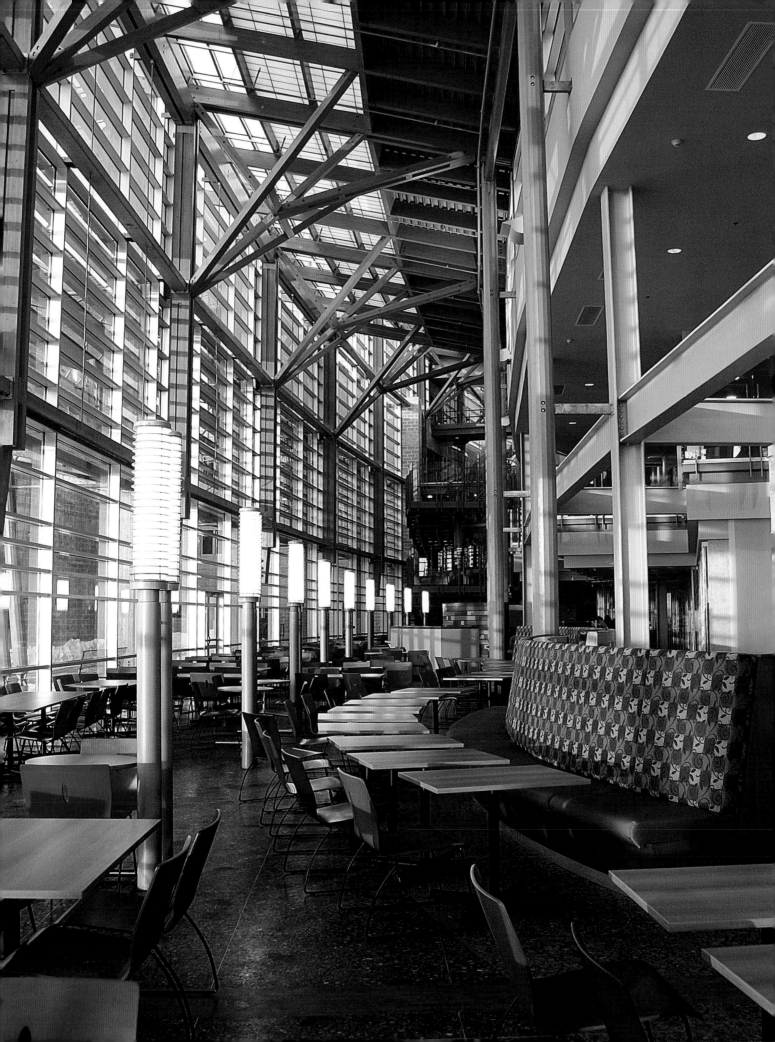

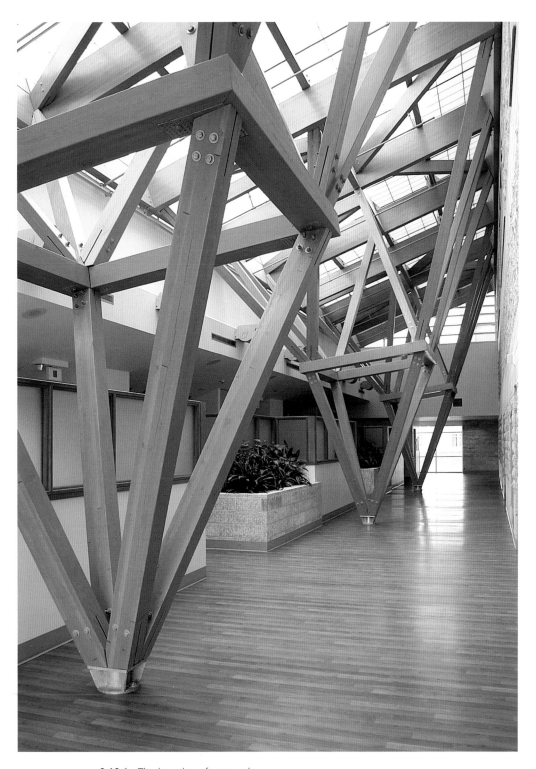

8.18.6 The *branches* of structural trees support the roof's translucent panels and function as sculpture

8.18.5 Horizontal sunscreens control daylight transmission, complementing the branches of structural *trees* as they ascend upward

deployed along a double-loaded corridor. The footprint is narrow, thereby allowing natural light to penetrate the envelope. The pediatric PCU is located at the end of the arrival axis to the patient housing realm, at the center of the three pods. On the ground level the bath/shower rooms are on the inboard side of the patient rooms. The functional brief was complex although, in all, the grand spirit and ingenuity of the public concourse was not extended into the main volume of the hospital.

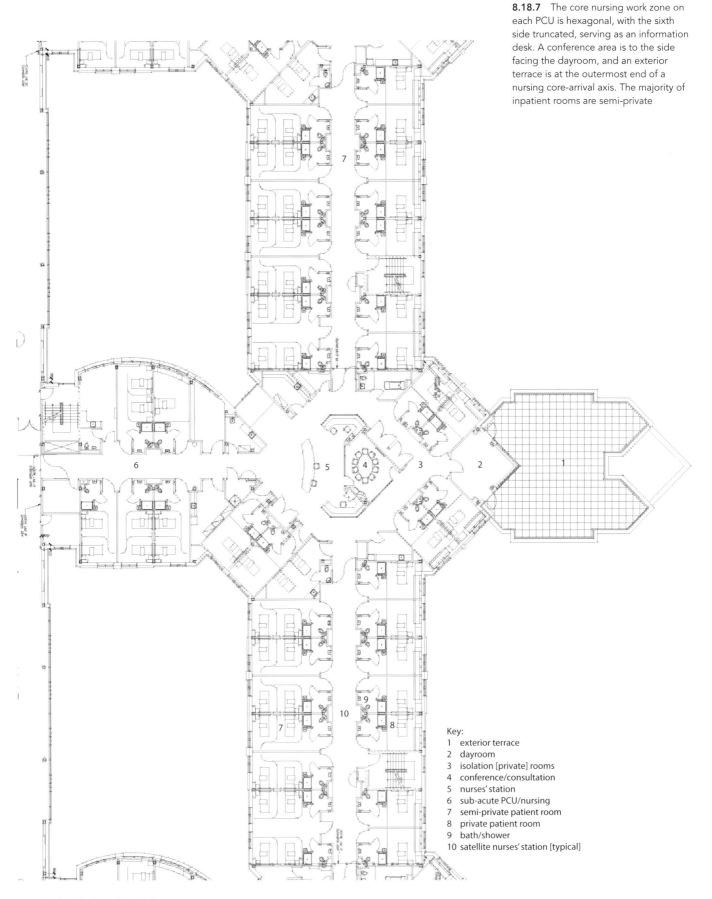

8.18.7 The core nursing work zone on each PCU is hexagonal, with the sixth side truncated, serving as an information desk. A conference area is to the side facing the dayroom, and an exterior terrace is at the outermost end of a nursing core-arrival axis. The majority of inpatient rooms are semi-private

Key:
1 exterior terrace
2 dayroom
3 isolation [private] rooms
4 conference/consultation
5 nurses' station
6 sub-acute PCU/nursing
7 semi-private patient room
8 private patient room
9 bath/shower
10 satellite nurses' station [typical]

Typical Patient Care Unit

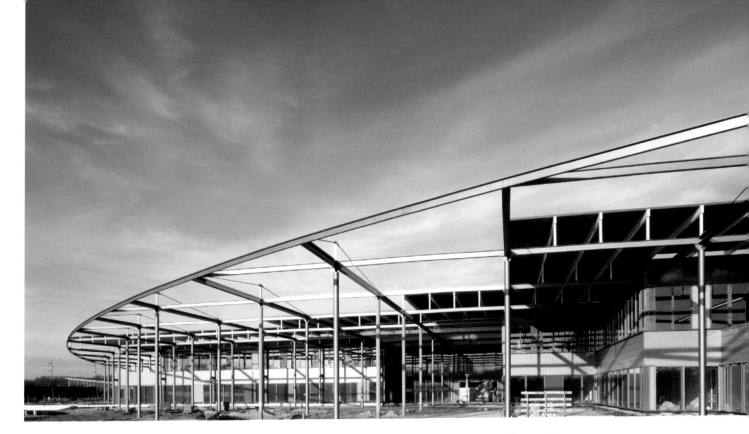

8.19.1 Deventer consumes 30 percent less energy than conventional hospitals and is a pioneering example of environmental sustainability for this building type

19 Deventer Ziekenhuis (Hospital), Deventer, the Netherlands

ARCHITECT: de Jong Gortemaker Algra, Amsterdam
LANDSCAPE ARCHITECT: Buro Poelmans Reesink
CLIENT: Dutch Care Federation (Nederlandse Zorgfederatie)
FEATURED MATERIALS: Cast-in-place concrete, wood, wood veneer panels, aluminum, stainless steel, stone, natural wood trim and interior finishes, accentuated thermal insulation, low-e exterior glazing
COMPLETED: 2007
INPATIENT BEDS: 380
SITE/PARKING: 45 acres/950 (50 percent in underground parking deck); racks for bikes
HOSPITAL SIZE: 592,015SF (main hospital) plus psychiatric center, radiation therapy clinic.

Context/site

This hospital was built on an open site outside Deventer, the Netherlands, in a metro area of 170,000. It replaced two older hospitals. The Dutch government mandated the new hospital consume 30 percent less energy on an annual basis compared to 1988 levels. Sustainable building design principles developed by the Dutch government (*duurzaam bouwen*, or DuBo) emphasize a building's total life-cycle operational costs. Deventer was chosen as one of the five initial European Union Hospital Demonstration Projects. As

a result, external consultants worked with the A/E team to model dozens of innovative massing configurations and site plan options. Early on it was decided to build the most compact footprint possible to preserve open space without compromising the hospital's complex programmatic requirements. Nearly 50 percent of the parking spaces are underground, pervious ground cover materials capture excessive storm-water runoff, and a system of swales and small drainage canals capture rainwater and store it for use during dry periods. The roof filters rainwater for use in landscaping. This is the most energy efficient hospital in the Netherlands, and the first in Europe to have a geothermal heating/cooling storage and retrieval system, including a system of heat pumps, ventilation heat recovery units, and a combined heat and power (CHP) plant. It is anticipated this system will reduce annual heating costs by as much as 70 percent, and cooling costs by half, versus comparable conventional systems. In addition, it is anticipated that annual electrical consumption will be 15 percent less than its conventional counterparts (Figure 8.19.1).

Building/unit

A major design goal was to break down the institutional scale of the typical regional hospital into a series of smaller elements – hospitals within a hospital, from the point of arrival on (Figure 8.19.2). A second functional planning goal was for the inpatient to receive as much

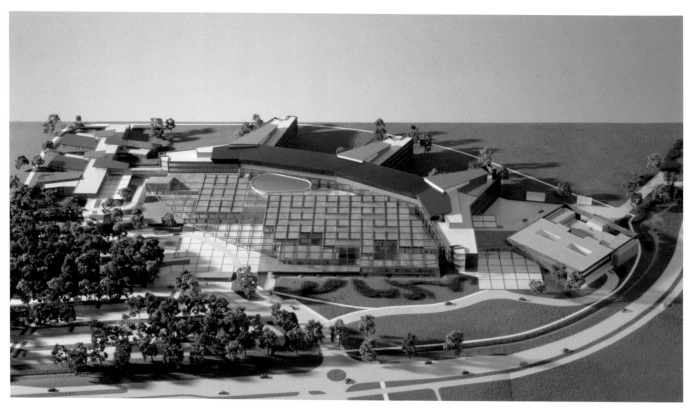

8.19.2 Functional requirements necessitated the articulation of multiple 'hospitals within a hospital', deployed around a central support platform. This grid-platform is composed of an interchangeable and expandable kit-of-parts

care as close in proximity to one's room. This led to decentralizing a percentage of diagnostic and treatment functions across a wider internal zone than would typically be the norm in a regional facility. A third goal was to maximize natural light and ventilation, resulting is a series of *fingers* that reach out on both sides from a staggered, curvilinear spine spanning nearly the entire length of the facility. The spine is its lifeblood, and is coordinated with the HVAC system and related building anatomical support. Spaces and departments with similar daily use–occupancy ratios were clustered together to improve thermal comfort and to reduce electrical use (Figure 8.19.3).

An egg-shaped building houses administrative and admitting functions. An elevator connects an arrival atrium with a parking deck immediately below. Adjacent spaces provide access to support areas on the main level (Figure 8.19.4 and Figure 8.19.5). The inpatient PCU environment 'fingers' (wings) are composed of a mix of private semi-private (2-bed) and semi-private suites (3-4 beds). These elements have footprints that narrow, tapering to their outermost endpoints (Figure 8.19.6). The windows are operable in patients' rooms and elsewhere within the PCU (and in much of the entire hospital). Interiors feature locally available species of woods in a variety of applications.

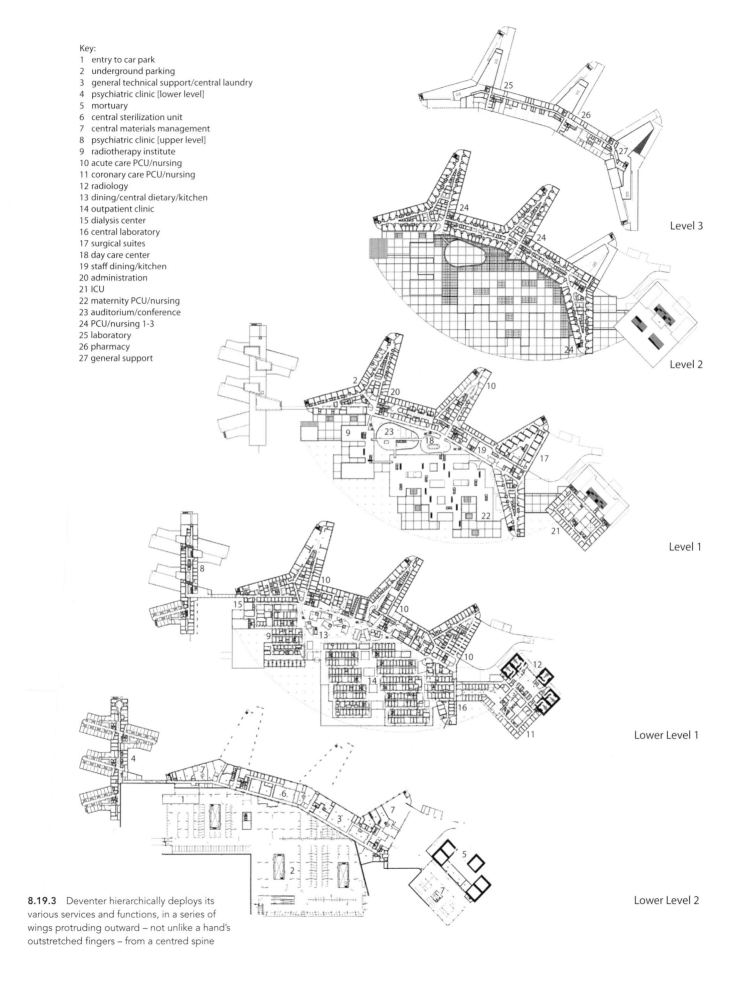

Key:
1 entry to car park
2 underground parking
3 general technical support/central laundry
4 psychiatric clinic [lower level]
5 mortuary
6 central sterilization unit
7 central materials management
8 psychiatric clinic [upper level]
9 radiotherapy institute
10 acute care PCU/nursing
11 coronary care PCU/nursing
12 radiology
13 dining/central dietary/kitchen
14 outpatient clinic
15 dialysis center
16 central laboratory
17 surgical suites
18 day care center
19 staff dining/kitchen
20 administration
21 ICU
22 maternity PCU/nursing
23 auditorium/conference
24 PCU/nursing 1-3
25 laboratory
26 pharmacy
27 general support

Level 3

Level 2

Level 1

Lower Level 1

Lower Level 2

8.19.3 Deventer hierarchically deploys its various services and functions, in a series of wings protruding outward – not unlike a hand's outstretched fingers – from a centred spine

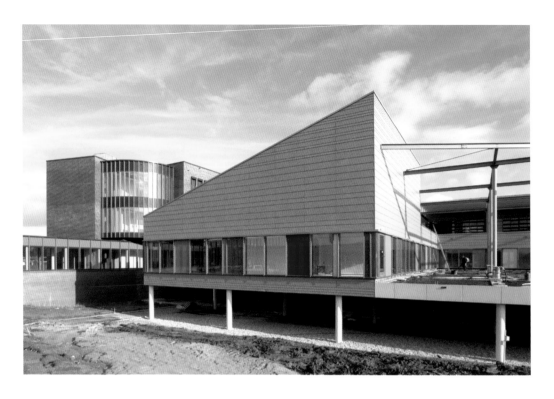

8.19.4 The main occupied floor level at Deventer is elevated in some parts of the campus as high as 4 meters above the floodplain

8.19.5 Individual cubes, or modules, within a central support grid are flexible and expandable, able to be plugged-in (or disengaged) without disrupting the overall structural aperture

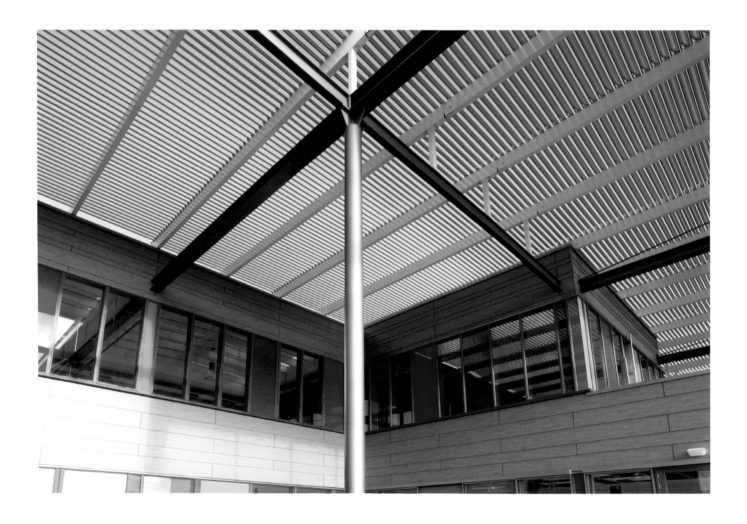

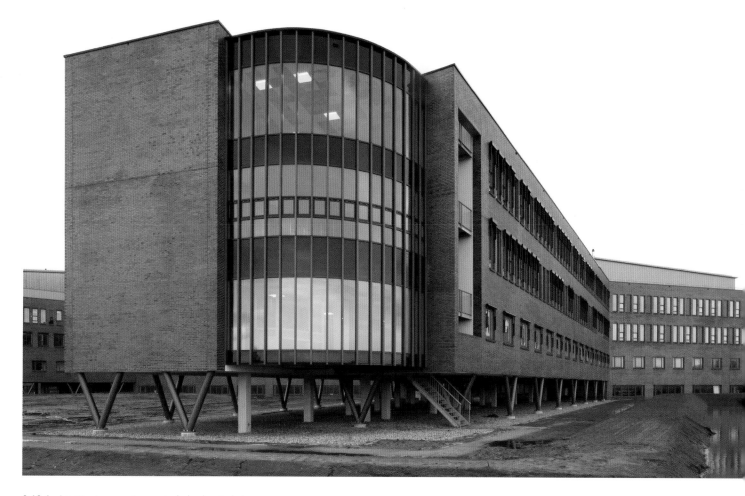

8.19.6 Inpatient care units are similarly elevated above the floodplain, a fundamental tenet of sustainable healthcare architecture – a cautionary note for twenty-first century medical institutions located in low-lying coastal areas globally in the face of rising sea levels

Wood doors and doorframes, windows frames, flooring, and wall systems are featured, and are complemented with a color scheme that is bold without being overpowering. Orange, yellows, bright green and pink are featured. The nursing station in the pediatric wing features a large tree that was brought to the hospital from France. This was a point of some contention during design development. Waiting rooms in this section have brightly painted wood boxes for children to play in as miniature playhouses.

The landscaped roof is accessible from numerous patient care areas, providing a degree of visual amenity and a place for outdoor seating. The bulk of the 139,000 square foot roof (situated above the outpatient clinics) is covered with decorative sedum. This is to filter rainwater and provide therapeutic amenity for patients housed in PCUs overlooking the roof. Deventer may best be described as an *autonomous village*: its scale and massing is such that individual main arteries and side 'streets' feature numerous landmarks, points of interest, and destination points not unlike walking though a small town, passing by the main square, park, shops, and houses. Urban life and experiences have specific, if metaphorical, counterparts on this campus – from the outdoor spaces, to the park where children play, the pediatric unit, to the inpatient rooms. In plan, however, Deventer may at first appear to be an airport, with one imagining planes parked at various gates around the perimeter of each inpatient housing wing. Finding an appropriate expression for a program this massive was the main challenge the architects faced combined with the client's mandate of innovation in sustainability. Deventer's sheer physical scale could easily overwhelm, even intimidate its occupants, and as such may be challenging for patients, visitors and staff. However, its hierarchy, massing, siting, person-nature connections, and attention to detail contribute to Deventer's overall success.

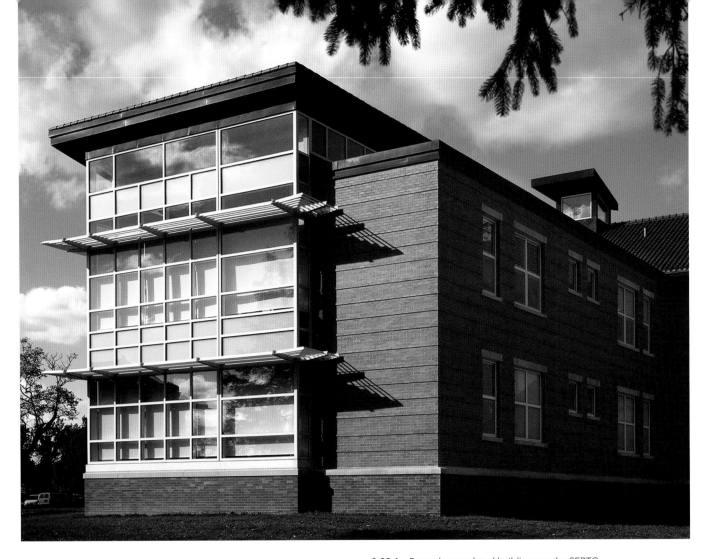

8.20.1 Recently completed buildings on the SERTC campus complement the original 1906 buildings with respect to their siting, footprint, aesthetic language, and reprise of pre-modern principles of sustainable design and construction

20 Southeast Regional Trauma Center (SERTC), Madison, Indiana

ARCHITECT: RATIO Architects, Inc., Indianapolis
LANDSCAPE ARCHITECT: RATIO Architects/Hellmuth, Obata + Kassabaum (HOK), Associate Architects
CLIENT: Madison State Hospital/Indiana State Office Building Commission
FEATURED MATERIALS: Laminate wood beams and interior veneer panels and finishes, low-e exterior glazing
COMPLETED: 2006
INPATIENT BEDS: 150
SITE/PARKING: 650 acres/345
HOSPITAL SIZE: 247,340SF

Context/site

This 150-bed regional treatment center is located on the 650-acre campus of the Madison Psychiatric Hospital, and provides 24/7 care for inpatients with mental illnesses and developmental disabilities. The Center, situated on the bank of the Ohio River, serves eighteen counties in southeast Indiana. The new buildings and renovations were limited to a 40-acre segment of the campus. Existing buildings on the campus are slated for restoration and adaptive use in the coming years as part of a phased renovation and upgrade of the entire campus. The State of Indiana, committed to environmental stewardship, now requires LEED (Silver Level, minimum) certification in all its new building initiatives. The charge given the design team was to renovate and restore the campus' historic core and augment these with new infill construction without significantly modifying or subverting the original campus master plan of 1906. Specifically, this consisted of improvements to four of the six early-twentieth-century buildings on the part of campus known as The Bluff (because it overlooks the town of Madison). Two small buildings were demolished and replaced with a new connector structure to enhance campus circulation and to reinforce *genius loci* within each of two core residential enclaves (Figure 8.20.1).

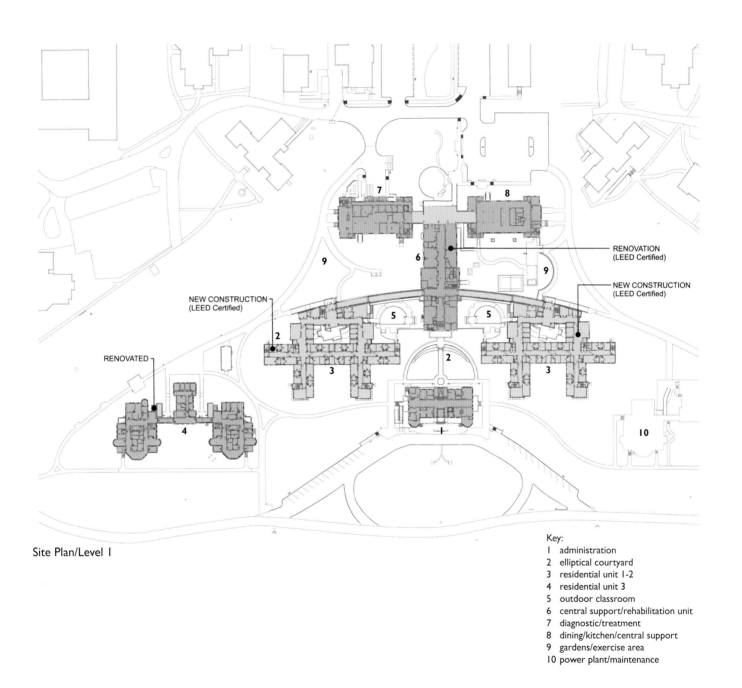

RENOVATION
(LEED Certified)

NEW CONSTRUCTION
(LEED Certified)

NEW CONSTRUCTION
(LEED Certified)

RENOVATED

Site Plan/Level 1

Key:
1 administration
2 elliptical courtyard
3 residential unit 1-2
4 residential unit 3
5 outdoor classroom
6 central support/rehabilitation unit
7 diagnostic/treatment
8 dining/kitchen/central support
9 gardens/exercise area
10 power plant/maintenance

8.20.2 Work on the SERTC campus consisted of a mix
of renovation, adaptive use, and new infill construction.
Two new residential enclaves were built

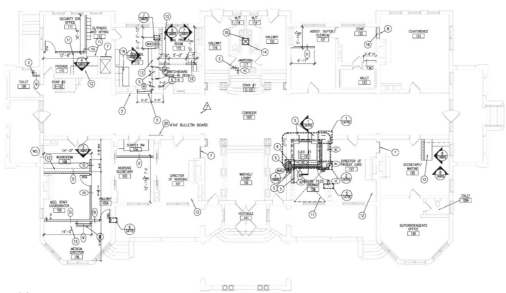

8.20.3a–c The 1906 administration building was retained and fully restored

Level 2

Level 1

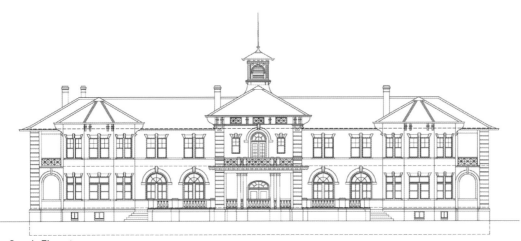

South Elevation

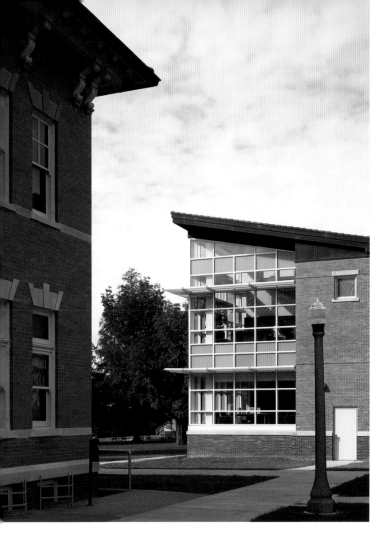

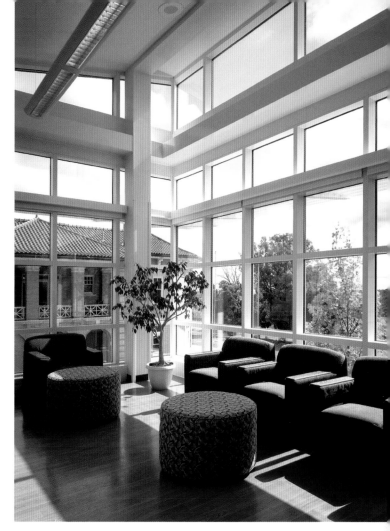

8.20.4 A sustainable balance between old and new was achieved at SERTC

8.20.5 Dayrooms in the new residential enclaves feature large expanses of glass, natural light, and views of the campus and its historic buildings

Building/unit

A large activity and support services building is located directly behind the 1906 Administration Building. Residential enclaves – called neighborhoods – are located to either side of the core buildings. Additional support buildings are located in the zone directly to the rear of the administration building. Existing courtyards were retained and new courtyards were created in two new enclaves. New additions to the existing residential dormitories flank buildings containing a mixture of enclaves and support spaces. These contain inpatient bedrooms and dayrooms, and spaces for social interaction and related activities. Each new *neighborhood* houses a dining area, an adjoining courtyard, and a group therapy room that also serves as a social space. A building known as The Cottage was also restored and adapted for ADL (activities of daily living) and for use as a semi-independent residential option for patients able to succeed in an autonomous living setting (Figure 8.20.2).

The 1906 Administration Building was fully restored (Figure 8.20.3a–c). The largest building on the campus, the T-shaped activity and support building was fully renovated and reconfigured. Level 1 houses a 'Main Street,' with therapy treatment areas and staff offices

housed on Level 2. This building also affords opportunities for both socialization and respite from the residential milieu. The new buildings constructed on the campus maximize natural light with clerestories, the aforementioned enclosed courtyards, and skylights. The footprints of the new structures are narrow, in keeping with those of the original buildings (Figure 8.20.4). Sunscreen devices are augmented with bands of Spandrel glass, thereby screening solar gain without sacrificing views. Indoor air quality was improved through the use of non-toxic interior finishes and materials. Dayrooms and social spaces provide full views and natural light (Figure 8.20.5). The innovative amenities at SERTC center on its strategic blend of preservation/adaptive use with new construction. Second, new and old buildings fit seamlessly together. The splayed roofs at the ends of the new buildings reach upward to maximize light transmission. In addition, patients are actively engaged in a campus-wide recycling program, with stations located within each residential enclave. These also serve as important places for social interaction. The project earned LEED certification (Silver Level) from the U.S. Green Building Council for its synthesis of environmental conservation with new architectural intervention. Perhaps most importantly, SERTC is exemplary for its reaffirmation of an historic American hospital campus.

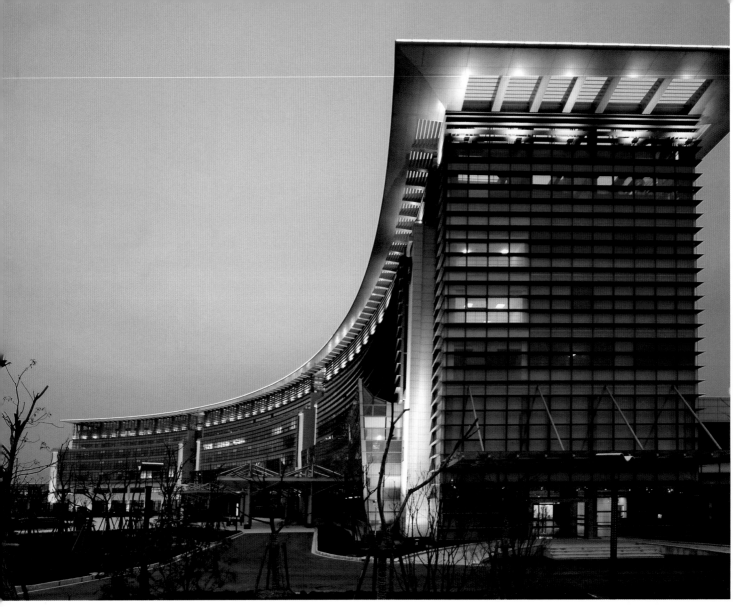

8.21.1 Shuguang Hospital's imagery is that of a high-tech medical center, and its services include traditional Chinese medical procedures used for thousands of years. On the exterior, a layered tripartite base/midsection/top is expressed

21 Shugaung Hospital, Shanghai, China

ARCHITECT: SmithGroup, Washington, D.C./CNA Architecture, Bellevue, Washington
LANDSCAPE ARCHITECT: SmithGroup, Washington, D.C.
CLIENT: Shanghai University of Traditional Chinese Medicine
FEATURED MATERIALS: Steel exterior panel system, aluminum, zinc, cast-in-place concrete, natural wood, low-e exterior glazing, wood interior surface, panel, and finishes
COMPLETED: 2005
INPATIENT BEDS: 728
SITE/PARKING: 72 acres/385
HOSPITAL SIZE: 883,000SF

Context/site

This comprehensive medical center opened in 2005 in a Newtown district in Shanghai. Shuguang Hospital is one of the first contemporary hospitals in China to fuse, through environmental design, Eastern and Western sensibilities in its healing philosophy. With its bold exterior, the hospital may appear imposing, even corporate, although the ancient Chinese practices of feng shui and its five elements of water, fire, wood, earth, and metal are promoted throughout the campus as a means to attain spiritual wholeness within the patient (Figure 8.21.1). Shuguang, commissioned by the Shanghai University of Traditional Chinese Medicine, equally emphasizes healing practices unique to China and the Far East, such as the provision of acupuncture treatment as an option in lieu of conventional surgery. Nonetheless, the hospital provides a full complement of surgical specialties not

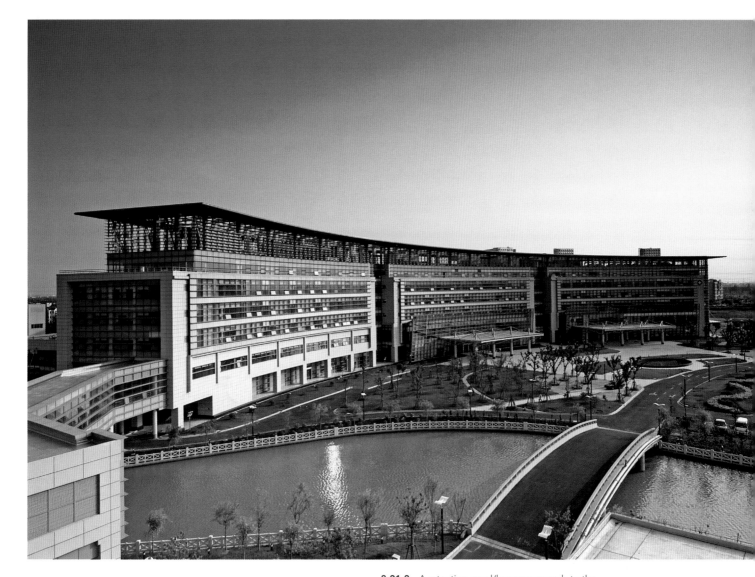

8.21.2 A retention pond/lagoon responds to the sweeping arc and horizontalism of the hospital. A landscaped plaza, paths, and pedestrian bridge is for use by cyclists and pedestrians in the community who commute to and from work

unlike those at large urban and suburban hospitals in the West. The hospital's central pharmacy stocks thousands of plant, animal, and mineral substances for the treatment of a multitude of illnesses and afflictions, in addition to a comprehensive inventory of conventional Western pharmaceuticals.

The site is circular, with access roads paralleling its perimeter on two edges. A large circular lagoon roughly follows the sweeping arc of the site; the footprint of the hospital conforms to the sweeping momentum resulting from this geometry (Figure 8.21.2). The diameter of the outermost circle determines the shape of everything within. This includes a series of circles of graduated, increasingly smaller diameters that define roadways, the water element, two bridges that pass over the lagoon, and a large park directly in front of the hospital. The park is situated in the arrival zone, and contains native species of trees and ground plantings. Large parking areas are located behind an adjacent medical arts office building, also housing the outpatient clinics (Figure 8.21.3).

Building/unit

The hospital's footprint conforms to the site's governing geometry. At first, as mentioned, it appears as if it might be the headquarters of a high-tech corporation although in point of fact the client merely sought a progressive, *global image*. As for hospitals, the grandeur of the main level is reminiscent of the Pei, Freed, and Cobb Mount

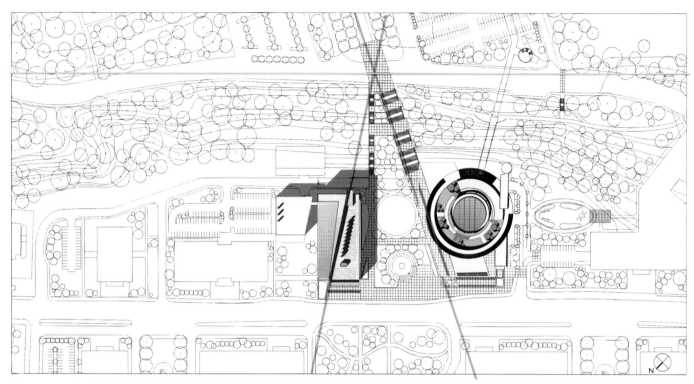

Site Plan

8.21.3 An early site plan called for a
semi-radial hospital footprint

Sinai Medical Center in New York City (1994–1996). As at Mount Sinai, high quality materials are in evidence throughout the main level at Shuguang. Two large canopies, fabricated of steel and translucent polycarbonate panels, are positioned at the two main points of arrival. One canopy is at the entry to the outpatient clinic and the other is at the main public entry (Figure 8.21.4). Upon entering, a large waiting room and the admitting area are encountered. The main public entry to the hospital is flanked by two oval elements, one housing a cafe and the other the main information desk and the central administration. Directly ahead is a large rectangular courtyard, with traditional Chinese gardens flanking both sides of a central circulation axis. This axis leads to departments beyond and eventually to the elevator core leading to the inpatient housing tower. A large oval-shaped auditorium is situated at the rear, to one side, connected by a single corridor. The exterior is articulated as a base, midsection, and top band. This tripartite facade treatment allows for various scale and material transitions and for contrasting light, shadows, texture, and proportions. The double-height ground level features expansive windows set deeply behind the structural columns.

Fenestration is regulated on the floors immediately above (Levels 2, 3 and 4) where the windows are operable; with the scale of individual inpatient rooms expressed on the exterior by means of an aperture/

box that projects beyond the facade. Acting as a sunscreen, this device relieves an otherwise imposing facade. These projecting window apertures also appear on the hospital's 'backside' facade. The elliptical geometry appears to want to thrust outward beyond the confines of the envelope itself and the suspended canopy further accentuates this. Mechanical apparatus housed on the roof is clearly visible as is the high-tech intent of the design team. The entrance to the emergency department, with its suspended canopy, is illustrated in the foreground (Figure 8.21.5). The penultimate exterior condition – its roof – is capped with a form that itself functions as a super-sunscreen. This giant steel screen dominates the composition from near and from afar. Finally, in terms of the hospital's formal vocabulary, its palette of materials and colors, though mostly white or closely related hues, are subdued yet elegant. This applies to exterior as well as throughout the interior spaces.

The first level houses the aforementioned public functions and the central administration (Figure 8.21.6). In the tower most inpatient rooms house 3-beds. There are three medical/surgical units per floor. Each PCU and its central nursing station supports sixty inpatients. Space for family members is minimal in the typical inpatient semi-private room. The bath/shower room is communal. The number of patients housed on a typical inpatient floor is so large (by current U.S. standards) that there are two full service elevator banks, with a circular

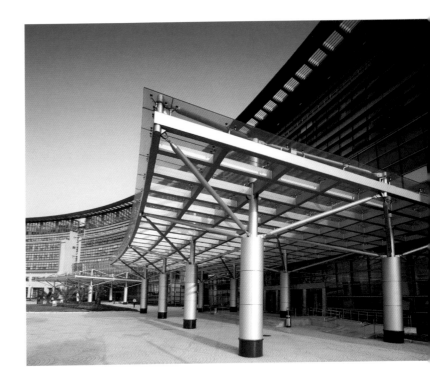

8.21.4 The vehicular arrival canopy is constructed of steel, with translucent panels providing protection from the elements, including excessive solar gain

8.21.5 Extruded cube-like window bays in inpatient rooms feature operable windows for natural ventilation. A cantilevered perforated sunscreen extension shields the uppermost level

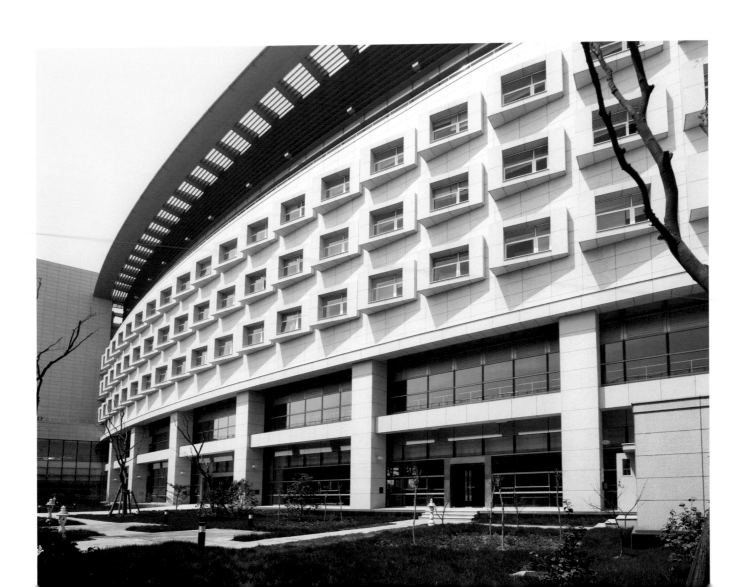

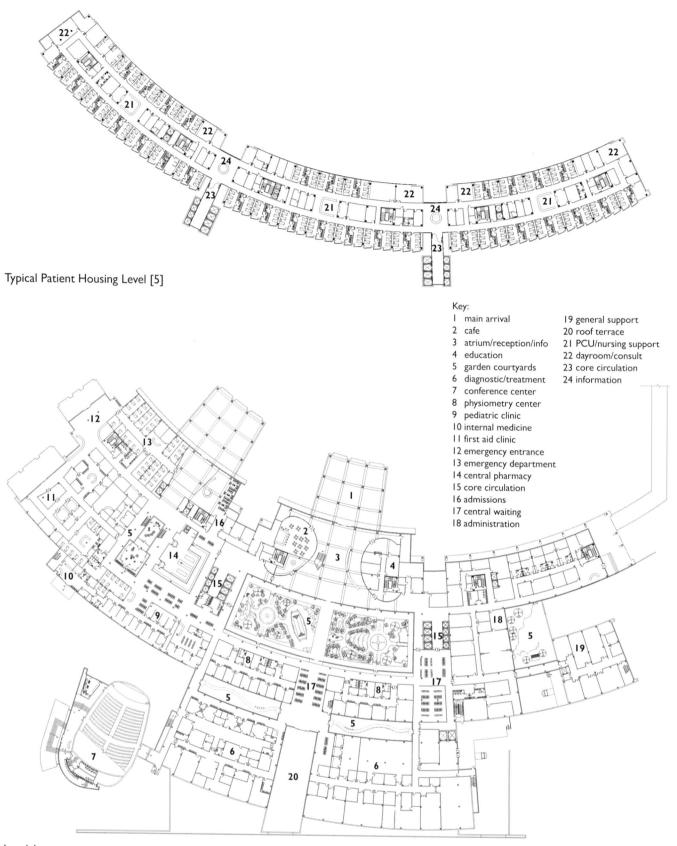

Typical Patient Housing Level [5]

Key:
1 main arrival
2 cafe
3 atrium/reception/info
4 education
5 garden courtyards
6 diagnostic/treatment
7 conference center
8 physiometry center
9 pediatric clinic
10 internal medicine
11 first aid clinic
12 emergency entrance
13 emergency department
14 central pharmacy
15 core circulation
16 admissions
17 central waiting
18 administration
19 general support
20 roof terrace
21 PCU/nursing support
22 dayroom/consult
23 core circulation
24 information

Level 1

8.21.6 Level 1 houses general support and therapeutic garden courtyard. The typical 3-bed semi-private inpatient room is deployed across three PCUs on each inpatient floor

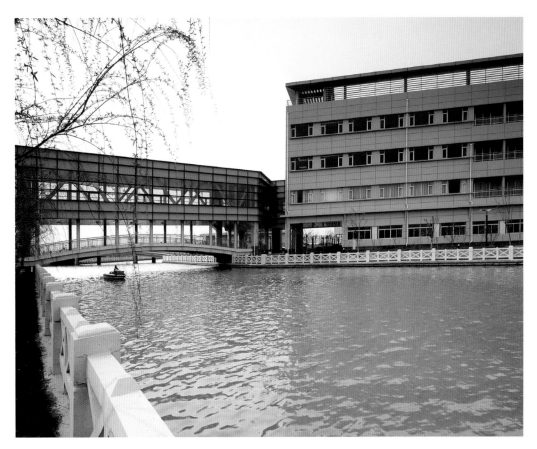

8.21.7 An all-weather pedestrian bridge is a central feature on the campus. The lagoon and adjacent green spaces are for use by patients, families, staff, and the local community

information desk located directly in front. Full height windows provide dramatic views. The circulation plan within each PCU is a racetrack, with support functions housed at the center, not unlike in hospitals in the West. The communal bath/shower rooms are positioned as buffers between alternate bedrooms in an A/B pattern.

To the extent possible in a high-tech medical institution of this size, traditional Chinese garden landscapes played a role in exterior landscaping and in the landscaping of the courtyards. Patients on the third level of the hospital can access a rooftop garden with traditional medicinal herbs including ginseng, ginkgo balboa, and ginger. Shuguang's ground level atrium and latticed glass curtain walls filter natural light throughout the interior and afford views to the park, side courtyards, and the man-made lagoon (Figure 8.21.7). The global aspirations of this hospital and its manicured campus match those of China's in the twenty-first century. This is evident in the quality of materials and overall imagery throughout the hospital campus as well as its exterior landscape (Figure 8.21.8). As a nation, China is striving to rapidly emerge as a world economic power. Yet for this to occur the nation's leaders are fully aware that sophisticated medical care must be available to its citizens, particularly in the nation's largest urban centers. Moreover, Shanghai is one of the fastest growing cities in the world and for these reasons the architecture of this hospital strives to express these goals to the fullest extent.

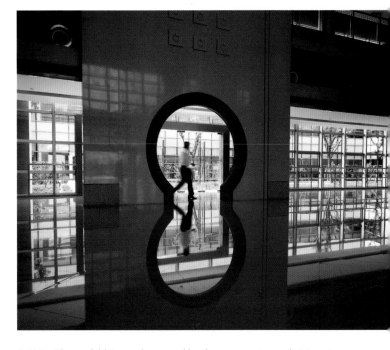

8.21.8 Elegant lobbies on the ground level connect various administrative, diagnostic, and treatment functions housed on upper levels

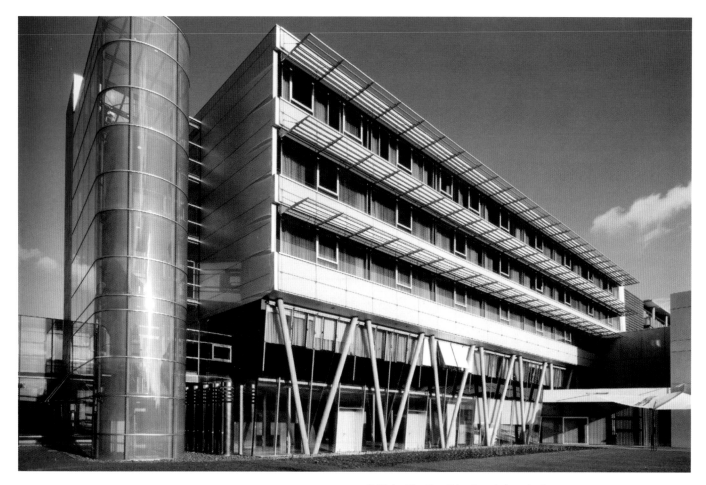

8.22.1 The Graz-West hospital was built to complement an existing regional healthcare network

22 Provincial Hospital of Graz-West (LKH Graz-West), Graz, Austria

ARCHITECT: Domenig Eisenköck Gruber Zinganel, Graz
LANDSCAPE ARCHITECT: Domenig Eisenköck Gruber Zinganel
CLIENT: Steiermärkische Krankenanstalten-gesellschaft m.b.H. (KAGes)
FEATURED MATERIALS: Cast-in-place concrete, low-e exterior glazing, wood veneer interior wall panels, finishes
COMPLETED: 2002
INPATIENT BEDS: 260
SITE/PARKING: 15 acres/195
HOSPITAL SIZE: 335,712SF

Context/site

The Austrian government is reinvesting at this time in its healthcare system and network of facilities. The country currently has the most hospitals per capita in the European Union (EU). This decade, the competition for patients has intensified dramatically due to a rise in alternative hospitals for patients increasingly opting for new, supplemental insurance. Simultaneously, the National Hospital Service commissioned architects and project management teams charged with the task of improving design quality while keeping capital improvement projects on time and on budget. Especially by public sector standards, the recently built Provincial Hospital Graz-West demonstrates that the public system in Austria is fully capable of delivering first-class hospitals that are both aesthetically elegant and highly functional (Figure 8.22.1). As part of an effort to build smaller, decentralized healthcare facilities in the region, the program brief called for functionally deconstructing the comprehensive University Hospital in Graz, located in the eastern part of the city. This new site in Graz's western outskirts largely consists of open fields. It shares its campus with a community-based hospital. Unbuilt greenfields were conserved, and unsightly surface parking areas were avoided, as occurs on so many American hospital campuses. An underground two-level parking deck was constructed. This freed up valuable acreage for undisturbed open space. This measure also allowed for retaining a far greater amount of storm-water runoff than would otherwise occur. The landscaping scheme is understated, in harmony with the massing, scale, and imagery of the building.

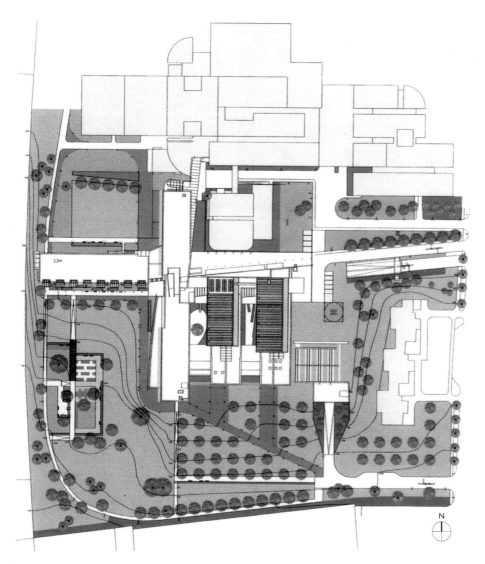

Site Plan

8.22.2 The campus site plan conserves open space while allowing for future expansion

Building/unit

Graz-West is a facility whose complex organizational parti' appears to be composed of many parts, with many permutations (Figures 8.22.2 and 8.22.3a–b). It may appear at first to be a hotel or similar building type, upon arrival. The hospital conveys an atmosphere of elegance, especially as judged against public sector EU standards. Its imagery is high-tech, with minimalist furnishings, artwork, materials, and lighting. The lighting at night is particularly stunning. The facades are composed of buffed, meshed, and ribbed stainless steel bands and panels, punctuated by concrete structural elements and finishes. All are well crafted and detailed, conveying an attitude of care and precision (Figure 8.22.4). The hospital features a two-level lobby that is playfully and colorfully accented by a series of blood-red sculptures. These installations, by the artist Hans Kupelwieser, evoke human organs, and are installed on the exterior approach to the main arrival, and in the lobby are suspended from various surfaces (Figure 8.22.5). The lobby houses a cafe, gallery, kiosk, and waiting areas.

Structurally, the facility is cross-shaped, a reinforced frame with curtain wall panels of lightweight design. A wing with elements resembling cubes is situated at the foreground, at a right angle. Towards the rear of the parti' a two-level private wing forms adjacent landscaped spaces, completing the form of a *cross*. The main entrance opens onto a circulation cross axis that connects the various wings. The

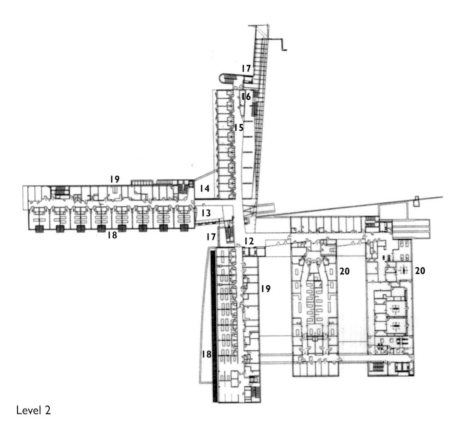

8.22.3a–b The site plan is bi-axial. Visitors arrive at the intersection of two principal axis, with services and treatment areas dispersed along three linear wings radiating as pinwheels from a hub. The lower right guardant contains inpatient care wings and nursing support

Key:
1 underground carpark entry
2 main entry atrium
3 reception/information
4 dining/kitchen
5 main waiting
6 admitting/administration
7 outpatient clinic
8 courtyard
9 central diagnostic/treatment units
10 central lab/pharmacy/administration
11 materials management
12 lobby/information
13 waiting
14 children's play room
15 ICU
16 nursing support
17 circulation
18 PCU/nursing
19 PCU support
20 diagnostic/treatment

Level 2

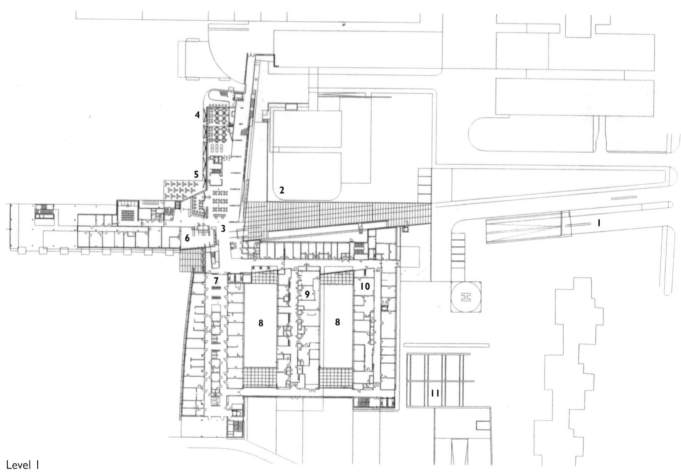

Level 1

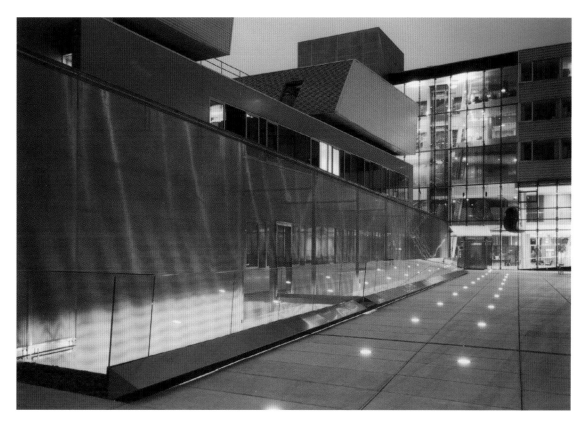

8.22.4 The arrival sequence and atrium recall an upscale hotel in terms of aesthetics and ambiance

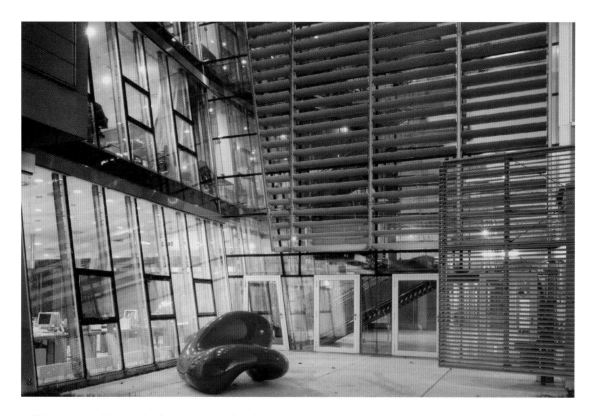

8.22.5 Horizontal louvered grills accentuate a glazed, angled window wall, and define the main public entrance

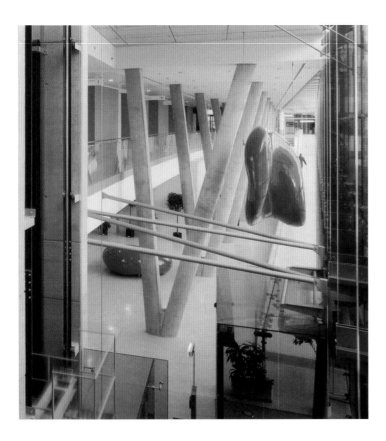

8.22.6 A series of blood-red, heart-like sculptures interplay with a diagonal column gird in the main arrival atrium

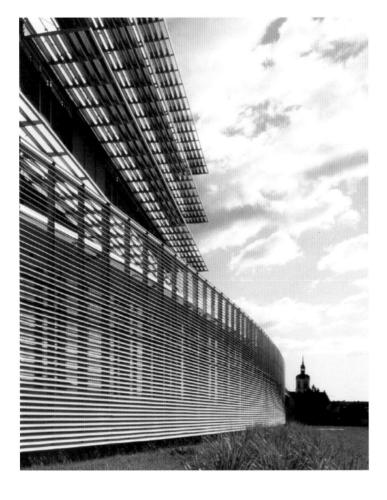

8.22.7 Horizontal sunscreens shield a parking deck, and provide shade for upper level inpatient care units

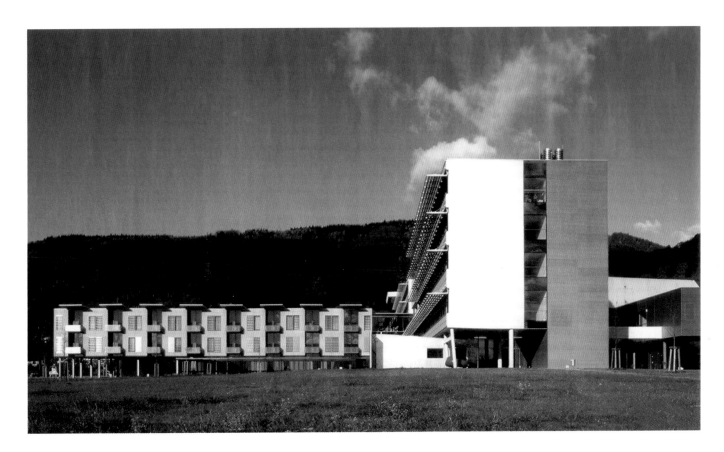

8.22.8 The massive A/B light and shadow rhythms of the inpatient care wing facades contribute to a residentialist imagery

dominant ward wing occurs at a right angle to the composition's main torso. The arrival entry leads into a two-level lobby. Natural materials and low-e exterior glass are featured on the exterior, and glass walls establish an interactive, layered transparency in the interior public zones, i.e. theraserialization.

A glass-encased elevator is transparent in its materiality and imagery. Slender white structural columns are splayed at 30 degree angles, providing spatial definition and scale in the lobby, and also serve as wayfinding orientation aids (Figure 8.22.6). The diagnostic and treatment wing is similarly appointed and transmits ample natural ventilation and light to the interior. This realm houses functions typically found only on the ground level of many American hospitals but at Graz-West the patients go up to the second and third levels for these services. Waiting areas are not unlike those in elegant contemporary EU boutique hotels.

Patient rooms are understated, by contrast, especially when compared to American counterparts in the private sector. Eighty percent of the 260 inpatient beds are in semi-private rooms (2-bed, 3-bed, and 4-bed) while a small complement of beds are deployed as isolation rooms throughout the PCU wings. Some wings house a higher proportion of 4-bed rooms than others. Natural light is emphasized throughout, made possible by the narrow footprint of the patient housing wings. Large operable windows are featured in patients' rooms. Vertical circulation is positioned at the endpoints of the upper level housing wings, and separate inpatient from outpatient treatment areas. Expansion options exist without unduly disrupting provisos for the preservation of open space. Layering, screening, and the judicious use of shade/shadow is applied throughout: the perimeter wall plane of the parking deck is buffered by a stainless steel, horizontally-slotted screen that allows light to enter yet blocks the view to within from the adjacent green space (Figure 8.22.7). The hospital's hotel-like qualities are expressed most visibly, aside from the main lobby, in the all-private room PCU wing (Levels 2 and 3) where each room has a private balcony and patients can directly experience fresh air and views of nature (or from a supine position from one's bed). This is possible due to the full height windows and the sliding glass door provided in each room (Figure 8.22.8).

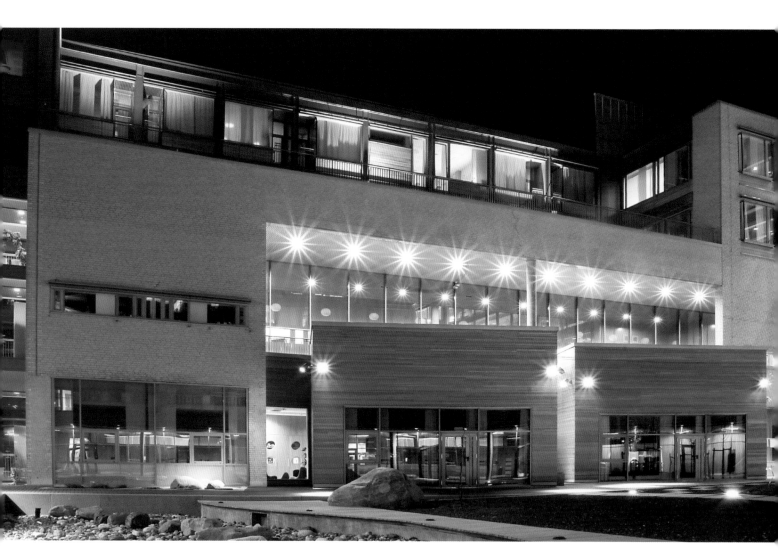

8.23.1   A pair of one-level wood-sheathed cubes is positioned in the auto frontcourt at the main entrance to the Women and Children's Hospital at St. Olav's

23 St. Olav's Hospital, Trondheim, Norway

ARCHITECT: Medplan AS arkitekter/COWI Denmar/Frisk Architects (Women and Children's Centre)
LANDSCAPE ARCHITECT: Various
CLIENT: Helse-Midt-Norge RHF (Central Norway Regional Health Authority)
FEATURED MATERIALS: Cast-in-place concrete, exterior stone cladding, low-e exterior glass, polycarbonate panels, stainless steel, natural and laminate wood
COMPLETED: 2005 (Women and Children's Centre), 2009 (Emergency Care Centre/Heart-Lung Centre)
INPATIENT BEDS: 1,187 (total: 2015)
SITE/PARKING:
HOSPITAL SIZE: 2,152,782SF (total campus)

Context/site

St. Olav's Hospital is the first hospital in Norway to fully integrate patient treatment, research, and teaching. This ambitious project, begun in 1998, will be fully completed in 2015. This university-based tertiary medical center is under construction in Øya in the central part of the city of Trondheim, near its historic downtown. More than 80 percent of the existing hospital campus is being demolished, replacing a century-old hospital on the site. The reinvented campus will serve a regional population of 650,000. This center will employ 7,500, admit 60,000, and serve 300,000 outpatients each year. The completed first phase consisted of the laboratory center, the Women and Children's Hospital (discussed below), the Centre for Neurotherapy, a central supply facility (Phase I), a 150-room hotel (opened in 2004), and the campus-wide power plant and related infrastructure. The on-campus hotel serves rural patients and their families who often face challenges in commuting across the rough terrain of the region (Figure 8.23.1).

In Phase II (2006–2015), the following facilities are being (or have been) built: the Emergency Care Centre/Heart-Lung Centre (discussed below), an abdominal research/treatment center, the second phase of the central facility, and a psychiatric hospital. The 1902 Old Main Building was restored and retained for use for the campus central administration and as the campus resource center/library. Norsk Form (The Foundation for Architecture and Form in Norway), an information and project-based institution in the fields of design, architecture and planning, in 2007 bestowed its annual National Honor Award to St. Olav's Hospital, cited it for an innovative, holistic integration of architecture with landscape design in an environment for healing. The project has thus far been an unusually interdisciplinary endeavor. The A/E team included transportation planners, specialists in sustainable design, medical experts, and representatives of local neighborhood advocacy groups. Sustainable design goals included the maximum reuse of all on-site construction waste materials, the life-cycle amenity of all materials selected, the maximum use of renewable resources such as wood, and the use of vertical landscaping.

Building/unit

The designs of the hospital already completed or under construction are based on the Planetree Model, which places the patient and the patient's family at the center of all care, rather than the traditional modus operandi of hospital/staff needs at the center of the caregiving equation. This symbolized a radical departure from how care had been provided in the past at St. Olav's. Research and teaching is now also fully integrated into the medical center's organizational culture. Structures feature narrow footprints and wings that reach outward to their neighboring buildings. Individual commissions for specific buildings have been awarded to a number of architectural firms. This was done for political correctness as much as to achieve diversity in aesthetic approaches while adhering to a set of consistent design and planning guidelines. The campus is being built in a six square block area. A landscaped boulevard is the main artery through the campus. The narrow wings of the various buildings allow for ample natural light transmission deep into the interiors. This is a critical consideration in Norway, where daylight is a scarce commodity during many months of the year. A network of elevated glazed pedestrian bridges, and underground tunnels, connect the buildings.

The arrival courtyard of the Women and Children's Pavilion features two cubes that establish an inviting image. An irregularly shaped plaza is at the center of this 'exterior room'. The cubes serve as the main entrance and are of the scale of a private residence. They are sheathed in a natural finish horizontal wood siding. This building is indicated at the lower right corner in the campus master plan (Figure 8.23.2). This six-level building is of masonry with wood accentuations, with a slatted screening device sheathing the facade of a pedestrian bridge

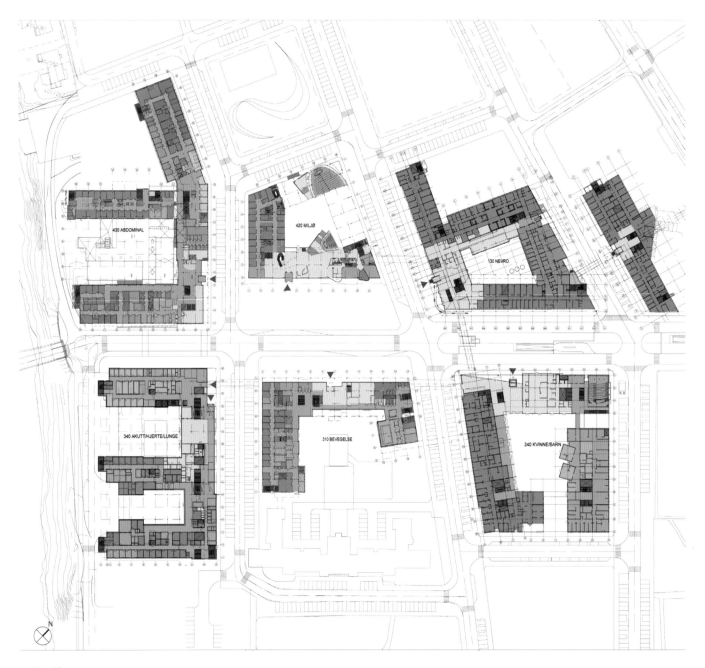

Site Plan

8.23.2 The St. Olav's replacement medical campus, when complete, will consist of six superblocks of new construction. The existing street grid was maintained with minimal changes

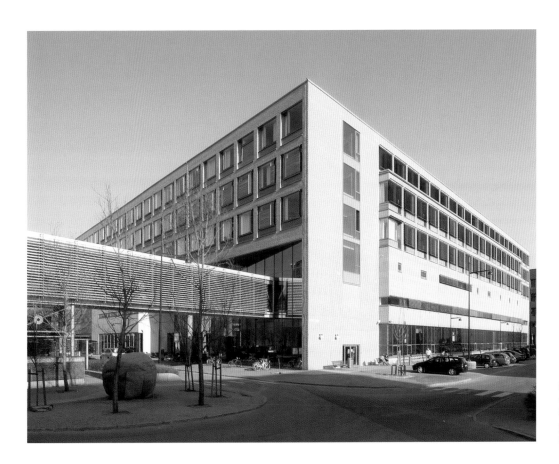

8.23.3 Extensive planning and design attention was devoted to campus coordinated bike, pedestrian, and vehicular networks

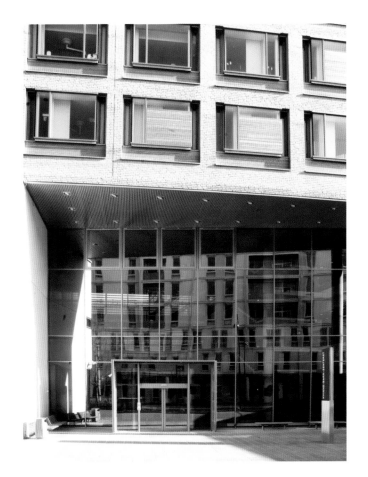

8.23.4 In the Women and Children's Pavilion, patient room bay windows are operable

linking this building with a research building. The patient rooms have operable windows, and they are configured as bay windows (Figure 8.23.3). The ground level features glass, patient care floors situated above (Figure 8.23.4). This level houses a large auditorium, the arrival lobby, cafe, gift shop, administration, admitting, and related public functions of the hospital. Diagnostic and treatment is housed on the second level, as is mechanical equipment. The third through fifth levels house PCUs. The cubes feature rooftop terraces; above this level are inpatient rooms. The hospital, as mentioned, consulted with local community organizations and patient advocacy groups. The inpatient pavilions and PCUs consist of six to eight private rooms. The Women and Children's Centre's only semi-private rooms are reserved for chemotherapy and dialysis patients.

In the nearby nine-level Emergency Care/Heart-Lung Centre, aforementioned narrow wings are reminiscent of the Hôpital Beaujon, near Paris (1932–1935), Charity Hospital in New Orleans (1935–1938), and similar high-rise Nightingale hospitals of the period (see Chapters 2 and 5). This building is located in the lower left corner of the campus site plan. The arrival level houses public functions, with upper levels housing diagnostic, treatment, and inpatient care units (Figure 8.23.5a–b). St. Olav's rejected the late-twentieth-century

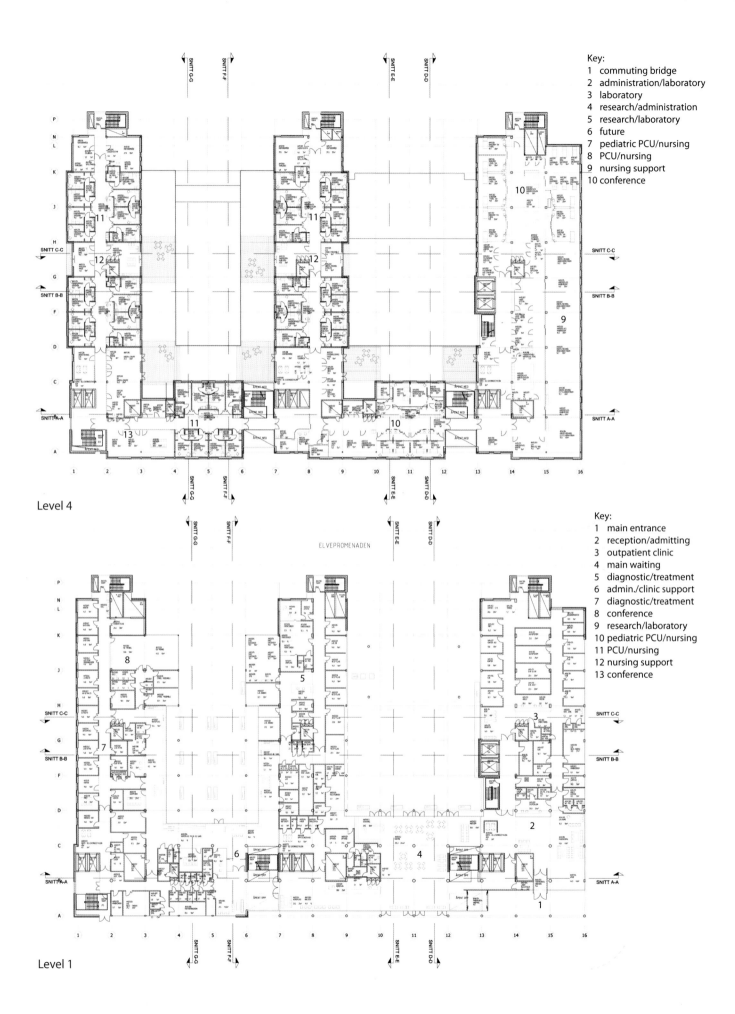

Key:
1 commuting bridge
2 administration/laboratory
3 laboratory
4 research/administration
5 research/laboratory
6 future
7 pediatric PCU/nursing
8 PCU/nursing
9 nursing support
10 conference

Level 4

ELVEPROMENADEN

Key:
1 main entrance
2 reception/admitting
3 outpatient clinic
4 main waiting
5 diagnostic/treatment
6 admin./clinic support
7 diagnostic/treatment
8 conference
9 research/laboratory
10 pediatric PCU/nursing
11 PCU/nursing
12 nursing support
13 conference

Level 1

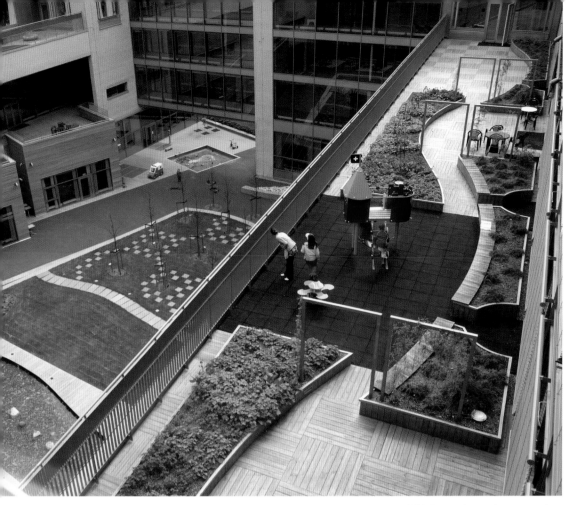

8.23.6 Landscaped terraces – theraserialized roofscapes – occur at the second through fourth levels. Wood decking, planters, bright colors, lay objects, and seating invite frequent use

megahospital's massive floor plan *block hospital* templates – with their large undifferentiated zones with myriad internal departments devoid of natural light and ventilation.

The stepped massing of the Women and Children's Pavilion Hospital is skillfully composed and executed. A pair of terraces – therapeutic garden roofscapes – occur at the fourth levels and each functions as an extension of the ground level arrival courtyard below. Wood decking, planters, gateways, bright colors, and playful geometries orchestrate these *places*. Play structures are provided for patients and their families, and a variety of materials are used, including wood decking. When viewed from above, the set of cubes appear as semi-autonomous from the hospital itself – not unlike two wooden play blocks of child's toys sitting beneath a table (Figure 8.23.6 and Figure 8.23.7). It will be interesting to experience the completed St. Olav's campus.

8.23.5a–b Sustainable design attributes at St. Olav's include narrow building footprints (daylight transmission), natural ventilation, and recycled materials. The decentralized campus is a radical break from the highly centralized, hermetically sealed, machine megahospitals of the late twentieth century

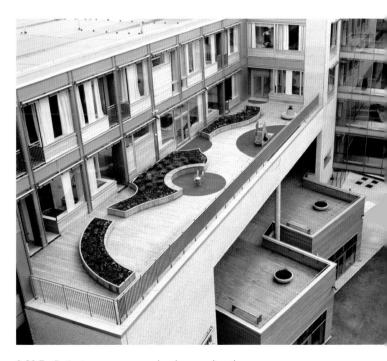

8.23.7 Patient rooms on upper levels open directly onto a roof terrace; other patient rooms are provided with small private balconies

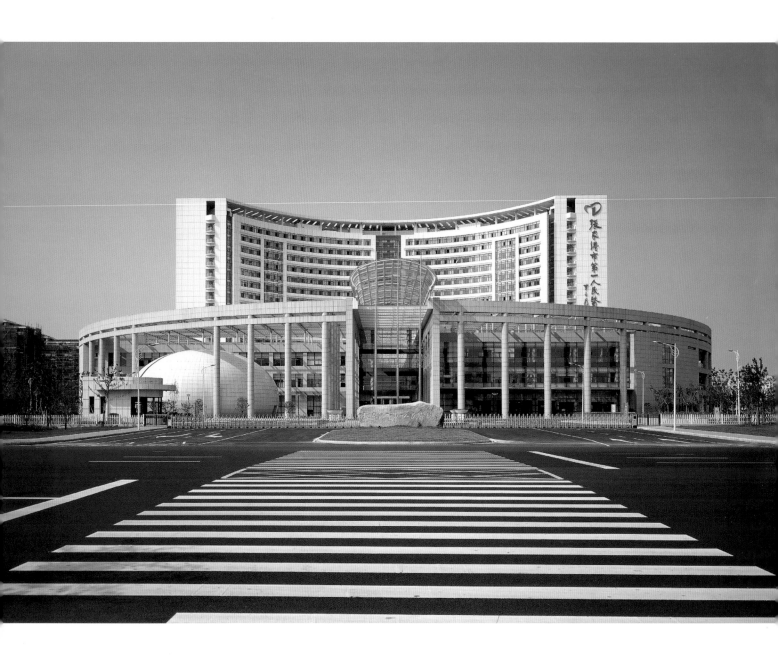

8.24.1   The symmetry and scale of the First People's Hospital is reminiscent of the European Palace Hospitals of the seventeenth and eighteenth centuries, as well as early-twentieth-century art deco skyscraper hospitals (see Chapter 5)

24 Zhangjiagang First People's Hospital, Zhangjiagang, China

ARCHITECT: Meng Jianmin, Hou Jun, Wang Iijuan, Tai Renji, Peng Ying, Wu Lianhua, Xia Changsong, Mu Li, Mai Xuanwei, Shanghai
LANDSCAPE ARCHITECT: Same as above
CLIENT: Ministry of Health, Beijing Province, China
FEATURED MATERIALS: Cast-in-place concrete, porcelain enamel exterior tiles, masonry, aluminum, exterior stone cladding and pavers, zinc, polycarbonate Plexiglas panels, natural and laminated wood interior finishes, doors, and millwork
COMPLETED: 2007
INPATIENT BEDS: 1,000
SITE/PARKING: 44 acres/325
HOSPITAL SIZE: 532,020SF

Context/site

This replacement hospital, located in a rapidly growing community in the Beijing metro area, is a large, comprehensive facility, providing 1,000 inpatient beds, outpatient facilities, and a research institute. More than 550,000 outpatients are served, and 8,000 surgical procedures are performed annually. This hospital features a paperless, digital medical records system, a first in China. An older hospital located nearby was demolished to make way for the new campus. The hospital at Zhangjiagang is an important addition to the medical services in the Beijing region for its sophisticated medical technology and range of services. A major concept was to provide a single-point care provider for a growing community, in a dignified care environment. Key goals were to be patient centered, to minimize life-cycle energy consumption costs, and to employ ecologically sound construction practices. Microclimate factors, prevailing winds, and sun orientation, in particular, were emphasized in building placement, orientation, and design (Figure 8.24.1).

A welcoming image, and navigable pedestrian and vehicular circulation systems were of priority, resulting in a north–south pedestrian street/axis spanning the length of the campus. With the hospital placed toward the front, four quadrants were established. The large size of the hospital called for an east–west/north–south cross axis. Logistical support buildings were placed in the northernmost quadrant of the site. Autonomous vehicular and pedestrian routes separate service, delivery, staff, and patient/visitor patterns of movement. Pathways pass through gardens leading into the hospital.

A semi-circular arrival frontcourt occurs at the main entry to the inpatient tower. Parking is provided on site, including a one-level underground parking deck.

Building/unit

The hospital and its exterior environs are based in radiality, symmetry, and their monumental expression. A sphere was chosen as the primary geometry as it symbolizes *holistic healthcare* – the circle of life. In Chinese culture, birth, sickness, wellness, spirituality, and death are recognized as fundamental – a hospital must equally and equitably care for the patient in every phase of one's life. A radial 16-level inpatient tower rises above a platform support structure. This base varies in height and volume according to its complex internal functions, with open spaces interspersed in between. These functions (including a lagoon) are screened by an overhead monolithic steel canopy sunscreen. This device covers the entire roof of this structure while also giving visual unity to the spaces below. Diagnostic and treatment services housed within this platform base structure include emergency care, research, and outpatient services. The horizontal central circulation axis terminates at the elevator core and then extends vertically up through the center of the inpatient tower (Figure 8.24.2).

A monumentally scaled steel and glass promenade functions as a ceremonial gateway to the campus. In its scale and articulation, this canopy is grandiose (Figure 8.24.3). Landscaped plazas, this gateway promenade, and the aforementioned lagoon are featured elements. To a first-time visitor, it is an impressive scene. In the case of the arrival/ceremonial axis, a second level pedestrian walkway parallels these paths on the hospital's backside with a vehicular access road in the center. The helipad is located near to the front entrance to the campus and its most ceremonial gateway (perhaps to impress visiting foreign dignitaries). By contrast, the typical U.S. hospital helipad is usually relegated to a purely rudimentary back-of-the-house location.

The entrances to the outpatient services and the emergency departments are located in side courts at the foot of a semi-radial inpatient tower, at its opposing endpoints. Each side court provides

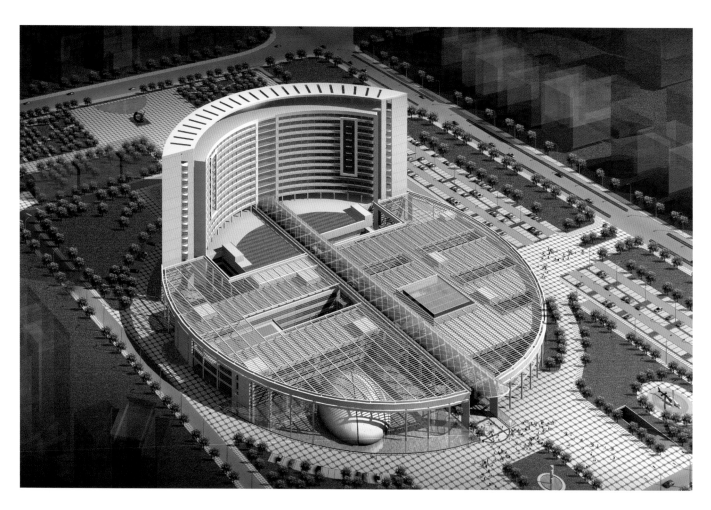

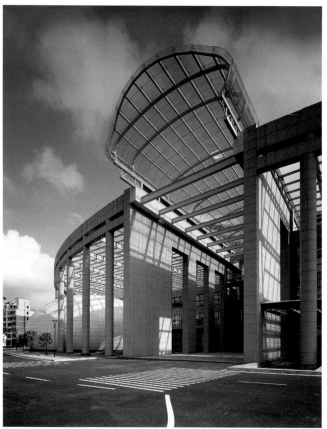

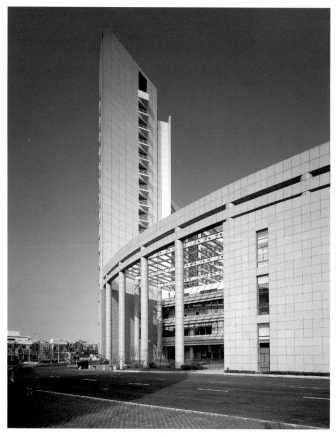

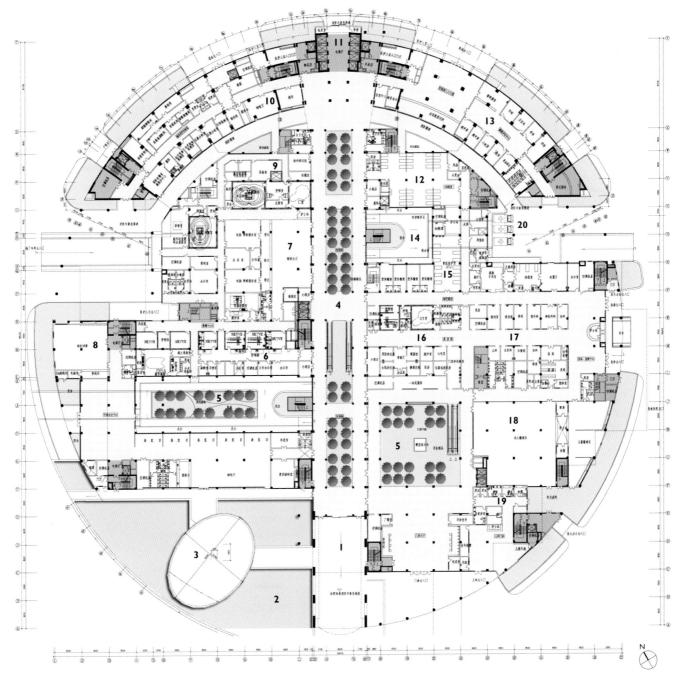

Level 1

Key:

1 hospital street extension/emergency	11 circulation
2 reflecting pond	12 emergency medicine/treatment
3 academic hall	13 health assessment
4 hospital pedestrian street	14 courtyard/garden
5 courtyard	15 ICU
6 radiology/administration	16 emergency medicine/administration
7 reception/waiting	17 outpatient services
8 medical records	18 adult intravenous injection/infusion
9 mechanical room	19 admitting/consultation
10 dining/market	20 emergency entrance/ambulance

8.24.2 The parti' consists of concentric rings and a biaxial orthogonal grid, defining a network of mass/void (support units) deployed beneath a monumental arrival canopy. Large green spaces mediate the zone between a platform base and an inpatient tower. The promenade/arrival axis, and an underground service road, function as two principal axis'. The inpatient tower occupies the outer ring to the rear of the parti

8.24.3 A dramatically glazed canopy announces the promenade – an egg-shaped academic lecture hall is to the left

8.24.4 The circular platform base is articulated as a series of consentric rings, further articulated by pedestrian and/or vehicular access, i.e. the below ground service drive

8.24.5 The platform base houses research and teaching facilities, administration, and general support

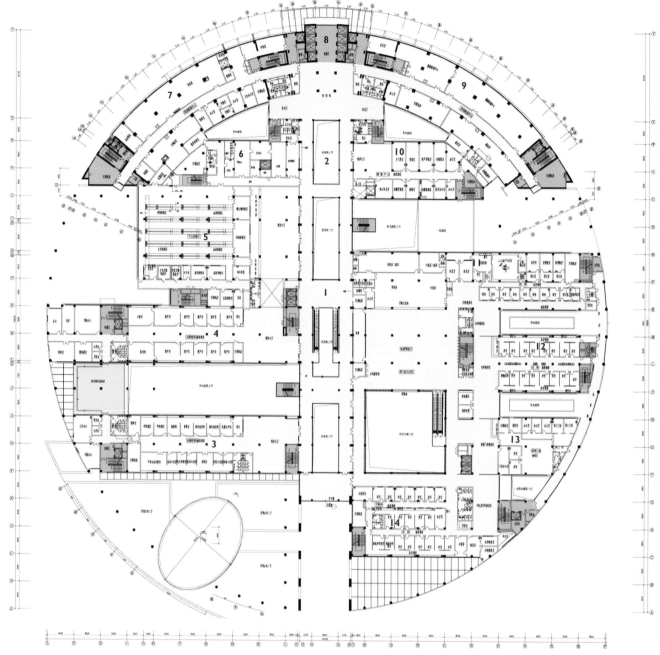

Level 2

Key:
1 hospital pedestrian street
2 atrium
3 central laboratory/support
4 lab/research unit
5 main lab testing
6 conference/administration
7 central pharmacy
8 circulation
9 central pharmacy/supplies/materials management
10 resonator mirror test center
11 gynecology/women's health
12 internal medicine unit
13 VIP clinic/cafe
14 traditional Chinese medicine center

8.24.6 The central arrival promenade established transition zones from exterior to interior space

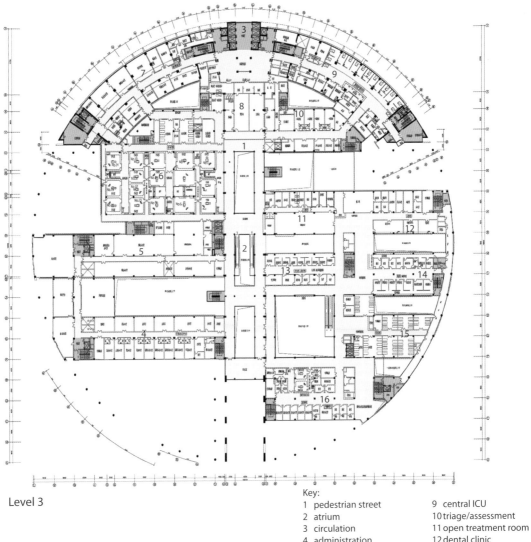

Typical Patient Care Level [Level 6]

Level 3

8.24.7a–b The thinness of the inpatient tower contrasts with the circumference and grid diagram of the medical center's support base

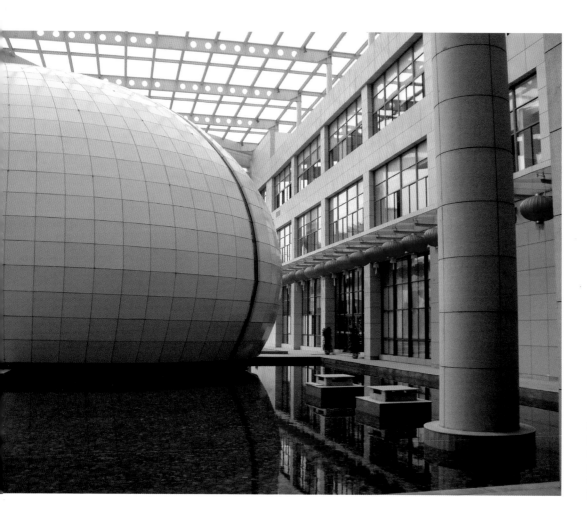

8.24.8 An academic lecture hall sits in a reflecting pond, anchored to the superordinate grid of the medical center's support platform by two footbridges

for vehicular and pedestrian access (Figure 8.24.4). The platform base, as mentioned, houses all non-inpatient care services and research facilities (Figure 8.24.5, Figure 8.24.6 and Figure 8.24.7a–b). Transverse and longitudinal sections through the hospital indicate a complex and yet clear diagrammatic relationship between the support platform and tower. The aforementioned large egg-shaped sphere is placed in the center of the lagoon (Figure 8.24.8). This 'Academic Hall' houses an auditorium and seminar rooms. Its main level is one level below the ground level. The five exterior courtyards within the platform base contain indigenous wooden footbridges over a narrow reflecting pond. Indigenous plant species are featured although patients are generally disallowed from using the courtyards.

The tower houses semi-private (a mix of 2-bed and 3-bed) rooms. Some isolation rooms are provided on each unit. The bath/shower rooms are communal and are located on the inboard side of the inpatient room. The windows in patients' rooms are operable, facilitating natural ventilation, and the slender footprint of the tower allows for maximum natural light to be transmitted to the interior. A nursing station is situated at the midpoint of each PCU. A key

planning concept was to provide decentralized waiting rooms near to the point of care, as opposed to the large monotonous waiting rooms endemic to the vast majority of post-World War II International Style hospitals in China. This hospital is a civic landmark for the community, insofar as it expresses the new, progressive attitude of the healthcare bureaucracy in twenty-first-century China. China, as is well known, is on a self-imposed fast track to a heightened global stature. To critics, it might appear, in this case, that a preoccupation with high-tech signature architecture outweighed fundamental principles of environmental stewardship per se. Nonetheless, this noteworthy hospital is located in the nation's capital, and China's Ministry of Health views it locally, nationally, and internationally as a symbol of China's future ambitions and potential on the global healthcare stage.

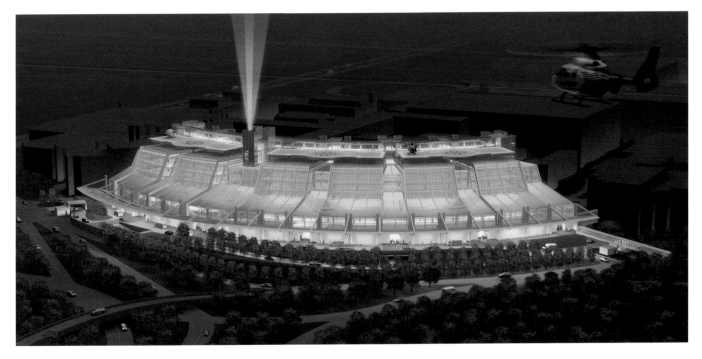

8.25.1 The ER One prototype was conceived in response to the 9/11 terrorist attacks in New York City and Washington. D.C. in 2001

25 ER ONE,
Washington, District of Columbia

ARCHITECT: HKS, Dallas/Pickard Chilton, New Haven
LANDSCAPE ARCHITECT: The Office of James Burnett
CLIENT: Washington, D.C. Hospital Center
FEATURED MATERIALS: Earthen berms, blast-resistant interior walls/
  panels
COMPLETED: Proposal 2003
INPATIENT BEDS: N/A
SITE/PARKING: 15 acres/200
HOSPITAL SIZE: 500,000SF

Context/site

The tragedy of the Al-Qaeda terrorist attacks on the Pentagon, in Washington, D.C., and the World Trade Center Towers, in New York City, on September 11 2001 vividly underscored the need for a rapid medical response capability in the U.S. It was immediately recognized that proactive measures were necessary to protect the nation's critical medical infrastructure in the aftermath of natural disasters, epidemics, and acts of terrorism. Beyond all else, the goal for post-disaster

trauma healthcare protocols would be that they would not in any way be construed as a source of breakdown in the delivery of care, or a source of response incapability. Any rapid response care systems must be fully operational and in an anticipatory posture, architecturally and otherwise, on a 24/7 basis. Most community hospitals in the U.S., however, and particularly their emergency departments, are not prepositioned to provide the necessary support, from a facility readiness perspective. A post-disaster trauma care center must adroitly manage the demand for high utilization in a very short span of time. At present, most American community hospitals are not designed to provide this level of support (Figure 8.25.1).

Project ER One originated at the Washington Hospital Center when it was awarded a contract from the U.S. Office of Emergency Preparedness, a unit of the Department of Health and Human Services (DHHS) in late September 2001, to study the feasibility and design of a fixed-site all-risk *scalable* emergency department on the campus of an existing urban medical center in the U.S. capital. In the study's first phase, the focus was on retrofit requirements for existing emergency departments. The second phase consisted of the development of a

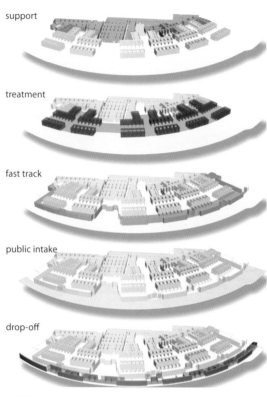

support

treatment

fast track

public intake

drop-off

3-D Diagrams 1-5

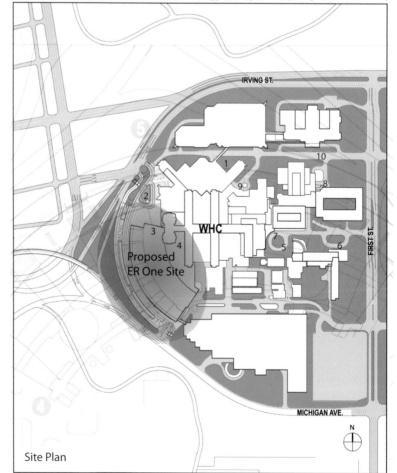

Necklace/HUB Plan

HUB Plan Key:
1 access control
2 HUB 1
3 HUB 2
4 HUB 3
5 waiting/information

Site Plan Key:
1 main entrance
2 emergency entrance
3 medSTAR entrance
4 service entrance
5 hyman building entrance
6 east building entrance
7 bus circle entrance
8 POB entrance
9 cancer institute entrance
10 national rehabilitation
   hospital entrance

Site Plan

8.25.2a–c Multiple lines of defense
are built into the site and structure

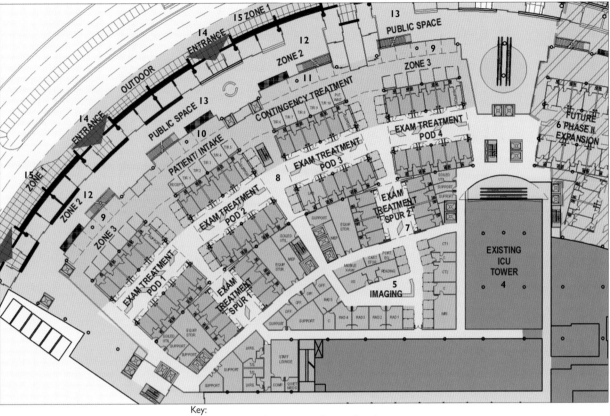

Level 1 [Phase 1]

Key:
1 therapeutic roofscape
2 main arrival/information
3 access road
4 existing ICU tower
5 diagnostic imaging
6 future phase II expansion
7 exam/treatment spur 2
8 exam/treatment pods 1-4
9 zone 3 intake
10 central patient intake
11 contingency treatment
12 zone 2
13 waiting/public area
14 ER entrance/triage
15 zone 1

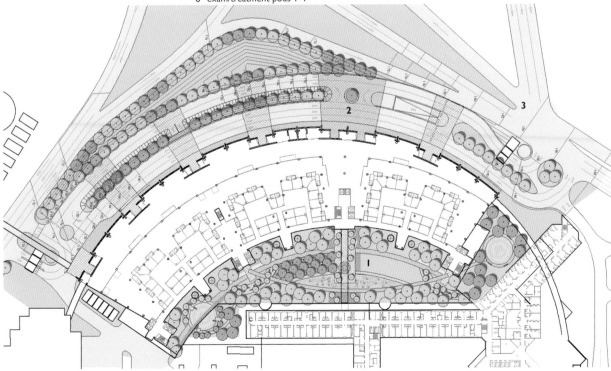

Site Plan/Landscape

8.25.3a–b The parti' is composed of semi-radial concentric rings, from outer arrival/triage to an innermost ring of treatment/surgical bays

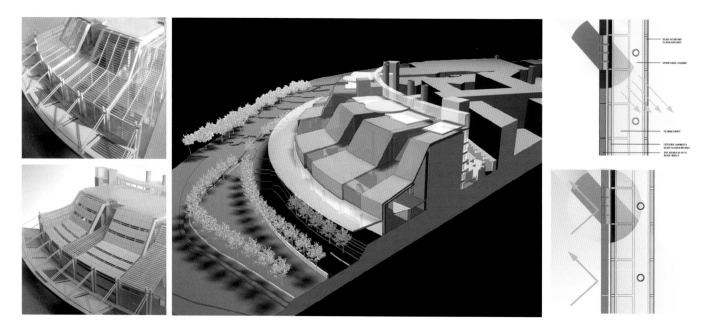

8.25.4a–e   A steel sunscreen/security grid can open or close as a means to fully lock down, or *armor* this trauma treatment center

prototype. ER One is a prototype for a crescent-shaped site at the edge of the existing campus of Washington Hospital. A risk assessment analysis was conducted and input was incorporated from a host of external consultants on blast engineering, decontamination processes, infectious disease mitigation, casualty modeling (with software provided by the U.S. Defense Threat Reduction Agency), and bomb-resistant structural and wall assembly systems. The prototyping process consisted of project definition and scope; operational needs assessment, aesthetic goals and concepts, risk assessment, timeline for implementation, alternate configurations, their testing, and refinement.

ER One is capable of assessing and treating thousands of injured persons in a matter of hours. An eight-level, 500,000 square foot trauma center features multiple ports of access for ambulances, cars, and buses at ground level, and heliport access. For persons in the immediate disaster strike zone, ER One provides self-check-in stations for immediate assistance and triage. In the event of a biological attack, or pandemic outbreak, intelligent scanning devices immediately identify a carrier and commence with decontamination of that individual in an isolation zone. Moveable walls in the various treatment bays provide staff and patients with needed functional support. Its bunker configuration is such as to minimize the possibility of the entire facility being shut down if subjected to a direct strike. The facility features a parkway, emergency vehicular access zone, and a roofscape garden with trees and ground plantings. Protective earthen berms shield the facility against vehicular-bomb attack.

Building/unit

The radial-shaped prototype conforms to its irregular site (Figure 8.25.2a–b and Figure 8.25.3a–b). Its massing is stepped, or tiered. This tiered concourse shields a mid-rise patient housing and support element that rises to eight levels above a three-level platform. The trauma center is comprised of five spatial zones: drop-off, public

intake, fast track, exam/treatment, and general support in a hub and spoke system, with Hub 1, Hub 2 and Hub 3 providing rapid response intake and triage assessment. Each hub is associated with its dedicated treatment zone. The main level houses routine care and yet is transformable into a high utilization unit capable of treating five times or more patients in the occurrence of a mass casualty event.

The facility is itself disaster resistant, with a sophisticated exterior louver system that armors the building against attack or airborne contamination in the atmosphere (Figure 8.25.4a–e). This shield can be sealed off in the event of an attack. The building envelope features a tamperproof air intake and exhaust system whereby air intake occurs on a lower roof and then it is exhausted from a vent on the uppermost roof. Patient intake occurs on the outermost radius and proceeds inward to the core treatment zone. Wide corridors and passages preclude bottlenecks. Multiple entry points are provided to facilitate inflow, outflow, and triage.

The three lower levels (basement) house general support and a fallout shelter. Level 1 is the drop-off and parking level (parking is provided on three levels below grade) intake/triage level, as well as emergency treatment. The main concourse (Level 1) houses Zones 1, 2 and 3 for triage and treatment. Level 2 is an interstitial floor, with Level 3 immediately above, housing the administration. Levels 4–6 house critical care units for inpatient care. A mechanical level is above (Level 7), with the helipads on the roof (Level 8).

A step-up Universal Treatment Room was developed that is readily convertible from a single to 3-bed treatment bay (Figure 8.25.5a–b). These treatment bays are acuity adaptable for use as post-trauma treatment *flex spaces*. The adjacent public concourse can also be used for triage and treatment. The bays are designed larger than the typical emergency room, and provide additional space for secondary treatment. Each room can be isolated from all adjacent spaces – functional autonomy – in terms of ER One's HVAC systems. When not in use, ultraviolet light decontaminates treatment zones on a continuous basis.

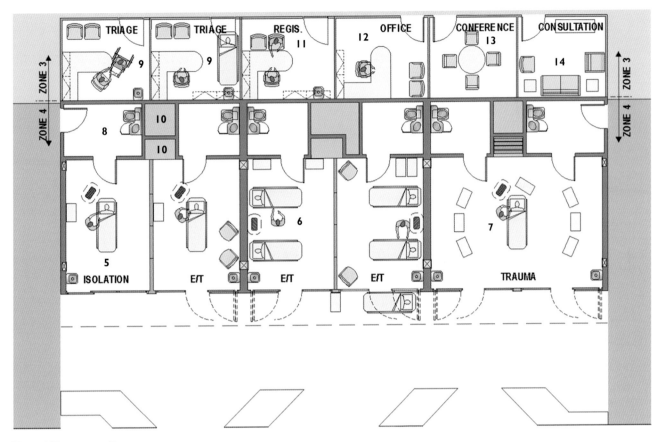

Typical Treatment Bay

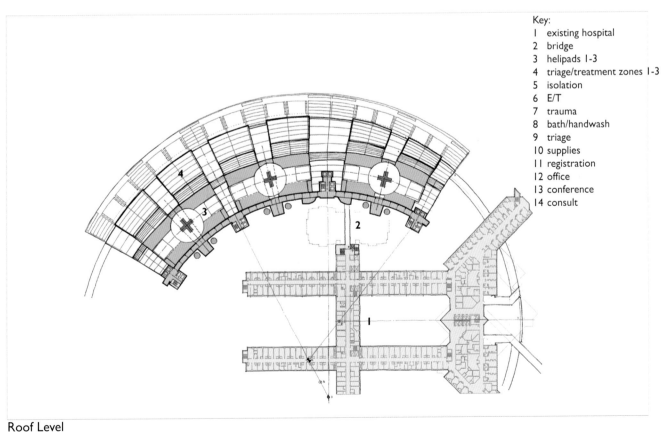

Roof Level

Key:
1 existing hospital
2 bridge
3 helipads 1-3
4 triage/treatment zones 1-3
5 isolation
6 E/T
7 trauma
8 bath/handwash
9 triage
10 supplies
11 registration
12 office
13 conference
14 consult

8.25.5a–b Treatment/surgical bays are transformational – wall partitions can be quickly relocated or removed based on rapidly changing needs

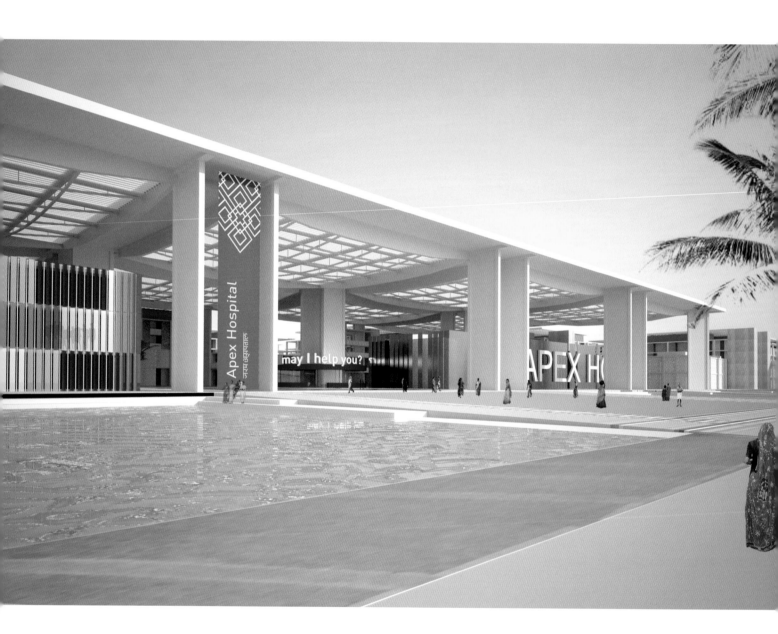

8.26.1 This scheme received second prize in an invited
international design competition for the master planning
and architectural design of six Apex Prototype medical
centers in India

26 Apex Prototype, Six All India Institutes of Medical Sciences, Jodhpur, India

ARCHITECT: Heinle, Wischer and Partners, Berlin
LANDSCAPE ARCHITECT: Heinle, Wischer and Partners
CLIENT: Indian Ministry of Health and Family Welfare (MoHFW)
FEATURED MATERIALS: Cast-in-place lightweight reinforced concrete, stone pavers, aluminum, wood, ceramic tile, precast concrete panels, wood interior finishes
COMPLETED: Proposal (2006)
INPATIENT BEDS: 450 beds (varies)
SITE/PARKING: 48 acres/350 (varies)
HOSPITAL SIZE: varies

Context/site

In the summer of 2006, the Indian Ministry of Health and Family Welfare announced an international design competition, the 'Six All-MS' (All India Institutes of Medical Sciences like Apex Healthcare Institutes). The objective was to build a network of new, high quality public healthcare campuses across the nation. The sites for construction of these new university-based medical centers are Rishikesh, Jodhpur (presented here), Bhopal, Raipur, Patna, and Bhubaneswar. The four principal program elements were to design a hospital complex, teaching complex and auditorium, public infrastructure, and residential facilities on each campus. Twelve international architectural firms were invited to submit proposals that were at once visionary, pragmatic, and constructible – each to be a state-of-the-art medical campus for the twenty-first century. This scheme is the second place winner in the competition. No first prize was awarded. The specific charge was to develop a prototype for a university medical center, including housing and infrastructure, and to demonstrate its adaptability to six very different site contexts, drawing upon the local vernacular cultural traditions of each geographic locale (Figure 8.26.1).

This competition submittal booklet included schematic campus plans for each of the six campuses to be built, and a detailed proposal for the Jodhpur campus. Jodhpur is situated at the edge of the Thar Desert. It is a hot, dry locale. Bhopal is a more tropical climate, with hot summers and temperate winters. The campus plan for Bhubaneswar was broken into two parts, with the residential campus separate for the other three core program components. Here, the summers are warm and rainy, and the winter months can be severe.

The campus at Patna is smaller by comparison to Jodhpur, and the climate is extreme and warm in the summer, with temperate winters, and monsoon rains occurring from June to September. The climate at Raipur is mostly tropical and humid, also with heavy monsoon rains. This campus was also subdivided with its three main components comprising a large square/grid with two nearby enclaves for residential housing. The proposal for the campus at Rishikesh was compact and contiguous because this region experiences a temperate climate much of the year.

This prototype is to be a patient and family-centered place, not merely an 'efficient' machine: 'The idea is to combine the modern concept of a hospital with established traditions while finding new forms of space and function by accommodating existing social structures, environmental requirements and the need for flexibility.' The campuses are each seen as autonomous urban villages interwoven

8.26.2 The complex and contradictory conditions of everyday urban life in India were the primary determinants – a high-tech yet outwardly traditional-appearing health village firmly rooted in the nation's indigenous vernacular architecture

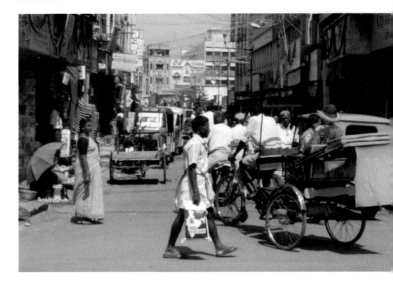

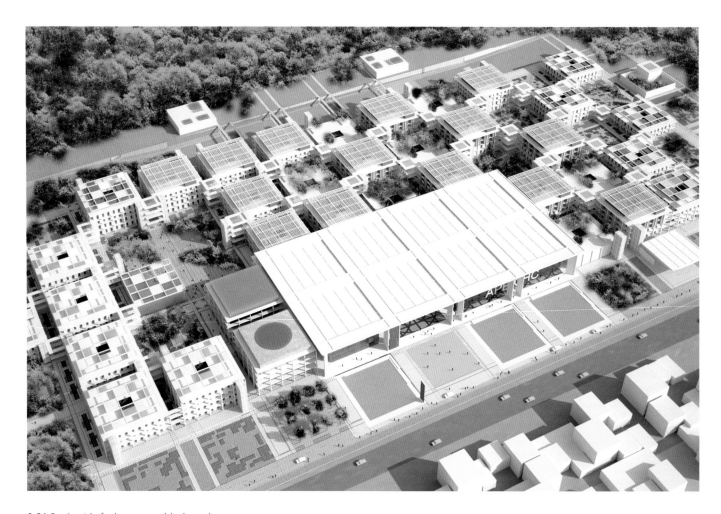

8.26.3 A grid of urban square blocks and open square was articulated as a means to create diverse zones and pockets – residential, arrival, nursing care, administration, diagnostic and treatment

into their surrounding community and its physical, often chaotic and random, urban fabric. The buildings at Jodhpur were arranged in a chessboard grid with an orthogonal network of pedestrian routes/paths articulating each campus/village as a network of interconnected, pedestrian-scaled city streets. The competition submittal included a photo of a chessboard in reference to the campus plan. An arrival gateway featuring a reflecting pool flanks a wide walkway with a large welcoming banner and a central information station (Figure 8.26.2). The campus is to be accessed and navigable by foot, bike, public transport, or auto. In this regard, each is a seamless expression of the often-chaotic urban life around it, while simultaneously referencing the necessity for the medical village's functional autonomy as a secure, specialized place.

Building/unit

The main entry portal is clearly visible from the street and establishes the medical center's civic presence. The campus wayfinding system, created by Kognito Gestaltung, of Berlin, was a highlighted feature of the competition submittal and is augmented by nature – ponds, groves of trees, trellises, hedges, and gardens interspersed as wayfinding devices and places for respite. Heat island effects are therefore minimized by means of natural ground plantings as opposed to concrete paths. A pictograph symbol-word system is used, with words keyed to various departments and buildings. As many as twenty blocks in the proposal for the Jodhpur campus are devoted to open or semi-enclosed spaces for use by patients, families, staff, and visitors.

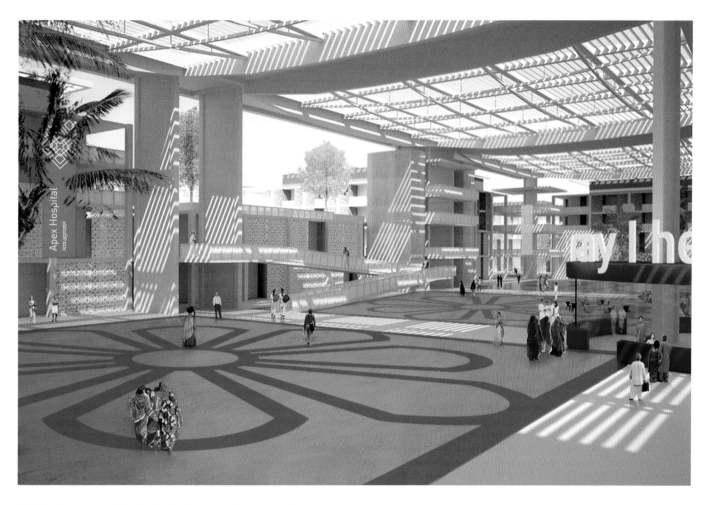

8.26.4 A monumentally scaled arrival concourse is the central civic gathering and orientation element in the 'health village'

Buildings are configured within the aforementioned orthogonal 6 x 12 square urban chessboard grid, with each resultant 'city block' identical in size. Building heights vary, as does the density of each block although no structure is more than four levels. Internal functions with each block vary widely as does their degree of transparency (Figure 8.26.3). The emergency department entrance is clearly identified and accessible. Natural daylight is filtered yet ample; windows are operable to transmit natural ventilation to within, and views are to overlook therapeutic gardens. Building footprints are relatively shallow and many have courtyards at their center:

From composition and proportion, to spatial transparency, orientation, material, light, color and greening, we have chosen

exactly those elements suitable for a modern hospital … the patient has to be respected by creating a relaxed and serene atmosphere. The conceptual design is similar to the traditional [Indian] urban layout featuring streets, courtyards, partial plantings and low buildings [and] is based on the rational pattern of the chessboard with an orthogonal grid of axis' oriented in two directions.

(Architects' brief)

The arrival pavilion is monumental, open air, screened from excessive sunlight, and is to be used for local civic events and ceremonies. The open-air roof functions as a sunscreen to shield occupants from the intense sun. Similarly, roof sunscreens are featured

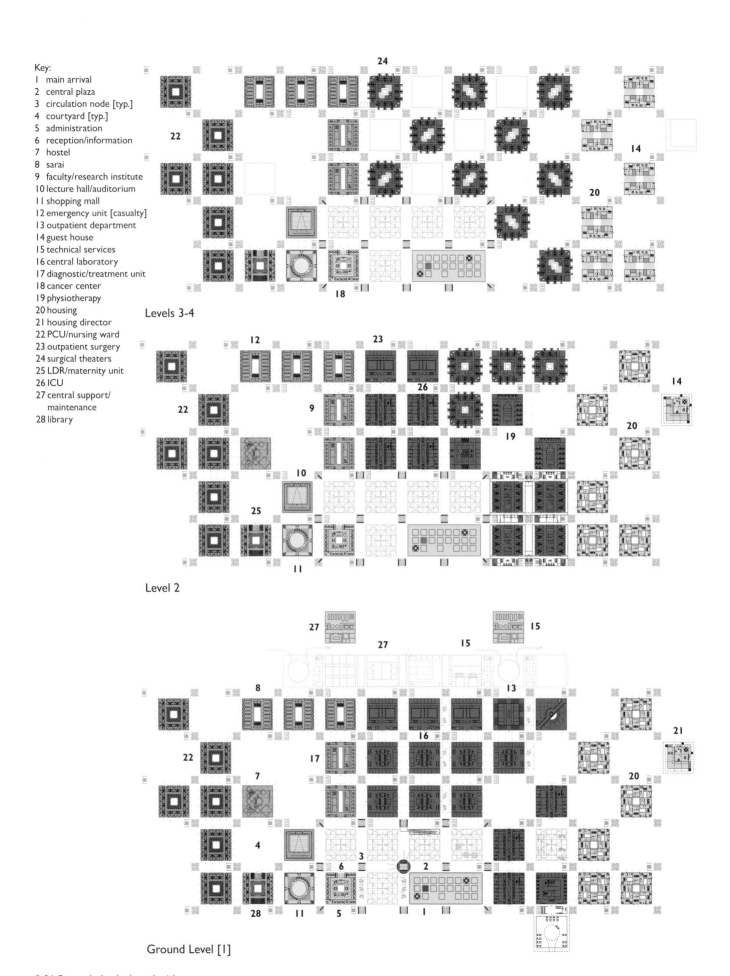

Key:
1 main arrival
2 central plaza
3 circulation node [typ.]
4 courtyard [typ.]
5 administration
6 reception/information
7 hostel
8 sarai
9 faculty/research institute
10 lecture hall/auditorium
11 shopping mall
12 emergency unit [casualty]
13 outpatient department
14 guest house
15 technical services
16 central laboratory
17 diagnostic/treatment unit
18 cancer center
19 physiotherapy
20 housing
21 housing director
22 PCU/nursing ward
23 outpatient surgery
24 surgical theaters
25 LDR/maternity unit
26 ICU
27 central support/
   maintenance
28 library

Levels 3-4

Level 2

Ground Level [1]

8.26.5a–c A checkerboard grid
of mass/void (open/built) spaces
characterizes the campus plan

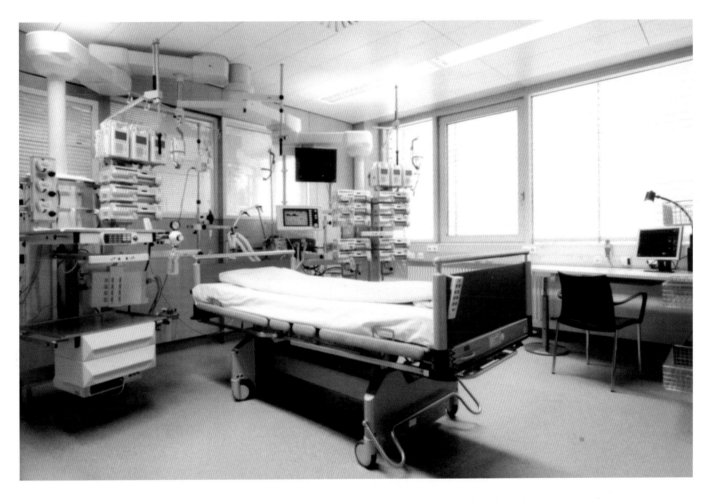

8.26.6 Natural daylight and ventilation is proposed as a key ingredient in diagnostic and treatment spaces, ranging from exam rooms to surgical theaters

in all buildings throughout the campus (Figure 8.26.4). Individual buildings are deployed within the grid to attain maximum functional affinities, including buildings devoted to research. Dormitories are provided on the site for staff and for the families of inpatients, as many families have to travel long distances (Figure 8.26.5a–c). Adaptable space is of high priority and a means to counter the depersonalizing aspects of the hospital experience. In the acute care hospital blocks, levels one and two are support floors with inpatients housed on levels three and four. In the inpatient wards, layout, natural light and ventilation, and furnishings reference local Indian vernacular traditions. Patient rooms in the ICU are to have a low balustrade to ensure that

the patient lying in bed stays in contact with the natural landscape and the world beyond (Figure 8.26.6). Public zones in the inpatient care realm are to have traditional Indian furnishings. All rainwater is captured and harvested for re-use on the site. Roof-mounted solar collectors are featured, perimeter walls are to be constructed with thermal air plenums to modulate changes in ambient temperature, and a campus-wide geothermal system is proposed.

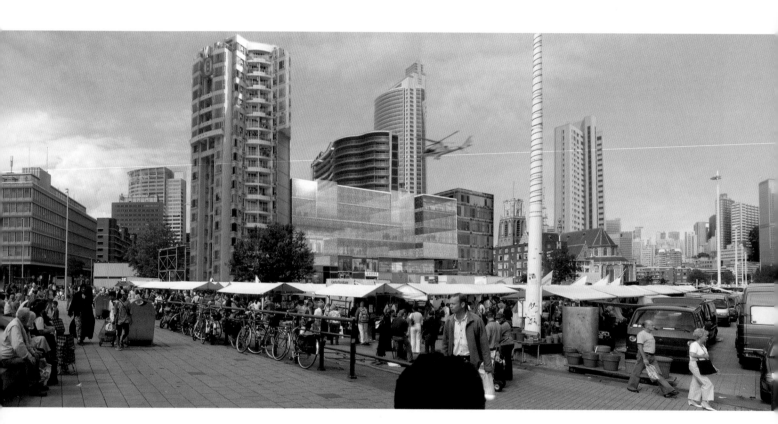

8.27.1 The Core Hospital is a sustainable urban infill prototype – an alternative to suburban fringe sites that are typically selected for new construction of healthcare facilities in North America and elsewhere

27 CORE Hospital Prototype, Rotterdam, the Netherlands

ARCHITECT: Itten + Brechbühl AG/Venhoeven C.S./BM Managers, Bern

LANDSCAPE ARCHITECT: Same

CLIENT: The Netherlands Board for Hospital Facilities

FEATURED MATERIALS: Cast-in-place concrete, polylaminate low-e 'breathing' glass, aluminum, modular building systems, wood interior panels and finishes

COMPLETED: Proposal (2004)

INPATIENT BEDS: 300

SITE/PARKING: 6 acres/200

HOSPITAL SIZE: variable

Context/site

This prototype for a 'Hospital of the Future' was the winning entry in a 2004 design competition sponsored by the Dutch Board for Hospital Facilities, based in Amsterdam. The site selected by the winning team was in the Randstad, near the center of Rotterdam. It focused on rethinking the urban 24/7 acute care hospital by first functionally deconstructing its parts in the vicinity of the 'hospital core'. It is premised on the argument that the urban hospital, as a typology composed of multiple internal typologies, must become a more flexible contributor to pulse of life in the city – with its sphere of civic engagement reconsidered to extend far beyond the traditional role of the hospital as a self referential, autonomous *island*. In so doing, it engages the surrounding urban fabric to an unprecedented extent. This prototype houses a commercial arcade, a pool/spa, numerous health-oriented shops, a hotel linked to the hospital, restaurants, a cinema, and vertical atrium gardens. These are to provide a source of income for the hospital. In further weaving it into its urban fabric, laboratories, outpatient clinics, health assessment centers, wellness care, pharmacy, and medical offices are dispersed to sites within walking distance from the 'mothership' inpatient facility. Other functions are distributed further afield, i.e. a geriatric care center, and freestanding outpatient centers for various specialized diagnostic and treatment services. It is to be a highly anticipatory and fluid entity in the face of evolving and often unpredictable political, socio-cultural, and techno-utopian realities (Figure 8.27.1).

The CORE Hospital is located in the center of a vibrant, walkable neighborhood, adjacent to a square containing a market, mid- and high-rise office structures, institutional buildings, churches, and a park, with direct proximity to public transport. This greatly minimizes the need for automobile dependency (Figure 8.27.2). The mothership hospital is to function within this urban fabric and its own fluid network of tightly coordinated care-dispensing nodes dispersed across the city.

Building/unit

The CORE Hospital is to be eminently adaptable. To this end, its structural aperture is modifiable as needs evolve. Components can be plugged and others unplugged. Mass/void relationships are malleable, indeterminate. This allows for an innovative use of open space, nature/ landscape, and rational transparency. Outsourcing various support and ancillary functions to off-site locations reduces total volume by 50 percent. This allows the focus to be entirely on acute care.

The parti' is configured as a horizontal/vertical grid, with interlocking, interchangeable parts. Parking is provided on two levels below the street; the street level contains shops and provides somewhat of a buffer (Figure 8.27.3). Various outpatient clinics are housed on Level 1. Level 2 houses technical support, interstitial space for centralized mechanical/HVAC apparatus, and clinic/ consultation units. Level 3 houses occupational and physical therapy, and inpatient care units including an ICU. Level 4 houses obstetrics and a pediatric inpatient care unit. Level 5 houses PCU/nursing support, and a restaurant. Level 6, the roof, contains a helipad and space for future expansion. The tiered, striated volume at the center is to be a tranquil refuge from the city. Semi-transparent walls transmit and filter natural daylight deep into the interior of this space. Gardens with orange trees, a pond, and a waterfall on the upper levels create an otherworldly ambiance. In section, the core hospital reveals an internal, multi-level *park* characterized by fluidity and vertical interaction, extending upward to the roof and sky (Figure 8.27.4a–b). The spatial configuration of the operating theatres is flexible, with walls and support space able to be reconfigured (Figure 8.27.5). The operating theatres are arranged in two decentralized pods of four and five theatres each. The inpatient rooms have operable windows, natural light and ventilation, full height windows affording views of the city, and a high level of patient and family amenities in comparison to the typical contemporary European urban hospital.

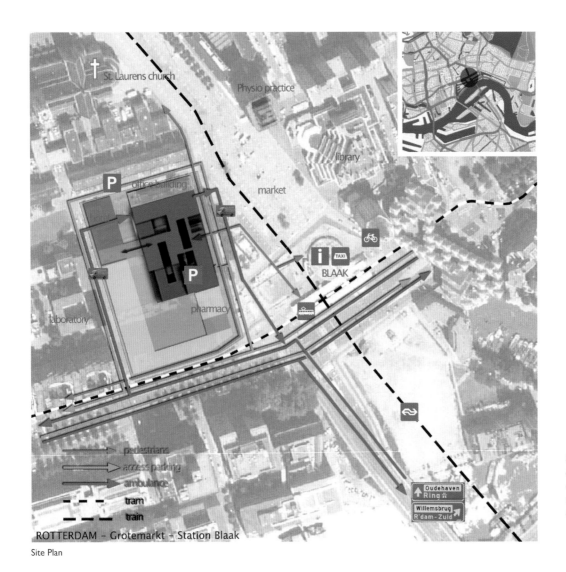

On the map:

† St. Laurens church

Physio practice

office building

library

market

P

P

BLAAK

i

TAXI

laboratory

pharmacy

pedestrians
access parking
ambulance
tram
train

Oudehaven
Ring
Willemsbrug
R'dam - Zuid

ROTTERDAM – Grotemarkt – Station Blaak

Site Plan

8.27.2 A network of community-based satellite clinics is tethered to a mothership within close cycling and walking distance

8.27.3 Places for healing warrant a high level of civic visibility in the twenty-first century – including prominent sites in city centers

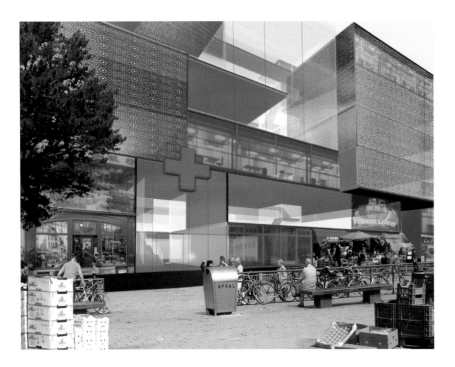

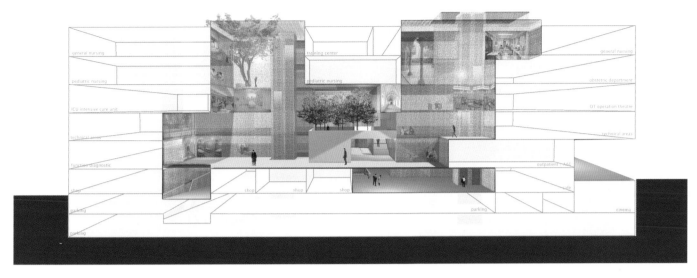

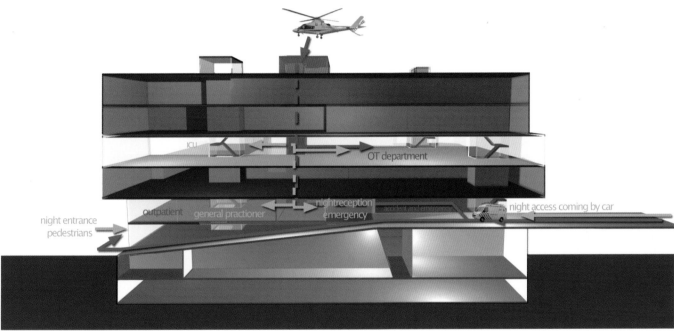

8.27.4a–b A series of horizontal trays and an atrium park are the primary formal elements in the Core Hospital prototype

8.27.5 Chameleon-like wall panels literally *breathe* as a means to ventilate and decontaminate the interior ambient environment

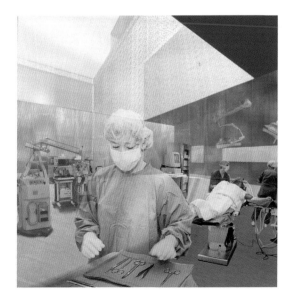

The Core Hospital prototype is a stripped-down, lean, deconstructed, *ecohumanist* hospital. Located in the urban core, it assumes a prominent civic role in the life and health of the city not by default but by design. Its primary focus is on emergency care, diagnostic care and treatment, and inpatient care, augmented by a coordinated network of off-site ancillary diagnostic and treatment nodes decentralized across the urban landscape. It is conceived for dense, infill sites, and yet the Core Hospital is equally envisioned as a vertical park and nature refuge.

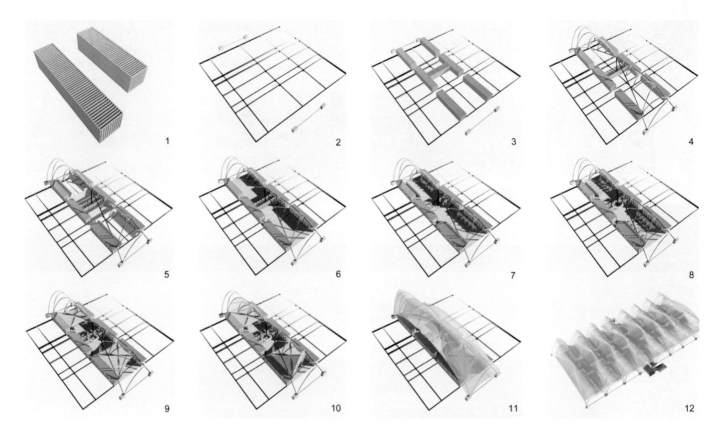

8.28.1a–d This modular trauma center prototype is transportable in standard intermodal shipping containers (ISOs) to sites globally in the aftermath of man-made and natural disasters

28 Transportable Trauma Center Prototypes for Global Deployment

ARCHITECT: Tulane University Rapid Response Studio and Clemson University Architecture + Health Graduate Program
COORDINATOR: Stephen Verderber
LANDSCAPE ARCHITECT: N/A
CLIENT: International Red Cross
FEATURED MATERIALS: Neoprene fabric roofs, lightweight aluminum tubular frames, adapted shipping containers, pneumatic foundation system, modular component systems
COMPLETED: Proposal 1 (2005)/Proposal 2 (2007)
INPATIENT BEDS: 60–280
SITE/PARKING: Multiple sites
HOSPITAL SIZE: 18,000–28,000SF

Context/site

Global expenditures for fixed-site healthcare facilities are escalating, and will rise dramatically in the coming decades. While a present fixed-site public health infrastructure will continue to be a critical component of the overall healthcare system, these facilities tend to be disproportionately concentrated in highly populated urban areas. However, with the onset of global warming the need for rapidly deployable non-fixed site facilities will gain in urgency (Figure 8.28.1). The world's population increases by nearly 9,000 people every hour. The Worldwatch Institute estimates that by 2050 between 9 and 9.5 billion people will be living on the planet. Suffice to say, unprecedented pressure will be exerted upon the conventional urban healthcare infrastructure, an infrastructure proven inadequate in the aftermath of recent disasters, most recently in the aftermath of Hurricane Katrina in the U.S. in 2005. Populations most in need of mobile, rapid response healthcare include those stricken by wars, and by natural and industrial disasters. Populations located in remote and medically underserved regions of the world are particularly vulnerable. This includes communities ravaged by HIV/AIDS, malaria, tuberculosis, plagues such as the virulent Ebola virus in Africa, and yellow fever. An increasing number of inhabitants reside in coastal zones, highly susceptible to the ravages wrought by hurricanes, monsoons, and tsunamis. Mobile medicine can provide one answer to this challenge to humanity.

Hurricane Katrina struck the U.S. Gulf Coast in August 2005. At $13.5 billion (U.S.), it ranks as the costliest disaster in United States

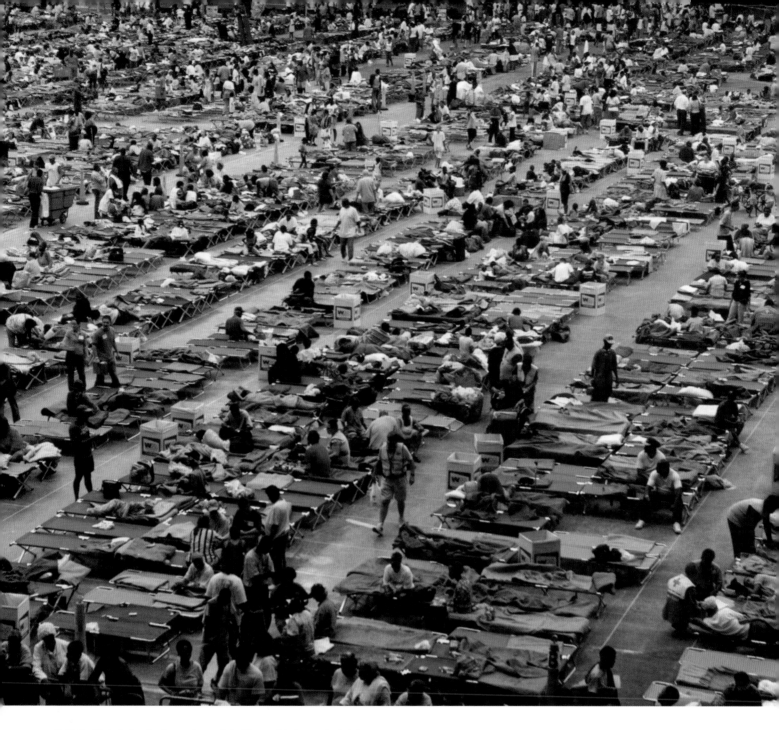

8.28.2 Global climate change is predicted to result in increasingly intense hurricanes. Hurricane Katrina resulted in nearly 1,800 deaths along the United States Gulf Coast in 2005. Shown here are just some of the tens of thousands who sought refuge in Houston's Astrodome sports stadium

history (Figure 8.28.2). More than one million people evacuated from the metro New Orleans area in the face of the hurricane, and the region's healthcare infrastructure completely collapsed. The aftermath of this intense Category 3 hurricane overwhelmed the infrastructure, including its hospitals and clinics. Katrina served as a national and international flashpoint. The outpouring of empathy and assistance was felt from nearly every corner of the world. This disaster galvanized the American public to take action in the wake of a

dismal governmental response at all levels. The profound pain, misery, and dislocation caused by natural disasters is predicted to become more widespread. The aftermath of disaster can be especially acute in communities with high concentrations of chemical and nuclear energy installations. Populations equally in need of rapid response architectural intervention now may be in Chicago, Omaha, Osaka, São Paulo, remote island nations in the Pacific, or Bangladesh. Rapid response architecture requires commitment, immersion, teamwork,

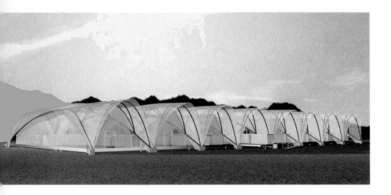

8.28.3 This hybrid, pneumatic fabric roof/structural panel system is erectable in a matter of hours upon arrival at the site. Multiple site layouts and facility plan configurations can be achieved

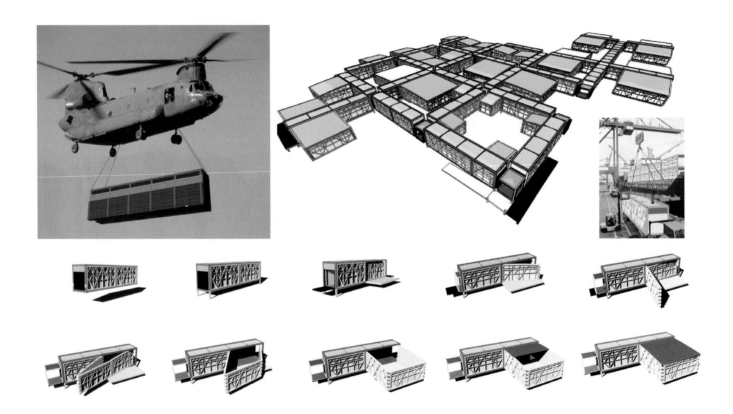

8.28.4a–l This prototype modular system is autonomous – rapidly shipped and deployed in clusters of modules, reconfigurable based on site dictates, local resources, and the needs of disaster victims

and resourcefulness. Correspondingly, the threat of future hurricanes of great ferocity is metastasized in the public psyche. Airports, schools, churches, housing, civic institutions, and hospitals were but a few of the building types where long-standing assumptions were rendered obsolete, literally overnight.

An innovative design studio at Tulane University in New Orleans (2005) focused on mobile medicine for rapid deployment globally. This endeavor, the Rapid Response Studio, centered on the design of a prototype transportable trauma center. In 2007, this studio was reprised at Clemson University, in its Architecture + Health Graduate Program. This portable hospital is designed for a baseline field deployment of 18,000SF up to 28,000SF. Non-site specificity was essential: a kit of parts responsive to four site variants – an urban street, i.e. lower Manhattan, an open field, i.e. a soccer field, a sandy shoreline condition, and a paved parking lot. The mission statement called for a flexible, adaptable trauma center for disaster victim assessment and treatment for rapid deployment to widely diverse cultural, geographic, and site contexts.

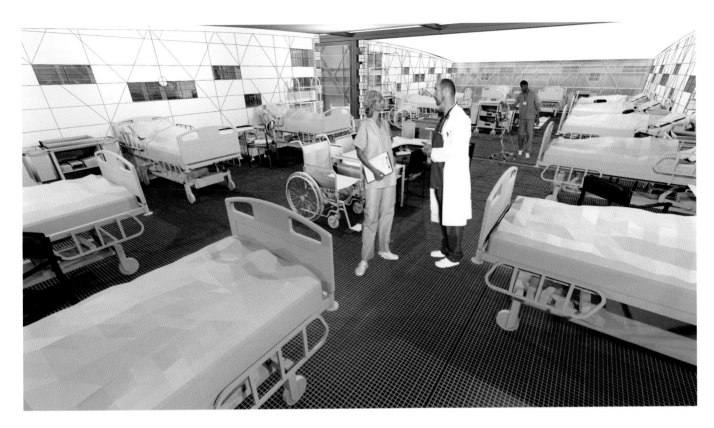

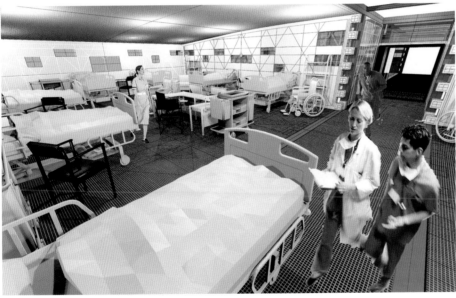

8.28.5a–b This redeployable modular prototype trauma center utilizes its ISC shipping containers as an integrated structural and circulation element, with fold out/plug-in side pavilions for the rapid delivery of emergency healthcare in the twenty-first century (continued overleaf)

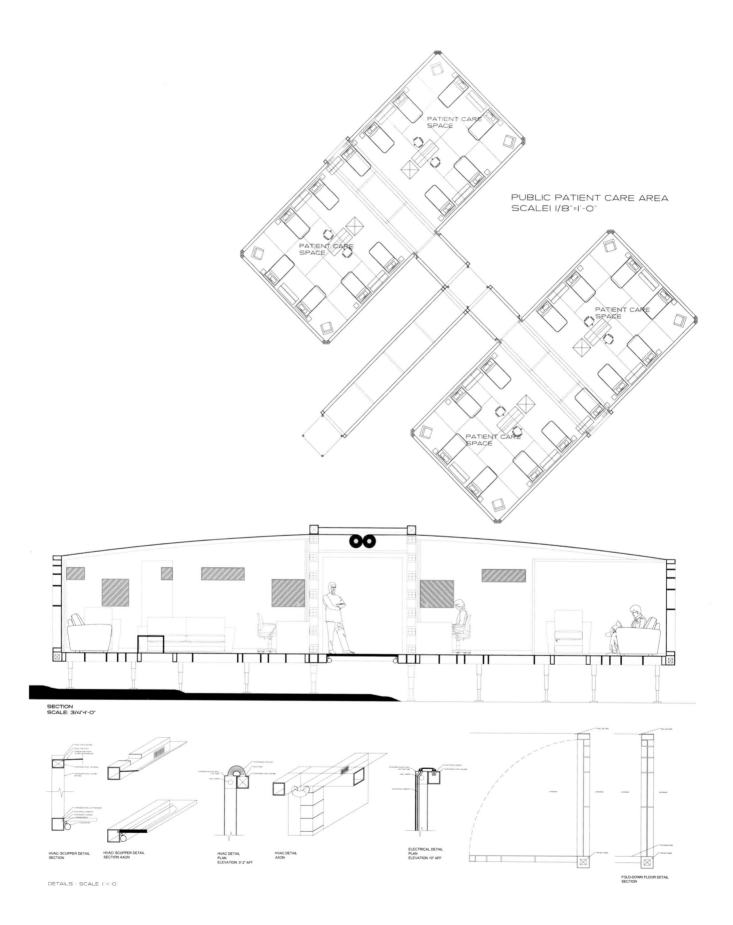

PUBLIC PATIENT CARE AREA
SCALE: 1/8"=1'-0"

PATIENT CARE SPACE

PATIENT CARE SPACE

PATIENT CARE SPACE

PATIENT CARE SPACE

SECTION
SCALE: 3/4"=1'-0"

HVAC/SCUPPER DETAIL
SECTION

HVAC/SCUPPER DETAIL
SECTION AXON

HVAC DETAIL
PLAN
ELEVATION: 9'-2" AFF

HVAC DETAIL
AXON

ELECTRICAL DETAIL
PLAN
ELEVATION 10" AFF

FOLD-DOWN FLOOR DETAIL
SECTION

DETAILS - SCALE 1"=1'-0"

Building/unit

Prototypes were designed premised on the five basic platonic volumes – the tetrahedron, octahedron, cube, dodecahedron, and icosahedron – as well as the ancient art of tent making. Additionally, the pioneering work of Buckminster Fuller and Frei Otto provided precedent, and precursors in lightweight portable buildings including case studies in pneumatic (air activated) structures with fabric sheathed roof/wall systems. The MASH tent hospitals of the Korean War through to the Iraq War were studied, as well as molecular structure and fractal geometry. The core program elements consisted of an exterior platform/staging area for triage, an intake zone, interior triage unit and admitting area, decontamination module, treatment bays, exam/consult rooms, waiting areas, inpatient PCU wards housing up to 30 beds each, up to four surgical theatres, pre- and post-operative units, housing for staff, an administration area, and hospital-wide support functions, including materials management, laboratory/central pharmacy, equipment sterilization unit, kitchen/dining unit, bulk storeroom, emergency generators (plus backup units), bath/shower facilities, and HVAC/mechanical support module(s). A helipad area is sited adjacent to the field hospital.

The standard Intermodal Shipping Container (ISC) served as the basic design module. Flat-pack and pre-formed modular variants on the standard ISC unit, and various site permutations were developed. The ISC units each were 10 feet wide by 10 feet in height and 30 or 40 feet in length. In Prototype 1 (Julia Ford/Claudia Foronda), the ISC units function as bookends within a flat-pack deployment and assembly strategy. The shipping container is the transport medium of all materials and its autonomous neoprene fabric roof system. The container becomes occupied space upon arrival at the site. The units become detached and reassembled as a contiguous row of units in a linear, radial, or grid site configuration, the latter condition with one or more open spaces in-between (Figure 8.28.3).

In Prototype 2 (Adam Missel/Shawn McKeever), extruded plastic pallet technology was adapted in a premanufactured modular container with unfolding wall panel system, fabricated with an extremely high impact polymer into self-contained units. Assembly components consist of a system of attenuated legs and moveable parts, with HVAC support provided through a network of modular ducts. Wall sections are unfolded from the core container, yielding habitable space to either side of a circulation spine. The units can become operational on site in any number of permutations, from as few as four modules to as many as forty modular units on a single site (Figure 8.28.4a–l). A typical PCU/nursing support care unit is depicted – each bay houses four beds plus required support amenities (Figure 8.28.5a–e).

Both Prototypes 1 and 2 are transportable via rail, plane, or from ship, or helicopter, then trucked to a site. They are then pre-positioned (staged) on site and readied for assembly. These systems are conceived to accommodate sophisticated medical technologies, HVAC, and electrical systems. Components are pre-packaged with the transport module prior to deployment. They are conceived to be equally responsive to extreme transport, assembly, and commissioning challenges likely to be encountered in the field.

There are compelling justifications for transportable, redeployable hospitals in the saving of lives. Beyond, they need to be conceived to tread lightly on the earth as they symbolize a collective purpose and spirit of community fundamental to a civilized, ecohumanist society. Transportability, rapid deployment, and social responsiveness, taken together, call for *lightness*. The metaphysics of lightness – minimization of weight and mass – in the abstract, together with transportability, poses an unprecedented opportunity for the designer. The challenges ahead may seem daunting, although the alternative is far worse. In a post-disaster situation, further loss of life often occurs from exposure to disease and traumatic conditions of far greater magnitude than the initial event itself. Complacency is equally unwarranted whether in government, the corporate boardroom, in organized religion, the art world, the global healthcare industry, or within the design professions. Nearly a century ago, Le Corbusier, Frank Lloyd Wright, Buckminister Fuller and others recognized the validity of modularization. Their arguments for the portable building are even more valid today in a world of increasingly scarce natural resources compounded by dramatic population increases. A critical reappraisal is called for at this time in order to harness the creative synergies necessary to advance the state of the art in transportable architecture for health.

Notes

1 Introduction

1 Verderber, Stephen (2009) *Delirious New Orleans: Manifesto for an Extraordinary American City*, Austin: The University of Texas Press.
2 Paul, Sara (2008) 'Nathan lost his job, and his health insurance', *The Charlotte Observer*, 31 March, p. 10A.
3 Engleman, Robert (2008) *More: Population, Nature, and What Women Want*, Washington, D.C.: Island Press. Nocks, Barry (2009) 'Healthcare policy', Lecture in Health 600 Seminar, Clemson University, Graduate Program in Architecture + Health. Also see Freking, Kevin (2009) 'Number of Americans without health insurance expected to grow by 9 million in next decade', *The Cleveland Plain Dealer*. Online. Available at http://blog.cleveland.com/medical/2009/02/number_of_americans_without_he.htm (accessed 27 May 2009).
4 Campbell, Carol A. (2009) 'Health outcomes driving new hospital design', *The New York Times*. Online. Available at http://www.nytimes.com/2009/05/19/health/19hosp.html (accessed 18 May 2009).
5 Newman, Peter (2008) *Cities as Sustainable Ecosystems*, Washington, D.C.: Island Press. Theories of sustainability are frequently based on a number of compelling but unreliable claims that condition the discourse and practice of green architecture (the cause of the energy crisis, the view that construction yields half the landfill waste and buildings consume half the energy in the U.S., the dominant role of technological determinism in professional practice, and the myths of vernacular and regional determinism). See Moe, Kiel (2007) 'Compelling yet unreliable theories of sustainability', *Journal of Architectural Education*, 60:4, pp. 24–30.
6 Frumkin, Howard (2004) *Urban Sprawl and Public Health*, Washington, D.C.: Island Press.
7 Krupp, Fred (2008) *Earth: The Sequel*, New York: W.W. Norton & Co.
8 Heinberg, Richard (2004) *Powerdown: Options and Actions for a Post-Carbon World*, Gabriola Island, British Columbia: New Society Publishers.
9 Ibid., p. 54.
10 Whitty, Julia (2008) 'March of the tourists', *Mother Jones*, 29:7/8. Online. Available at http://www.motherjones.com/politics/2008/07/march-tourists (accessed 10 October 2008). Also see Sample, Ian (2008) 'Final Warning', *New Scientist*, 198:2662, 32–8; and Simmons, Matthew R. (2008) 'Time to go cold turkey', *New Scientist*, 198:2662, 22. Also Pearce, Fred (2008) *The Last Generation: How Nature Will Take Her Revenge for Climate Change*, London: Eden Project Books.
11 Anon (2008) *Princeton Carbon Mitigation Initiative*. Online. Available at http://www.princeton.edu/~cmi/ (accessed 12 May 2009).
12 McDonough, William and Michael Braungart (2002) *Cradle to Cradle: Remaking the Way We Make Things*, New York: North Point Press. Also see Sinclair, Cameron (2006) *Architecture for Humanity – Design Like You Give a Damn: Architectural Responses to Humanitarian Crises*, New York: Metropolis Books.

13 Steffen, Alex (2006) *Worldchanging: A User's Guide to the 21st Century*, New York: Abrams.

14 Intergovernmental Panel on Climate Change (IPCC) (2001) *Global Warming: Early Warning Signs*. Online. Available at http://www.climatehotmap.org/ (accessed 4 January 2009). In 2004 more than 300 healthcare leaders from 28 countries met in Vienna and agreed to far-reaching reforms for the delivery of 'environmentally responsible' healthcare. Participants included Health Care Without Harm, the International Council of Nurses, the World Health Organization, the Health Promoting Hospitals Network, the European Environmental Agency, and UNIDO. This document is known as the *Vienna Declaration of Environmental Standards for Healthcare*. Online. Available at http://www.inges.at/viennadeclaration/vd_english. pdf (accessed 28 April 2008).

15 Weller, Kin (2006) 'The top 10 green hospitals in the U.S.: 2006', *National Geographic Green Guide*. Online. Available at http://www.thegreenguide. com/doc/113/top10hospitals (accessed 2 February 2008). In 2006, the top ten green hospitals in the U.S. were chosen on the following twelve criteria, none of which specifically relate to aesthetics: siting, water efficiency, energy conservation and air pollution control, materials and natural resources conservation, indoor environmental quality, hospital food and nutrition protocols, waste reduction education and recycling, procurement of green supplies and equipment, contaminant reduction regimens, use of green housekeeping chemicals, waste reduction measures, and healing gardens.

16 Block, Dustin (2008) 'Critics say LEED building program puts popularity before planet', *New Orleans City Business*. Online. Available at http:// www.neworleanscitybusiness.com/ (accessed 27 September 2008).

17 Carr, Robert F. (2008) 'Health care facilities', *Whole Building Design Guide*. Online. Available at http://www.wbdg.org/design/health_care. php (accessed 27 September 2008).

18 Johnson, Linda A. (2008) 'Hospitals suffering from economic meltdown', *The Greenville News*, 28 December, 8A.

19 Klare, Michael T. (2008) 'Barreling into recession', *Mother Jones*. Online. Available at http://www.motherjones.com/ (accessed 18 February 2008). Also see Farrar, Lara (2008) 'Is America's suburban dream collapsing into a nightmare?', *CNN*. Online. Available at http://www.cnn.com/2008/ TECH/06/16/suburb.city/index.html?iref=newssearch (accessed 22 June 2008), and Karp, Jonathan (2008) 'Suburbs a mile too far for some', *The Wall Street Journal*. Online. Available at http://online.wsj.com/article/ SB121366811790479767.html (accessed 22 June 2008).

20 Andersen, Kurt (2009) 'The reset', *Time*, 173:13, 32–8. The subtitle for this essay was 'Don't pretend we didn't see this coming for a long, long time'.

21 Wagenaar, Cor (ed.) (2005) *The Architecture of Hospitals*, Rotterdam: NAi Publishers.

2 Architecture for health: a brief history of sustainability

1 Thompson, John D. and Grace Goldin (1975) *The Hospital: A Social and Architectural History*, New Haven, CT: Yale University Press.

2 Montague, Joel (1984) 'Hospitals in the Muslim Near East: a historical overview', *MIMAR 14: Architecture in Development*. Singapore: Concept Media, Ltd, 52–69.

3 Chadwick, John and W.N. Mann (eds) (1983) 'The Oath', in *Hippocrates: Hippocratic Writings*, London: Penguin Group, p. 67.

4 Ibid., pp. 148–9.

5 Ibid., pp. 168–9.

6 Loudon, Irvine (ed.) (1997) *Western Medicine: An Illustrated History*, New York: Oxford University Press.

7 Ibid., p. 32.

8 Thompson and Goldin: p.4. A large 'incubation hall' for patient-dreamers was situated at the center of the open courtyard. The latrines were at the lower left corner. The temple at the center of the fourth side was a miniature replica of the Pantheon (built some twenty years earlier), plus a room for the Emperor, which also served as a library. A large semicircular outdoor amphitheater was located immediately behind the treatment halls. On the opposite side nearer to the temple was a circular, two-level treatment hall. This building contained stairs that adjoined the interior of the courtyard as well as the exterior grounds. It contained six large apses, each expressed on the exterior, and which were housed on the second floor. Each contained a large therapeutic water basin.

9 Ibid., p. 27.

10 Vitruvius (1931, trans. Frank Granger) 'The site of a city', in *Vitruvius: De Architectura*, Cambridge, MA: Harvard University Press. Also see Rowland, Ingrid D. and Thomas Noble Howe (1999 translation) *Vitruvius: Ten Books on Architecture*, Cambridge: Cambridge University Press; and Gwilt, Joseph (1826 translation) *The Architecture of Marcus Vitruvius Pollio*, London: Priestly and Weale.

11 Vitruvius, 'Book VI', p. 174.

12 Loudon, p. 39.

13 Thompson and Goldin, p. 42.

14 Vitruvius, 'Book VI'.

15 Public Broadcasting Service (2008) '*NOVA: Secrets of Lost Empires: Roman Bath*'. Online. Available at http://www.pbs.org/wgbh/nova/lostempires/ roman/ (Accessed 6 August 2008).

16 Peck, Harry T. (1898) 'Balneae', in *Harpers Dictionary of Classical Antiquities*, New York: Harper and Row Co.

17 Smith, William (1870) 'Balneae', in *Dictionary of Greek and Roman Antiquities*, New York: W.W. Norton and Co.

18 Ibid., p. 98.

19 Ibid., p. 99.

20 Peck: 'Suet', p. 82.

21 Ibid., *Pallad i.* 40, v8. Service areas consisted of various back passages, the spaces that serviced the large furnaces and the rooms where the fires were stoked. At Pompeii there were three boilers, one of which held the hot water, a second the tepid water, and a third the cold water. A complex lead-piping system transported the three types of water to the various baths and pools throughout the complex. At Pompeii the boilers themselves no longer remain, but the impressions they left in the mortar are still visible. These impressions allow for the accurate estimates of their size and position. Such coppers and the boilers were called *miliaria*, from their similar appearance to a milestone.

22 Richmond, Irving A. and J.M.C. Toynbee (1955) 'The Temple of Sulis-Minerva at Bath', *The Journal of Roman Studies*, 45(4), 97.

23 Anon (2002) *City of Bath World Heritage Site Management Plan*. Bath and Northeast Somerset, U.K. Online. Available at http://www.bathnes.gov.uk/worldheritage/1.Introduction.htm (accessed 1 August 2008). The earliest humans to gather around the hot springs at Bath were Neolithic hunters 7,500 years ago. In prehistoric times the steamy water gushed up out of the round continuously, and this made the immediate area extremely marshy. Much of the valley where the baths were subsequently constructed was at one time heavily wooded in the vicinity of the spring. The hot spring was seen as a work of supernatural forces. In pre-Roman times people came to the site to worship *Sulis* and worshipped in a comparatively primitive shrine.

24 Anon (2008) *Sacred Spring*. Roman Baths Museum (Home Page). Online. Available at http://www.romanbaths.co.uk/walkthrough/sacred_springs.aspx (accessed 20 August 2008). At Bath, hot water has for thousands of years been at a temperature of 46 degrees Celsius (114.8F) and has flowed from a geological fault. The Romans had no rational explanation for the hot spring. To them, it was the work of gods, i.e. a sacred place. When the first structure was built, statues of various gods were placed in the pool. It was at first a dark and somewhat foreboding place. It remains possible today to toss offerings through the arched openings and to enter the building by the original steps from the ancient temple courtyard. The bath complex was modified over the centuries, including in the twelfth and sixteenth centuries. By the early nineteenth century the city had literally grown over the site, at a height of nearly 5 meters above the original city. Wet, moist conditions chronically present in the buildings above – including a number of row houses – and when examined by means of excavations conducted by the city, the original baths were found to lie directly below a by-then Victorian era city. This led to a series of archaeological excavations by teams from Oxford University and the original site was partially uncovered and restored. Various Victorian era architectural additions to the site include a museum, restaurant, and statues. The entire structure above the level of the pillar bases and some partial columns is an interpretative reconstruction.

25 Richmond and Toynbee, p. 97.

26 Anon (2008), 'Sacred Spring'.

27 Thompson and Goldin, p. 54.

28 Ibid., p. 56.

29 Goldin, Grace (1994) *Work of Mercy: A Picture History of Hospitals*, Erin, Ontario: The Boston Mills Press.

30 Ibid., p. 22.

31 Thompson and Goldin, pp. 59–62.

32 Montague, p. 58.

33 Ibid., p. 60.

34 Ibid., p. 61. In the Islamic world, the therapeutic amenity of nature in healthcare settings has undergone a reappraisal to some degree in recent years. This trend is predicted to continue, as Islamic fundamentalists increasingly disavow Western high-tech medical ideologies and practices. In truth, it is likely that ideologies and practices associated with the architecture of the high-tech Western hospital and attempts to transport this template to locales in the Muslim world will be similarly viewed with suspicion and contempt, if not rejection.

35 Thompson and Goldin, pp. 79–81.

36 Ibid., pp. 57–8.

37 Ibid., p. 53.

38 Goldin, pp. 182–5.

39 Nightingale, Florence (1858) *Notes on Nursing: What It is and What It is Not* (1976 edition), Philadelphia: J.B. Lippincott Company. See Chapter 1. Also see Burdett, Henry C. (1891) *Hospitals and Asylums of the World: Volumes I-V*, London: Westminster.

40 Nightingale, Florence (1859) *Notes on Hospitals*, London: Parker and Son. Also see Nightingale, Florence (1864) *Notes on Hospitals*, Third Edition and Enlarged, *Journal of Mental Science*, 10(2), 403–16.

41 Goldin, pp. 200–1.

42 Ibid., pp. 188–97.

43 Ibid., p. 94.

44 Rosenberg, Charles (1987) *The Care of Strangers: The Rise of America's Hospital System*, New York: Basic Books, pp. 15–16, 139.

45 Ibid., pp. 122–41.

46 Hancock, Trevor (1993) 'The evolution, impact and significance of the healthy cities/communities movement', *Journal of Public Health Policy*, 49, Spring, 5–18.

47 Yenni, Carla (2007) *The Architecture of Madness: Insane Asylums in the United States*, Minneapolis: University of Minnesota Press.

48 Ibid., pp. 1–12.

49 Thompson and Goldin, 77–9.

50 Ibid., p. 78.

51 Tomes, Nancy (1984) *A Generous Confidence: Thomas Story Kirkbride and the Art of Asylum-Keeping, 1840–1883*, Cambridge: Cambridge University Press. Additional sections of his book were as follows: Water Supply (Chapter XV), Drainage (Ch. XVI), Character of Proposed Plans (Ch. XX), Size of Buildings and Number of Patients (Ch. XXI), Position and General Arrangement of the Building (Ch. XXII), Form of Building (Ch. XXIII), Height of Hospitals (Ch. XXIV), Temporary or Wooden Structures (Ch. XXV), Number of Patients in a Ward (Ch. XXVI), Natural Ventilation

(Ch. XXVII), Cellars (Ch. XXVIII), Material of Walls (Ch. XXIX), Plastering (Ch. XXX), Security From Fire in Construction (Ch. XXXI), Roofs (Ch. XXXII), Size of Rooms and Height of Ceilings (Ch. XXXIII), Floors (Ch. XXXIV), Doors (Ch. XXXV), Locks (Ch. XXXVI), Windows and Window Guards (Ch. XXXVII), Inside Window Screens (Ch. XXXVIII), Stairs (Ch. XXXIX), Associated Dormitories (Ch. XL), Infirmary Wards (Ch. XLI), Bath Rooms (Ch. XLII), Water Closets (Ch. XLIII), Ward Drying Rooms (Ch. XLIV), Water Pipes (Ch. XLV), Railroad (Ch. XLIX) and Heating and Ventilation (Ch. L). These chapters were followed by the presentation of a prototype hospital design case study.

52 Yenni, pp. 79–104.

53 Ibid., pp. 145–58.

54 Thompson and Goldin, pp. 79–93.

55 Tomes, pp. 95–114.

56 Lawrence, Henry W. (1983) 'Southern spas: source of the American resort tradition', *Landscape*, 27(2), 1–12. Also see Severens, Kenneth (1981) *Southern Architecture: 350 Years of Distinctive American Buildings*, New York: E.P. Dutton; and Frary, L.T. (1950) *Thomas Jefferson: Architect and Builder*, Richmond, VA: Garrett and Massie.

57 Addison, William (1951) *English Spas*, London: Batsford. Also see Bridenbaugh, Carl (1946) 'Baths and watering places of colonial America', *William and Mary Quarterly 3rd Series*, Vol. III, No. 2, 151–81; Cohen, Stan (1981) *Historic Springs of the Virginias: A Pictorial History*, Charleston, West Virginia: Pictorial Histories Publishing Co.; Huth, Hans (1957) *Nature and the American: Three Centuries of Changing Attitudes*, Berkeley: University of California Press.

58 Lawrence, p. 10.

59 Ibid., p. 6.

60 Ibid., p. 3.

61 Ibid., p. 10. In the pre-Civil War (antebellum) American South the plantations were built and staffed by African-American slaves. In time, a National American style would emerge east of the Mississippi River. Many spa/retreats would later de-emphasize their regionalist origins.

62 Bullard, Loring (2004) *Healing Waters: Missouri's Historic Mineral Springs and Spas*, Columbia and London: University of Missouri Press.

63 Ibid., p. 99.

64 Fowler, Gene (1991) *Crazy Water: The Story of Mineral Wells and Other Texas Health Resorts*, Fort Worth: Texas Christian University Press, pp. 237–9.

65 Kaysing, Bill (1974) *Great Hot Springs of the West*, Santa Barbara: Capra Press.

66 Lawrence, p. 12.

67 Gallup, Joan W. (1999) *Wellness Centers: A Guild for the Design Professional*, New York: John Wiley. Also see Holms, Karin B. (2000) *101 Vacations to Change Your Life: A Guide to Wellness Centers, Spiritual Retreats, and Spas*, Boston: Citadel Press; and Minton, Melinda M. (2003) *Medical Spas to Wellness Centers: The Next Wave*, Self Published.

68 Caldwell, Mark (1988) *The Last Crusade*, New York: Macmillan Publishing Company.

69 McBride, Deborah L. (1998) 'American sanitoriums: landscaping for health, 1885–1945', *Landscape Journal*, 44(3), 26–41.

70 Ibid., 29–32.

71 Lynch, Charles, Joseph H. Ford, and Frank W. Weed. (1925) *The Medical Department of the United States Army in the World War, Volume 8: Field Operations*. Washington: D.C.: U.S. Army Surgeon General's Office. Online. Available at http://www.archive.org/stream/WW1ArmyMedDeptHistV8#page/n1/mode/2up (accessed 2 February 2009).

72 Ginn, Richard V. (1997) *The History of the U.S. Army Medical Surgical Corps*. Washington, D.C.: Office of the Surgeon General and Center of Military History.

73 Ibid., p. 313.

74 Kopchinski, Bernard J. (2000) 'Trauma patient outcome in an army deployable systems environment compared with a medical center', *Military Medicine* 47(4), 58–74.

75 McMurtie, Douglas C. (1920) 'Work of the Crippled Children's Hospital School', *The Modern Hospital*, 25(5), 424–5.

76 Thompson and Goldin, pp. 195–7.

77 Verderber, Stephen and David J. Fine (2000) *Healthcare Architecture in an Era of Radical Transformation*, New Haven and London: Yale University Press.

78 Guenther, Robin and Gail Vittori (2008) *Sustainable Healthcare Architecture*, New York: John Wiley & Sons, Inc.

79 Hornsby, John A. and Richard E. Schmidt (1913) *The Modern Hospital: Its Inspiration, Its Architecture, Its Equipment, Its Operation*, Philadelphia and London: W.B. Saunders Company.

80 Currie, John Michael (2007) *The Fourth Factor: A Historical Perspective on Architecture and Medicine*, Washington, D.C.: The American Institute of Architects Academy of Architecture and Health.

81 Nasatir, Judith (1993) 'Alvar Aalto', *Interior Design*, 24(8), 84–7.

82 Verderber and Fine, pp. 101–4.

83 Ibid., pp. 95–6.

84 Frank, Lawrence D., Peter Engelke, and Thomas L. Schmid (2003) *Health and Community Design: The Impact of the Built Environment on Physical Activity*, Washington, D.C.: Island Press.

85 Verderber, Stephen (2008) 'Evidence-based design for healthcare in post-Katrina New Orleans: current dilemmas', *Health Environments Research & Design Journal*, 1(2), 71–6. In the case of post-Katrina New Orleans, historic Charity Hospital – symbolizing the intersection of landmark pre-World War II hospital design, intrinsic environmental sustainability, health inequities, race and class distinctions, and urban cultural history – merits renovation and reuse because it is an undeniable part of the city's cultural mosaic. Its intelligent reuse and rebirth can serve as a lesson in sustainable hospital architecture for hospitals and communities elsewhere.

86 Anon (2009) 'Newberry, South Carolina: Newberry Senior Apartments', *The Landmark Group*. Online. Available at http://www.landmarkdevelopment. biz/cmt/111.html (accessed 15 January 2009). Also see Anon (2008) 'Redevelopment of historic hospital facilities – Fort Sam Houston, San Antonio, Texas', *Weston Solutions*. Online. Available at http://www. westonsolutions.com/projects/project_ftsamhouston_eul.htm (accessed 25 June 2008).

87 Simon, Peter (2002) 'Passavant Memorial Hospital, 1865–1972', *Northwestern Memorial Hospital* (Home Page). Online. Available at http://www.nmh.org/nm/about+us+history+timeline (accessed 12 January 2009).

88 Verderber, p. 74.

89 Moe, Richard (2007) 'The 11 Most Endangered Places', Washington, D.C.: *The National Trust for Historic Places*. Online. Available at http://www. preservationnation.org/issues/11-most-endangered/listings.html?place_ status=&threat=&listed=2007&related_region=&related_state= (accessed 12 December 2007). Also see Moe, Richard (2009) 'Disaster for St. Elizabeth's', *The Washington Post*, 8 January. Online. Available at http://www.washingtonpost.com/wp-dyn/content/article/2009/01/07/ AR2009010702977.html (accessed 12 January 2009). Also see Yenni (pp. 66–8) for a detailed discussion of the history of St. Elizabeth's. St. Elizabeth's Hospital (1852–1860) was the first and only federally funded asylum, and was intended to be a model institution. The hospital was a pet project of Dorothea Dix, who had proposed a nationwide system of charitable instructions for the mentally ill. This program was scuttled by a presidential veto. Regardless, the hospital was a model for many state-built asylums in subsequent years and it fully expressed the most advanced theories of treatment for the insane.

90 Vitullo-Martin, Julia (2008) 'Expanding a hospital in historic territory', *The Manhattan Institute*, Online. Available at http://www.manhattan-institute. org/email/crd_newsletter05-08.html (accessed 25 June 2008). Also see letter sent to the New York Landmarks Commission. Online. Available at http://209.86.165.104/search?q=cache.html (accessed 25 June 2008). Also Amateau, Albert (2008) 'Group gets top attorney to help battle St. Vincent's', *The Villager*. Online. Available at http://www.thevillager. com/villager_248/groupgets.html (accessed 25 June 2008).

3 The evolving role of site, landscape, and nature

1 Ralph, Edward (1976) *Place and Placelessness*, London: Pion.

2 Anon (2008) 'Flexible healthcare', *worldarchitcturenews.com*, Online. Available at http://www.worldarchitecturenews.com/index. php?fuseaction=wanappln.projectview&upload_id=10263.html (accessed 24 November 2008).

3 Kellert, Stephen R. (2008) 'Dimensions, elements, and attributes of biophilic design', in Kellert, Stephen R., Judith H. Heerwagen, and Martin L. Mador (eds.) (2008) *Biophilic Design*, New York: John Wiley & Sons, Inc.

4 Rheims, Maurice (1988) *Hector Guimard*, New York: Harry N. Abrams.

5 Bassegoda, Juan and Melba Levick (2001) *Antonio Gaudi: Master Architect*, Boston: Abbeville Press.

6 Hoffman, Donald (1984) *Frank Lloyd Wright's Robie House: The Illustrated Story of an Architectural Masterpiece*, New York: Dover Publications.

7 Jencks, Charles (1995) *The Architecture of the Jumping Universe*, London: Academy Editions.

8 Ibid., p. 102.

9 Nickl, Christine (2007) *Hospital Architecture*, Berlin: Braun.

10 Jencks, p. 109.

11 In Aalto's buildings, curves, undulations natural forms were nearly always limited to small-scale interior elements such as doors, ceiling recesses, and stairs.

12 Jencks, pp. 110–11.

13 Kent, Cheryl, David Gordon, and Jeff Millies (2005) *Santiago Calatrava: Milwaukee Art Museum Quadracci Pavilion*, New York and London: Rizzoli.

14 Jencks, p. 49.

15 Marrin, West (2002) *Universal Water: The Ancient Wisdom and Scientific Theory of Water*, Maui: Inner Ocean Publishing. Also see Schwenk, Theodora and Wolfram Schwenk (1989) *Water, the Element of Life*, Herndon, VA: Arthroscopic Press, and Wylson, Anthony (1986) *Aquature: Architecture and Water*, London: Architectural Press.

16 Mador, Martin (2008) In *Biophilic Design*, 43–57.

17 Anon (2007) 'Bon Secours St. Francis Cancer Institute', *Healthcare Design*, 8(9), 118–20.

18 Anon (2005) 'Banner Estrella Medical Center', *Modern Healthcare*, 26 September, 78(9), 27.

19 Guenther, Robin and Gail Vittori (2008) *Sustainable Healthcare Architecture*, New York: John Wiley & Sons, Inc.

20 Sala, M., A. Trombadore, and G. Alcamo (2006) 'Energy-saving strategies for the new design: Meyer Children's Hospital in Florence', in *Design and Health IV: Future Trends in Healthcare Design*, A. Dilani (ed.), Huddinge, Sweden: International Academy for Design and Health. Also see Williams, J.M., I.P. Knight and A.J. Griffiths (1999) 'Hospital energy performance: new indicators for UK National Health Services Estate', *Building Services Engineering Research & Technology*, 20(1), 9–12.

21 Guenther and Vittori, pp. 261–2.

22 Ibid., p. 321.

23 Marcus, Clare Cooper, (2007) 'Healing gardens in hospitals', *Interdisciplinary Design and Research e-Journal*, 1(1), 1–27, Online. Available at http:// www.idrp.wsu.edu/Vol_1/Cooper_Marcus.pdf (accessed 23 February 2009). Also see Ulrich, Roger (1992) 'Effects of interior design on wellness: theory and recent scientific research', *Journal of Healthcare Design*,

3(2), 97–109, and Horsburgh, C.R. (1995) 'Healing by design', *The New England Journal of Medicine*, 11(333), 735–40. The first post-occupancy evaluations of healing gardens were reported in Cooper Marcus, Clare and Mimi Barnes (1995) *Gardens in Health Care Facilities: Uses, Therapeutic Benefits, and Design Considerations*, Martinez, CA: The Center for Health Design. Also see Cooper Marcus, Clare and Mimi Barnes (eds.) (1999) *Healing Gardens: Therapeutic Benefits and Design Recommendations*, New York: John Wiley & Sons, Inc.

24 Thompson, John and Grace Goldin (1975) *The Hospital: A Social and Architectural History*, New Haven, CT: Yale University Press, p. 169.

25 Cooper Marcus, pp. 4–5. Also see Cooper Marcus, Clare (2001) 'Hospital oasis', *Landscape Architecture*, 47(10), 36–41, 99.

26 Ulrich, Roger (1999) 'Effects of gardens on health outcomes: theory and research', in Cooper Marcus and Barnes, *Healing Gardens*, 27–86. Possible outcomes from exposure to a healing garden include a reduction in stress among patients, reduced pain in patients, reduction in level of depression, a higher reported quality of life among chronic and terminally ill patients, improvements in wayfinding capabilities, reduced length of stay for certain types of patients, increased patient mobility levels and independence, higher levels of patient satisfaction, and higher levels of job satisfaction among caregivers.

27 Cooper Marcus, p. 6.

28 Giella, B. (1995) 'Buena Shore Club', in March, Lionel and Judith Sheine (eds.) *R.M. Schindler Compositions and Construction*, London: Routledge. Also see Pfeiffer, B.B. (ed.) (1992) 'Architect, architecture, and the client' (1896), by Frank L. Wright, in *Frank Lloyd Wright: Collected Writings*, Rizzoli: New York.; and Wright, Frank L. (1954) *The Natural House*, Doubleday: New York.

29 Leatherbarrow, David (2002) 'Sitting in the city, or the body in the world', in Dodds, George and Robert Tavernor (eds.) *Body and Building: Essays on the Changing Relation of Body and Architecture*, Cambridge and London: The MIT Press.

30 Ibid., pp. 287–8. Leatherbarrow writes 'Given Schindler's acceptance of the basic principles of Wright's built and written work, it is not surprising that he invoked the concept of the organic in explanation of his buildings. What is more, the outcome of organic composition was described as a unified ensemble, a synthesis. Having circled back to this ambition, after considering the counterarguments for Loos and Frank, it is now possible to turn to the problem of unity or wholeness itself in an attempt to indicate the ethical and philosophical implications of its different meanings … In design, architects are always concerned with bounded settings. Consequently we tend to see the field around them as a background, the darkness needed in the theater to show up our performances.'

31 Cooper Marcus, p. 21.

32 Verderber, Stephen (1986) 'Person-window transactions in the hospital rehabilitation environment', *Environment and Behavior*, 18(4), 450–66. Also see Heerwagan, Judith (1990) 'Affective functioning, light hunger and

room brightness preference', *Environment and Behavior*, 22(5), 608–35, and Heerwagan, Judith H. and G.H. Orians (1993) 'Humans, habitats and aesthetics', in *The Biophilia Hypothesis*, by Kellert, Stephen R. and E.O Wilson (eds.) Washington, D.C.: Island Press, Shearwater Books.

33 Malkin, Jain (2008) *Visual Reference for Evidence-based Healthcare Design*. Concord, CA: Center for Health Design.

34 Ibid., pp. 132–3.

35 Ibid., p. 133.

36 Verderber and Fine, p. 167.

37 Ibid., pp. 174–7.

38 Ibid., pp. 167–8.

39 Ibid., p. 58–9.

40 Ibid., pp. 134–43. The International Style failed at the level of site, landscape and nature, particularly in the hands of lesser architects, because it choked any remaining tattered fragments of locality and local culture from the life of healthcare architecture. Indigenous expression is an alien concern in most franchise healthcare architecture. Wall Street healthcare was an utter failure in this regard. Corporate healthcare bureaucracies of America failed to give expression to locality, to place, to local traditions. Why not *both/and* rather than either/or? Must the outpatient surgicenter always be in a suburban strip mall next to the Wendy's and Wal-Mart?

41 Sloan, David C. and Beverlie Conant Sloane (2003) *Medicine Moves to the Mall*. Baltimore & London: The Johns Hopkins University Press.

42 Frampton, Kenneth (1983) 'Prospects for a critical regionalism', *Perspecta: The Yale Architectural Journal*, 20 January, 147–62.

4 The evolving patient room and PCU

1 Kaplan, Stephen and Rachael Kaplan (1983) *Cognition and Environment: Functioning in an Uncertain World*, New York: Praeger.

2 Ibid., pp. 77–80.

3 Ulrich, Roger S., Craig Zimring, Xuemei Zhu, Jennifer DuBose, Hyun-Bo Seo, Young-Seon Choi, Xiaobo Quan, and Anjali Joseph (2008) 'A review of the research literature on evidence-based healthcare design', *Health Environments Research & Design Journal*, 1(3), 61–125.

4 Yenni, Carla (2007) *The Architecture of Madness: Insane Asylums in the United States*, Minneapolis: University of Minnesota Press.

5 Ibid., p. 122. Nightingale herself praised the Hospital Laribrosiere in Paris for its two parallel rows of pavilions situated on either side of a rectangular courtyard. These allowed for abundant ventilation and daylight and connecting corridor spines that efficiently allowed for the movement of people and supplies.

6 Ibid., p. 123.

7 Ibid., p. 124.

8   Verderber, Stephen and David J. Fine (2000) *Healthcare Architecture in an Era of Radical Transformation*, London and New Haven: Yale University Press. See Chapter 4. Expansion necessitated expropriation of land and often the destruction of the surrounding neighborhood. The older neighborhoods surrounding these hospitals, such as was the case with the Michael Reese Hospital in Chicago, consisted of dwellings, churches, schools, and small business establishments.

9   Yenni, p. 124.

10 Ibid., p. 125.

11 Ibid., pp. 126–7. The administration building at Johns Hopkins was highly ornamented and larger in size than the other buildings on the campus. This was also the case at the Kirkbride asylums. These institutions straddled a curious balance between grandeur and functionalism.

12 Thompson, John and Grace Goldin (1975) *The Hospital: A Social and Architectural History*, London and New Haven: Yale University Press, p. 207.

13 Ibid., p. 208. Goldin believed that not everyone wants or needs a private room though it was and is an extension of the American obsession with privacy in all aspects of everyday life. One may extrapolate from this that Americans' love affair with the private auto and the single family detached dwelling were similar expressions of this national trend during throughout the post-World War II years and especially since 1980.

14 Ibid., p. 209.

15 Ibid., p. 211.

16 This created two smaller wards on either side of from six to ten beds each. By the 1960s the dilemma that confronted healthcare planners and architects was how to design an inexpensive private patient room without overextending the length of the corridor within the nursing unit.

17 Thompson and Goldin, p. 216. The replacement Guy's Hospital in London (1958–1961) contained two L-shaped 12-bed wards with the nursing station at its intersection.

18 Ibid., p. 249.

19 Nickl-Weller, Christine and Hans Nickl (eds.) (2007) *Hospital Architecture*, Berlin: Braun.

20 Anon (2008) *Southwest Washington Medical Center's E.W. and Mary Firstenburg Tower*, Project narrative provided to the Author by NBBJ Seattle Office, WA., 27 October.

21 Ibid.

22 Spohn, John (2007) 'Imagining a better hospital room', *Healthcare Design*, 12(11), 58–70. The Adopt-a-Room prototypes were copyrighted and were constructed at a total cost of $1.8 million although this figure also included all retrofit costs.

23 Allison, David (2006) *Patient Room Prototype*, Clemson, SC: Clemson University Architecture+Health Graduate Program and Carleton University Industrial Design Program.

24 Ibid., pp. 17–18.

25 Ibid., pp. 23–4.

26 Malkin, Jain (2008) *Visual Reference for Evidence-Based Design*, Concord, CA: The Center for Health Design, p. xii.

27 Frampton, S.B., L. Gilpin, and P.A. Charmel (2003) *Putting Patients First: Designing and Practicing Patient-Centered Care*, New York: Jossey-Bass (John Wiley imprint).

28 Malkin, p. 88. Although the terms 'patient-centered care' and 'patient-focused care' are often used interchangeably, they are quite different. Patient-centered care is based on evaluating all ideas in terms of what is most convenient and comfortable for the patient. Patient-focused care, by contrast, denotes a top to bottom re-engineering of hospital operations to achieve higher institutional performance. In the end, however, not all 'improvements' made in hospital operations had a direct net positive benefit for patient care. Also see Lathrop, P. (1993) *Restructuring Health Care: The Patient Focused Paradigm*, San Francisco: Jossey-Bass, Inc.

29 Malkin, pp. 5–6.

30 DeBuono, R. (2007) 'What is health literacy?' *Partnership for Clear Health Communication*, Online. Available at http://www.npsf.org/pchc/health-literacy.php (accessed 12 February 2009). Also see the special issue on this topic published in *Advances in Family Centered Care* (2002). 8(1): 1–37.

31 This trend has been at the core of the New Residentialism movement of the past two decades and the evidence-based research movement has reinforced this trend in healthcare design.

32 Malkin, p. 24.

33 Ibid., p. 25. In 2009 the Pebble Project was incorporated into the Global Health Safety Initiatives (GHSI) RIPPLE database. The GHSI is a sector-wide collaboration to transform the way healthcare environments are designed, built, and operated, and also focuses on products used within. The GHSI was launched in October 2007 and the RIPPLE database was in beta testing at the time of writing. The Pebbles case study data was also scheduled to participate in a study conducted by the Agency for Healthcare Research and Quality (AHRQ). The study 'Safety and Quality in Healthcare: A Framework for Evaluating Evidence-based Design' is being conducted for the AHRQ by Batelle, the Center for Health Design and the MANILA Consulting Group. Also see Taylor, Ellen M. (2009) 'The Pebble Project: the year in review', *Healthcare Design*, 9(1), 20–6. Contact Mark Goodman at http://www.healthcaredesignmagazine.com/ ME2/dirmod.asp?sid=9B6FFC446FF7486981EA3C0C3CCE4943&nm= Articles&type=Publishing&mod=Publications%3A%3AArticle&mid=8F 3A7027421841978F18BE895F87F791&tier=4&id=002D5FF8A0A54E0 A9DC83E9D13C2C4E1. Topics of Pebble case studies have included master planning, NICU, ICU, and PCU settings, staff engagement, the use of gardens and nature as therapeutic intervention, philanthropy, and outpatient care settings. Additional research carried out under the umbrella of the Pebble Project addresses overall healthcare quality, staff performance, patient safety, and cost-benefit trade offs. This research is focused on lighting, noise, satisfaction, perceived anxiety, art as therapy, and workplace safety. Many of these initiatives can be

categorized in multiple categories. In the case of Dublin Methodist Medical Center (2005–2008), in Ohio, many evidence-based design amenities were incorporated: accessible roof gardens, acoustic abatement, acuity-adaptable rooms, artwork, bathrooms on headwalls, equipped with handrails, decentralized nursing workstations, internal courtyards, accentuated thresholds to bath/shower rooms and to the patient room from the adjoining corridor, large windows, lighting options, same-handed patient rooms, operable windows in patient rooms, a water feature in the main lobby, and well located, highly visible handwash stations. The Planetree initiative and the Pebble Project have aided the growth and influence of evidence-based design research, and are now considered part of its canon.

34 Ulrich et al., p. 123.

35 de Verneil, Christine and Lindsay Todd (2008) Re-considering The Semi-Private Patient Room: A Review of Where We Have Come From and Where We Are Going. Unpublished Research Report, Clemson, SC: Clemson University, Graduate Studies in Architecture+Health.

36 Burnette, Tonia (2006) 'Is "semiprivate" always an oxymoron?' Healthcare Design, 6(1), 45–51.

37 Chaudhury, Habib, Atiya Mahmood and Christine Valente (2005) 'Advantages and disadvantages of single versus multiple occupancy rooms in acute care environments: a review and analysis of the literature', Environment and Behavior, 37(6), 760–86.

38 Anon (2002) 'Maternity hospital', Japan Architect, 87:6, 23–7.

39 Van de Glind, I., S. de Roode and A. Goossensen (2007) 'Do patients in hospitals benefit from single rooms? A literature review', Health Policy, 84(2–3), 153–61.

40 Dettenkofer, M., S. Seegers, G. Antes, E. Motschall, M. Schumacher, and F.D. Daschner (2002) 'Does the architecture of hospital facilities influence nosocomial infection rates? A systematic review', Infection Control and Hospital Epidemiology, 25(1), 21–5. Also see Ben-Abraham, Ron, Nathan Keller, Oded Szold, Amir Vardi, Marius Weinberg, Zohar Barzilay and Gideon Paret (2002) 'Do isolation rooms reduce the rate of nosocomial infections in the pediatric intensive care unit?' Journal of Critical Care, 17(3), 176–80.

41 Kohn, Linda, Janet Corrigan and Molla Donaldson (eds.) (2000) To Err is Human: Building a Safer Health System. Washington, DC: Institute of Medicine and the National Academy Press.

42 Tarkan, Laurie (2008) 'Arrogant, abusive and disruptive – and a Doctor', The New York Times, 2 December. Online. Available at http://www.nytimes.com/2008/12/02/health/02rage.html (accessed 5 December 2008).

43 Ulrich et al., pp. 107–9.

44 Calkins, Margaret and Christne Cassella (2007) 'Exploring the cost and value of private versus shared bedrooms in nursing homes', The Gerontologist, 47(2), 169–83. Also see Cahnman, Samuel F. (2006) 'Key considerations in patient room design, Part 1', Healthcare Design, 6(2), 24–30.

45 Dowdeswell, Barrie, Jonathan Erskine, and Michael Heasman (2004) Hospital Ward Configuration: Determinants Influencing Single Room Provision, A Report for NHS Estates, London: The European Health Property Network.

46 Ulrich et al., p. 112.

47 Ulrich, p. 47.

48 Chaudhury, p. 49. Also see Chaudhury, Habib, Atiya Mahmood and Maria Valente (2006) 'Nurses' perception of single occupancy versus multi-occupancy rooms in acute care environments: An exploratory comparative assessment', Applied Nursing Research, 19(3), 118–25.

49 Malcolm, Helen A. (2005) 'Does privacy matter? Former patients discuss their perceptions of privacy in shared hospital rooms', Nursing Ethics, 12(2), 156–66.

50 Newell, Patricia Brierley (1998) 'A cross-cultural comparison of privacy definitions and functions: a systems approach', Journal of Environmental Psychology, 18(3), 357–71.

51 Malcolm, 164–6. Also see Romano, Michael (2005) 'Personal space', Modern Healthcare, 35(31), 20.

52 Kaya, Naz and Margaret Weber (2003) 'Cross-cultural differences in the perception of crowding and privacy regulation: American and Turkish students,' Journal of Environmental Psychology, 23(4), 301–9.

53 Dowdeswell et al., pp. 27–34.

54 Ulrich et al., p. 124.

55 Malcolm, p. 20.

56 See the home page of The United States Green Building Council, Washington, D.C., Online. Available at http://www.usgbc.org/.

57 Malkin, pp. 127–34.

58 Ulrich et al., p. 125.

59 Joint Commission on the Accreditation of Healthcare Organizations (2002) Healthcare at the Crossroads: Strategies for Addressing the Evolving Nursing Crisis, Oakbrook Terrace, IL: Joint Commission on the Accreditation of Healthcare Organizations.

60 Morrissey, John (2003) 'JCAHO to require stepped-up infection control', Modern Healthcare's Daily Dose, 14 November. Online. Available at https://home.modernhealthcare.com/clickshare/authenticateUser Subscription.do?CSProduct=modernhealthcare-web&CSAuthReq= 1:37336616244058O:AIDIIDAID=20031114/PREMIUM/311140304 IID=:B0D9025C30D5B0DD6E0FC5D68F774F9B&AID=20031114/ PREMIUM/311140304&title=JCAHO%20to%20require%20stepped%20 up%20infection%20control&ID=&CSTargetURL=http%3A%2F%2F www.modernhealthcare.com%2Fapps%2Fpbcs.dll%2Flogin%3FAssign SessionID%3D37336616244058O%26AID%3D20031114%2FPREMIUM %2F311140304 (accessed 30 November 2008).

61 Thompson and Goldin, pp. 215–16. This can be achieved not unlike how the open Nightingale wards at the Rigshospital in Copenhagen were redesigned in 1910 into a series of patient bed zones subdivided with partitions, albeit fixed partitions, that still allowed air to circulate freely below and above a moveable partition or storage device. Such

devices allow for visual privacy without impeding staff supervision requirements.

62 Babwin, Donald (2002) 'Building boom', *Hospitals and Health Networks*, 76(3), 48–54.

63 Malkin, p. 109.

64 Nickl, Christine-Weller and Hans Nickl (eds.) (2007) *Hospital Architecture*, Berlin: Braun, pp. 150–3.

5 The evolving role of memory, place, and sustainability

1 Farr, Douglas (2008) *Sustainable Urbanism: Urban Design With Nature*. New York: John Wiley & Sons, Inc. Also see Ewing, Reid and Richard Kreutzer (2006) *Understanding the Relationship Between Public Health and the Built Environment: A Report Prepared for the LEED-ND Core Committee*. Washington, D.C.: United States Green Building Council, May 2006, Online. Available at http://www.usgbc.org/ShowFile. aspx?DocumentID=1480 (accessed 12 May 2008).

2 Verderber, Stephen and David J. Fine (2000) *Healthcare Architecture in an Era of Radical Transformation*, New Haven and London: Yale University Press.

3 Ibid., pp. 96–9.

4 Ibid., pp. 116–18.

5 Ibid., p. 119.

6 Ibid., p. 122.

7 Ibid., pp. 124–9. This innovation was conceived in response to the period's hyper-accelerated rate of change in medical science.

8 Ibid., pp. 120–2.

9 Verderber, Stephen (2008) 'Evidence-based design for healthcare in post-Katrina New Orleans: current dilemmas', *Health Environments Research & Design Journal*, 1(2), 71–6.

10 Eaton, Lewis (2007) 'New Orleans' recovery is slowed by closed hospitals', *The New York Times*, 24 July. Online. Available at http://www.nytimes. com. (accessed 15 November 2007). Nearly 125,000 former residents continue to live elsewhere, forced away in the largest Diaspora in U.S. history. For most Americans it continues to be difficult to comprehend the sheer magnitude of the upheaval caused by Katrina. The U.N. refers to the dislocated as internally displaced persons (IDPs). Since Katrina, the metro area's remaining hospitals have lost nearly $75 million in the provision of uncompensated care for the uninsured. The metro areas healthcare network was decimated. Ninety percent of its mental health professionals were lost at a time when suicides and chronic depression rates rose significantly more than those of the rest of the U.S. Major health facilities were permanently closed, including the Lindy Boggs Medical Center in the Mid-City neighborhood in New Orleans, Chalmette Medical Center, Charity Hospital, a number of nursing homes, including

the venerable Maison Hospitaliere in the Vieux Carré, dating from 1843. Nearby a dozen neighborhood outpatient clinics were ruined in addition to scores of private physicians' offices, counselors' offices, and dental clinics. See De Gregorio, James (2007) 'Victory developers seek demolition permit for Lindy Boggs Medical Center', 26 November, *The Times-Picayune*, Online. Available at http://www.noloa.com. (accessed 26 November 2007).

11 Katz, Alan (1992) 'Big Charity: a history of emergencies', *Tulane Medicine*, 87(1), 13–22.

12 Moller, Jan (2007) 'VA decides to put hospital in New Orleans', *The Times-Picayune*, 21 August. Online. Available at http://www.nola.com. (accessed 24 August 2007).

13 The Foundation for Historical Louisiana (2008) *Medical Center of New Orleans Charity Hospital Feasibility Study, RMJM Hillier*, 15 September. Online. Available at http://www.fhl.org/FHL/News/PresvAlerts/Charity Hospital.html (accessed 15 December 2008). Also see the extensive field research reported by Karen Gadbois and others at http://www. squanderedheritage.com.

14 Groth, Paul and Todd Bressi (eds.) (1997) *Understanding Ordinary Landscapes*, New Haven and London: Yale University Press.

15 Verderber, p. 72.

16 Katz, pp. 19–20. It is considered a classic high-rise interpretative Nightingale hospital for its open wards, its long, narrow ward configurations, its large, operable windows, its natural ventilation, its abundant natural daylight, its high (17 foot) floor to floor heights, and its site plan configuration. It was a peer to and influenced by the aforementioned Hospital Beaujon in France, which opened three years earlier (see Chapter 2). Charity's main lobby is exquisite. At street level, its large physical volume seems human-scaled due to its massing and amenities.

17 Moe, Richard (2008) '11 Most Endangered Historic Places for 2008', Washington, D.C.: *The National Trust for Historic Preservation*. Online. Available at http://www.preservationnation.org/travel-and-sites/sites/ southern-region/charity-hospital-neighborhood.html (accessed 6 February 2009).

18 Gallas, Walter (2008) 'National Trust 11 most endangered places: Charity Hospital and the adjacent neighborhood', *Preservation Nation*. Online. Available at http://www.preservationnation.org/travel-and-sites/sites/ southern-region/charity-hospital-neighborhood.html (accessed 20 February 2009).

19 Nossiter, Adam (2008) 'Plan for New Orleans hospitals draws outcry', *The New York Times*, 25 November. Online. Available at http://www. nytimes.com/2008/11/26/us/26hospital.html (accessed 20 February 2009).

20 Ed Blakely garnered a reputation for ineffectiveness. He has also stated he was in favor of saving the historic modernist St. France Cabrini Church (1960–1963), in the Gentilly area of the city, from demolition. However, his office stood idly by while FEMA, the city, and the Archdiocese of New Orleans conspired to allow the Holy Cross Boys' School to

destroy this landmark church in June 2007. See Verderber, Stephen (2008) *Delirious New Orleans: Manifesto or an Extraordinary American City*, Austin: University of Texas Press. Blakely resigned his post as the Director of the Office of Recovery Management and left the city in June 2009.

21 This Internet site emerged as a powerful voice of the grassroots movement to hold public officials accountable for their actions in post-Katrina New Orleans. Houses illegally slated for demolition by FEMA and the city were posted on the site. Countless meetings were attended to reinforce the concerns of still-displaced residents whose homes were slated for demolition. *Squandered Heritage* was featured in an article in *The New York Times* (2008). See http://www.squanderedheritage.com.

22 These updates were authored by Walter Gallas, the head of the New Orleans field office of the National Trust for Historic Preservation. See various updates posted by Gallas online at http://www.preservationnation.org.

23 The RMJM Charity Hospital Report to *The Foundation for Historical Louisiana* (2008), 6–12.

24 Ibid., pp. 10–11.

25 Ibid., pp. 92–8.

26 Ibid., p. 99.

27 Ibid., p. 101.

28 Tyler, William (2000) *Historic Preservation: An Introduction to its History, Principles, and Practice*, New York: W.W. Norton & Co.

29 Advisory Council for Historic Preservation (2002) *Protecting Historic Properties: A Citizen's Guild to Section 106 Review*. Washington, D.C. Online. Available at http://www.achp.gov/citizensguide.pdf. (accessed 12 August 2008). Also see Irvin, Norman (2003) *Historic Preservation Handbook*, New York: McGraw Hill.

30 Verderber, Stephen (2009) 'The Un-building of historic neighborhoods in Post-Katrina New Orleans', *Journal of Urban Design*, 18(4), 257–77.

31 See http://www.squandredheritage.com for updates on reactions to the controversial LSUHSC/DVA Memorandum of Understanding from October 2006.

32 Morgan, Denise W., N.I. Morgan, and B. Barnett (2008) 'Finding a place for the commonplace: Hurricane Katrina, communities, and preservation law', *American Anthropologist*, 108(4), 706–18. Also see Moran, Kate (2008) 'Plans for LSU-VA complex stir resentment', *The Times-Picayune*, 21 February. Online. Available at http://www.nola.com. (accessed 10 March 2008).

33 Stokes, Sandra (2008) 'Letter to Legislative Appropriations Subcommittee on Health and Human Services', *Foundation for Historical Louisiana*, 4 December. Online. Available at http://www.squanderedheritage.com (accessed 19 February 2009).

34 Verderber, Stephen (2008) *Delirious New Orleans: Manifesto for an Extraordinary American City*, Chapter 6, pp. 203–34.

35 Lombardi, John (2009) 'Leaders back new LSU hospital', *The Times Picayune*, 29 January. Online. Available at http://www.nola.com. (accessed 1 February 2009).

36 Barrow, Bill (2009) 'Tempers flare over new LSU Medical Complex', *The Times-Picayune*, 2 February. Online. Available at http://www.nola.com/news/index (accessed 2 February 2009). Also see Moller, Jan (2009) 'Legislators weigh price tag for new LSU teaching hospital in New Orleans', *The Times-Picayune*, 22 January. Online. Available at http://www.nola.com/news/index.html (accessed 23 January 2009).

37 Barrow, ibid. Also see Gill, James (2009) 'Unhealthy attitude infects LSU', *The Times Picayune*, 20 March. Online. Available at http://www.nola.com. (accessed 21 March 2009). Gill attacked LSU for being far less than transparent in its public statements on its reasons for pursuing the replacement hospital. To him, the LSU strategy was an act of self-aggrandizement, an embarrassment to the University's integrity, and a cover-up of the facts. His article fueled hundreds of online comments of which the vast majority sided against LSU. In June 2009 the LSU public relations position deteriorated even further when a radio ad it placed stated that LSU would move its entire medical school and health sciences center to Baton Rouge unless its new hospital was built. See Barrow, Bill (2009) 'Ad warns of LSU moving medical school out of New Orleans', *The Times Picayune*, 5 June, p. A-1. Online. Available at http://www.nola.com. (accessed 6 June 2009). Within 24 hours this article had fueled more than 200 online posts, with 90 percent against the LSU position. Also see Gill, James (2009) 'LSU trying hard to save city from itself', *The Times Picayune*, 2 June, p. A12. Online. Available at http://www.nola.com. (accessed 7 June 2009).

38 Verderber (2008), *Delirious New Orleans*, Chapter 6, pp. 207–12.

39 Groth and Bressi, pp. 104–16.

40 Moller, Jan (2008) 'Charity Hospital can be restored, report says', *The Times-Picayune*, 20 August. Online. Available at http://www.nola.com/news/index. (accessed 5 September 2008). Also see Gallas, Walter (2008) 'Nationally recognized architectural firm says Charity Hospital "structurally sound" and ready for transformation to state-of the-art modern medical facility', *The National Trust for Historic Preservation*. Online. Available at http://www.preservationnation.org (accessed 5 September 2008).

41 Verderber (2008), *Health Environments Research & Design*, pp. 74–5.

42 Guillet, Jamie (2007) 'Stafford Act behind slow moving recovery funds', *New Orleans City Business*, 1 April. Online. Available at http://www.neworleanscitybusiness.com.html (accessed 17 January 2007).

43 Verderber, Stephen (2008) 'Emergency housing in the aftermath of Hurricane Katrina: An assessment of the FEMA travel trailer program', *Journal of Housing and the Built Environment*, 23(4), 367–81.

44 Hayden, Dolores (1995) *The Power of Place: Urban Landscapes as Public History*. Cambridge, MA: MIT Press.

45 The Louisiana Superdome was repaired within twelve months after the hurricane in order for the city's National Football League (NFL) team to return (the New Orleans Saints). Charity Hospital is no less revered than that iconic building. Why was the sports facility fully restored (and improved, at a total cost of $185 million) while Charity would sit abandoned without any proposed new use on the horizon?

46   Mallory, Keith (1973) *The Architecture of War*, New York: Pantheon.

47   Verderber (2008) *Delirious New Orleans*, pp. 209–12.

48   MacCash, Doug (2007) 'Architectural soul of the city at stake', *The Times-Picayune*, 27 August. Online. Available at http://www.nola.com (accessed 28 August 2007).

49   Charlesworth, Esther (2006) *Architects without Frontiers: War, Reconstruction, and Design Responsibility,* Oxford: Architectural Press/ Elsevier.

50   To critics, the apparent public relations strategy was to refute critics as out of touch and unrealistic.

51   Margolis, Mac (2006) 'Travel: the world's most endangered destinations', *Newsweek International*, 10 April. Online. Available at http://www. globalheritagefund.org/news/conservation_news/newsweek_vanishing_ acts_7_endangered_wonders.asp (accessed 17 January 2008). Also see Sutter, John D. (2009) 'Five places to go before global warming messes them up'. Online. Available at http://www.cnn.com/2009/ TRAVEL/02/17/global.warming.travel/?iref=mpstoryview (accessed 23 February 2009).

52   Verderber and Fine, pp. 147–54.

53   Francis, Susan, Rosemary Glanville, Ann A. Noble, and Peter Scher (1999) *50 Years of Ideas in Health Care Buildings*: *Report to the Nuffield Trust*, London: The Nuffield Trust.

54   From the advent of cost containment legislation in the U.S. they fell out of favor with politicians and the general public because they were seen as too costly to build, and required so much land. By 2010, many megahospitals in developed nations were staffing less than half the number of beds they were built for. In Houston, this happened at the U.S. Department of Veterans Affairs, when it demolished its 1935 Nightingale hospital and built a 950-bed megahospital.

55   Bafna, S., R. Choudhary, and C. Zimring (2007) *Rebuilding New Orleans Hospitals – Task 2: A Working Resource Guide for Clinic Redesign*, Atlanta: Georgia Institute of Technology. This team developed a protocol to bring research into the planning and design of a Charity replacement facility, versus the renovation of the existing hospital. They focused on patient outcomes, safety, satisfaction, staff retention, and service delivery efficiencies.

56   Groth and Bressi, pp. 97–9.

57   Farr, p. 36.

58   Verderber (2008) *Health Environments Research & Design*, p. 74.

59   Verderber, Stephen (2005) *Compassion in Architecture: Evidence-based Design for Health in Louisiana*, Lafayette, LA: Center for Louisiana Studies.

60   Verderber (2008) *Health Environments Research & Design*, p. 75.

61   Singletary, Mark (2009) 'LSU/VA complex set for Mid-City – end of story', *New Orleans City Business*, 23 February. Online. Available at http:// www.neworleanscitybusiness.com (accessed 25 February 2009).

62   Barrow, Bill (2009) 'Citizens argue against state's FEMA appeal on Charity Hospital', *The Times Picayune*, 17 April. Online. Available at http//:
www.nola.com (accessed 17 April 2009). By the summer of 2009 the growing grass-roots effort to restore Charity had gained additional steam. In August, a second line rally and processional march of 1,200 persons occurred at the site of the shuttered hospital campus in downtown New Orleans. Brass bands accompanied the chanting marchers, and the event was broadly covered by the local media. *The Times Picayune*, in a series of articles and in two editorials, finally began to question the motives behind the abandonment of Charity. See Barrow, Bill (2009) 'Critics fear LSU hospital site could end up half-empty,' 9 May, *The Times Picayune*. Online. Available at http://www.nola.com (accessed 15 May 2009); Gill, James (2009) 'LSU trying hard to save city from itself', 2 June, *The Times Picayune*. Online. Available at http://www.nola.com (accessed 4 June 2009); Editorial (2009) 'Resolving the impasse over New Orleans' proposed teaching hospital', 25 June, *The Times Picayune*. Online. Available at http://www.nola.com (accessed 27 June 2009); and Barrow, Bill (2009) 'Group says poll shows support for rebuilding in the shell of Charity Hospital,' *The Times Picayune*, 5 August. Online. Available at http://www.nola.com (accessed 8 August 2009). The local daily newspaper published an Op Ed piece by a well-known local author. See Piazza, Tom (2009) 'House thieves, on a grand scale', 5 September, *The Times Picayune*. Online. Available at http://www.nola.com. (accessed 6 September 2009). Also see http://www.savecharityhospital.com for detailed information on the fight to restore Charity, including numerous *You Tube* videos detailing the grass-roots effort.

63   American Institute of Architects (2009) 'Campus revitalization: transforming 1950s hospitals into modern health care environments', *Healthcare Design*. Online. Available at http://www.hcdmagazine.com. (accessed 21 April 2009). This is a webinar on the topic. Meanwhile, the U.S. architectural press had taken note of the ongoing battle. The editor of *Architectural Record* magazine wrote an editorial on the subject of the senseless destruction of twentieth-century architectural landmarks. See Ivy, Robert (2009) 'What will happen to Charity Hospital and other endangered projects? – A fresh look at the state of historic preservation', June, *Architectural Record*. Online. Available at http://www.architecturalrecord. com (accessed 12 July 2009).

6   Prognostications

1   World Health Organization (1998) *District Health Facilities: Guidelines for Development and Operations*, Geneva: World Health Organization. Also see World Health Organization (2000) *Global Water Supply and Sanitation Assessment 2000 Report*, Geneva, World Health Organization.

2   Verderber, Stephen (2003) 'Architecture for health – 2050: an international perspective', *The Journal of Architecture*, 8:3, 281–301. This chapter is an expanded version of the basic argument presented in this paper.

3   Lynas, Mark (2008) *Six Degrees: Our Future on a Hotter Planet*, Washington, D.C.: National Geographic Books, pp. 186–8.

4   Brown, Valerie A., John Grootjans, Jan Ritchie, Mardie Townsend, and Glenda Verrinder (2005) *Sustainability and Health: Supporting Global Ecological Integrity in Public Health*, Crows Nest, New South Wales: Earthscan/Allen & Unwin. Also see McDowell, Christopher (2002) 'Involuntary resettlement, impoverishment risks, and sustainable livelihoods', *The Australasian Journal of Disaster*, 22:2, 117–34.

5   Andersen, Kurt (2009) 'The reset', *Time*, 173:13, 32–8.

6   Kunstler, James Howard (2005) *The Long Emergency: Surviving the End of Oil, Climate Change, and Other Converging Catastrophies of the Twenty-First Century*, New York: Grove Press, pp. 248–9.

7   Woods, Lebbeus (2008) 'Delirious Dubai'. Online. Available at http://lebbeuswoods.wordpress.com/2008/03/05.html (accessed 7 January 2009). Also see Kamin, Blair (2008) 'Chicago architects plan more towers in Dubai', *The Chicago Tribune*, 7 October, pp. B-4, and Alter, Lloyd (2008) 'Is the architecture fun over or just getting started', *Toronto Globe and Mail*, 22 December, p. A-12. In a letter published a few weeks later in *The New York Times* by the founders of *Architecture for Humanity*, Cameron Sinclair and Kate Stohr, they refuted the piece by Alter, claiming he completely failed to cite the many talented design-oriented architects whose work is devoted to helping the poor, and marginalized segments of society. Online. Available at http://www.treehuger.com/files. (accessed 7 January 2009).

8   Kunstler, pp. 250–70.

9   Benjamin, David (2003) 'Hopefuls cite preservation of open space as key issue', *News Transcript*. Online. Available at http://www.newstranscript.gmnews.com (accessed 15 March 2003). Also see Calthorpe, Peter (1993) *The Next American Metropolis: Ecology, Community, and the American Dream*, New York: Princeton Architectural Press. Also Brooks, David (2002) 'For Democrats, time to meet the exurban voter', *The New York Times*, Sunday, November 10, p. WK 3. He wrote: 'Before 1980, only a quarter of all office space was in the suburbs. But about 70 percent of the office space created in the 1990s was in suburbia, and now 42 percent of all offices are located there. You have a tribe of people who don't live in cities, or commute to cities, or have any contact with urban life. Mesa, Arizona, another quintessential exurb east of Phoenix, already has more people than St. Louis. Extrapolate out a few years, and some of these sprawling suburbs will have political clout equal to Chicago. Their motto: More Highways, Less Growth.'

10 Duany, Andres, Elizabeth Plater-Zyberk, and Jeff Speck (2002) *Suburban Nation: The Rise of Sprawl and the Decline of the American Dream*, Boston: North Point Press, p. 47.

11 Hopkins, Jim (2003) 'Wal-Mart's influence grows', *USA Today*, Wednesday 29 January, Section B, 1–2. Wal-Mart alone accounted for as much as 25 percent of U.S. productivity gains from 1995–1999. With 1.3 million workers, it became the world's largest private employer in 2003, employing one in every 123 U.S. workers and nearly one in every twenty retail employees. This empire was built at a dizzying pace. At the same time, the giant's relentless price wars decimated historic town centers. In terms of facilities, the expansion of the company's stores from first generation Wal-Mart's into metamorphosed Super-Wal-Mart's had deleterious consequences in terms of environmental and social health, with many unanticipated consequences on the quality of everyday life. One consequence is that the chain often built a far larger, second generation store only a few blocks away from the first generation one, and then let the older one sit empty, rotting, lest a competitor get their hands on it.

12 Piquepaille, Roland (2008) 'Smart holograms to monitor our health?', *EmergingTech*. Online. Available at http://www.ZDNet.com. (accessed 26 May 2009). Also Quinn, Valens (2009) 'Plasma and LCD TVs time warp: Back to the future?' *Gadget Guy*. Online. Available at http://www.gadgetguy.com.au/time-warp.html (accessed 26 May 2009).

13 Peach, Laurie A. (1997) 'Holography finds a home in medicine', *Laser Focus World*, 33:1212, 131–5. Online. Available at http://www.laserfocusworld.com (accessed 21 May 2009). Also see Anon (2006) 'Preliminary study finds holographic imaging system promising for cancer treatment planning', *Bio-Medicine*. Online. Available at http://www.bio-medicine.org (accessed 26 May 2009).

14 Vterrain (2002) *Artificial Terrain Tools and Software Packages*. Online. Available at http://www.vterrain.org (accessed 12 July 2002).

15 Bentley, P.J. (2002) *Digital Biology: How Nature is Transforming Our Technology and Our Lives*, New York: Simon and Shuster.

16 Calmenson, D.W. (1999) 'Participatory healing', *ISdesignet Magazine*, March. Online. Available at http://www.isdesignet.com/magazine (accessed 12 July 2002).

17 Wellnessllc (2002) 'The wellness room'. Online. Available at http://www.wellnessllc.com (accessed 12 August 2002).

18 Nitsche, Michael (2008) *Video Game Spaces*, Cambridge: MA: MIT Press.

19 Verderber, Stephen and Refuerzo, Ben J. (2005) *Innovations in Hospice Architecture*, London: Routledge/Taylor & Francis, pp. 176–80.

20 Rowland, Christopher (2006) 'Digital divide widens in medicine', *The Boston Globe*. Online. Available at http://www.boston.com/business/globe/articles/2006/02/10/digital_divide_widens_in_medicine/.html (accessed 24 May 2009). Also see Hesse, Bradford, W., David E. Nelson, Gary L. Kreps, Robert T. Croyle, Neeraj K. Arora, Barbara K. Rimer, and Kasisomayajula Viswanath (2005) 'Trust and sources of health information', *Archives of Internal Medicine*, 165:12/26, 2618–2624.

21 Kreps, Gary L. (2006) 'Communication and racial inequities in health care', *American Behavioral Scientist*, 49:6, 760–74.

22 Ashton, James (2002) 'From sickness treatment … to sustainable development', *Green Futures*, 34:5, 32–4.

23 Adcox, Seanna (2008) 'Nuclear waste piles up at hospitals', *The Greenville News*, 26 September, p. 14A.

24 Thurgood, Michael (2002) 'Waste future – 2020 visions – and a zero waste world?', *Green Futures*, 35:7, 32–8.

25 Anon (2001) 'Managing biomedical waste', *Express Healthcare Management*, 4:8, 31 April, 21–5.

26 Connor, Stephen (2002) 'Hospitals for a healthier planet', *Green Futures*, 34:5/6, 43–7.

27 The Nuffield Trust (2003) *Building a 2020 Vision: Future Health Care Environments*. Report. London: South Bank University/Royal Institute of British Architects. Also see Global University Programs in Healthcare Architecture (GUPHA), (2005). *Global Hospitals in the Year of 2050*, Tokyo: University of Tokyo/Japan Ministry of Health.

28 Waibel, Markus (2007) 'Architecture and robotics', *Robots.net*. Online. Available at http://www.robots.net/article/2249.html (accessed 27 May 2009).

29 Verderber and Fine, p. 351.

30 Lang, Jon T. (1987) *Creating Architectural Theory: The Role of the Behavioral Sciences in Environmental Design*, New York: Van Nostrand Reinhold.

31 Robinson, Julia W. (2001) 'The form and structure of architectural knowledge: from practice to discipline.' In Robinson, Julia W. and Alan Piotrowski (eds.) *The Discipline of Architecture*, Minneapolis and London: University of Minnesota Press. This is a main reason why the disciplinary knowledge base of the field advances at such a glacial pace compared to the health sciences.

32 Verderber, Stephen, Julia Fauerbach, and Brandon Walter (2008) 'On the value of stewardship and sustainability in health administration education', *The Journal of Health Administration Education*, 26:3, 248–68.

33 Tuxworth, Brian (2002) 'Sit still while I empower you … ', *Green Futures*, 35:7/8, 24–32.

34 Kramer, S. (2001) *The Continuance of Existence*, Santa Barbara, CA: Creations in Consciousness. Also see Kramer, S. (1997) 'Agelessness', *Self Help Magazine*, August, 42–9.

35 More, M. (2001) 'On Becoming Posthuman'. Online. Available at http://www.maxmore.com (accessed 12 July 2002).

36 Uldrich, J. (2002) 'Eleven reasons why nanotechnology will arrive sooner than expected', *Futures Research Quarterly*, 18:1, 54–62.

37 Vikhanski, L. (2001) *In Search of the Lost Cord: Solving the Mystery of Spinal Cord Regeneration*, Washington: Joseph Henry Press.

38 Stewart, Alan (2002) 'A silver lining?', *Japan Inc.*, 29:3, 6–8.

39 Dent, Harry S. Jr. (1999) *The Roaring 2000s Investor: Strategies for the Life You Want*, New York: Simon and Schuster.

40 Dossey, Larry (1999) *Beyond Mind-Body to a new Era of Healing*, San Francisco: Harper Collins.

41 Carme, Sara and Seymore M. Glick (1996) 'Compassionate-empathic physicians: personality traits and social organizational factors that balance or inhibit this behavior pattern', *Social Science and Medicine*, 43:8, 1253–61.

42 Allgood, Lawrence (1997) 'Architects have been shopping their visions for 2,500 years', *Emory Report*, 50:8, 38. Also see Toy, Maggie, and Charles Jencks (eds.) (2000) *Millennium Architecture*, New York: John Wiley and Sons.

43 Freking, Kevin (2009) 'Number of Americans without health insurance expected to grow by 9 million in next decade', *The Cleveland Plain Dealer*. Online. Available at http://www.blog.cleveland.com/medical/2009/02.html (accessed 27 May 2009).

44 Bingman, A. L. Sanders, and R. Zorach (eds.) (2002) *Embedded Utopias: Gender, Social Change, and the Modern Metropolis*, London: Routledge. Also see Verderber, Stephen (2008) 'Evidence-based design for healthcare in post-Katrina New Orleans: Current dilemmas', *Health Environments Research & Design Journal*, 1:2, 71–8.

45 Verderber, Stephen (2005) *Compassion in Architecture: Evidence-based Design for Health in Louisiana*, Lafayette: Center for Louisiana Studies.

46 Verderber, Stephen (2003) 'Compassionism and the design studio in the aftermath of 9/11', *Journal of Architectural Education*, 56:3, 60–74.

47 Brenner, Lynn 'How did you do?' *Parade Magazine*, 2 March, 4–5.

48 Allsopp, Bruce (1974) *Towards a Humane Architecture*, London: F. Muller.

49 Verderber, Stephen, and Refuerzo, Ben J. (1999) 'On the construction of research-based design: a community health center', *Journal of Architectural and Planning Research*, 16:3, 225–41.

50 Gans, Herbert J. (1978) 'Towards a human architecture: a sociologist's view of the profession', *Journal of Architectural Education*, 31:2, 26.

51 Garrott, Jay S. (1983) 'Interpreting value system milieus', pp. 21–9 in Peter G. Burgess, (ed.) *The Role of the Architect in Society*, Pittsburgh: Carnegie Mellon University.

52 Gans, 26.

53 Peterson del Mar, David (2006) *Environmentalism*, Harlow, U.K.: Pearson.

54 Rokeach, Milton (1979) *The Nature of Human Values*, New York: McGraw-Hill. Personal constructs are the unstable and are constantly being modified to respond to the ever-changing influences within one's life. Institutional value constructs such as education, religion, government, are more stable in nature and one responds to these societal influences more slowly. The third type, societal value constructs, while being the most stable of the three, are the most deterministic, as they affect both personal and institutional value constructs.

55 Garrott, p. 24.

56 Burgess, Peter, Elliott Littman, and James Mayo (1981) 'Political knowledge and the architectural studio', *Journal of Architectural Education*, 34:3, 24–8.

57 Garrott, p. 27.

58 Too many 'healthcare firms' chase only those clients with the deepest pockets at the expense of so-called 'poorer' clients. Second, few architects who specialize in this area proactively engage in shaping public governmental policy to influence the quality of the built environment for health. Case in point: architects working for healthcare clients over

the ten-year period from 1990 to 2000 were increasingly obsessed with private sector corporate clients. The largest number of awards (48) was bestowed upon private sector corporate projects. Across the decade a clear upward trend occurred in the number of corporate-built winners, with a corresponding downward trend in the number of not-for-profit public governmental sector award-winning buildings. Perhaps not surprisingly, only eight (5.4 percent) awards were bestowed on architects who had designed and built publicly financed community outpatient clinics.

59 Belcher, John R., and Frederick A. DiBlasio (1990) *Helping the Homeless: Where Do We Go From Here?*, New York: Lexington Books.

60 McClam, Erin (2002) 'NYC looks at retired cruise ships as shelters', *The Times-Picayune*, 16 November, p. A-12.

61 Portable Building Research Unit (1997) *Portable Architecture Conference and Symposium*, Liverpool: University of Liverpool. Also see Kronenburg, Robert (1995) *Houses in Motion: The Genesis, History and Development of the Portable Building*. London: Academy Editions.

62 International Red Cross (2002) *Response Preparedness in Bangladesh*, Geneva: International Red Cross. Online. Available at http://www.ifrc. org. (accessed 12 December 2002). Also see *Principles of Disaster Mitigation in Health Facilities: Preparedness and Relief Coordination* (2000), New York: Pan American Health Organization, 2000.

63 Sinclair, Cameron (2002) *Architecture for Humanity: Building a Better World: Mobile HIV/AIDS Health Clinic Design*, Architecture for Humanity. Online. Available at http://www.architectureforhumanity.org (accessed 12 December 2002).

64 Duby, Peter (2002) *Flood Adaptive Housing in Bangladesh*. Online. Available at http://www.archnet.org. (accessed 12 December 2002). Also see Comerio, Mary C. (1998) *Disaster Hits Home: New Policy for Urban Housing Recovery*, Berkeley: University of California Press.

65 Goldhagen, Sarah W. (2003) 'Our degraded public realm: the multiple failures of architecture education', *The Chronicle of Higher Education*, 10 January, B1-2. On the fractured relationship between clients and their architects, Goldhagen asserts that postmodernism's influence, as reappraised in the aftermath of 9/11, has had both positive and negative consequences for the learning and the practice of architecture.

66 Anderson, Stanford (1991) 'Postscript: regrounding architecture'. In Malcolm Quantrill and Bruce Webb (eds.) *Constancy and Change in Architecture*, College Station: Texas A&M University Press.

7 Designing for hospital-based care

1 American Hospital Association (2007) *Fast Facts on U.S. Hospitals*, Chicago: American Hospital Association. Online. Available at http://www.aha.org/aha/resource-center/Statistics-and-Studies/fast-facts.html

(accessed 4 May 2009). Hospitals are classified by type of ownership (public hospitals, federal hospitals, voluntary not-for-profit hospitals, and proprietary, or for-profit, hospitals). As of 2007 there were 221 federal government-run hospitals. In this same year there were 2,919 nongovernmental not-for profit community hospitals, and 889 for-profit community hospitals. A second classification system in the U.S. is by length of stay. Most hospitals are short-stay facilities where the average length of stay is less than 30 days. These patients suffer from acute conditions. By contrast, a patient in a facility for 30 days or longer is housed in a long-term care hospital. These facilities provide extended medical and rehabilitative care to patients with clinically complex acute and chronic conditions. Rehabilitation and children's hospitals provide specialized care. There are also cancer, women's care, surgical, heart, and orthopedic specialty hospitals. As of 2007, Medicare had certified 129 long-term care hospitals in the U.S. Third, classifications exist according to the type of service. General acute care hospitals provide a variety of services, including general and specialized medicine, general surgery and specialized surgery, and obstetrics. Most U.S. hospitals are general acute care institutions. By contrast, specialty hospitals admit only certain types and ages of patients or those with specific illnesses and conditions. Behavioral health or psychiatric hospitals provide diagnostic and treatment services for persons with mental health disorders. In 2007 there were 451 such institutions nationally.

Community hospitals are non-federal, short stay; acute care general, or specialty hospitals whose facilities and services are available to the general public. As of 2007 there were 4,927 community hospitals in the U.S. Non-community hospitals include hospitals operated by the Department of Veterans Affairs (DVA), prison hospitals, college infirmaries, and long-term care institutions. Classification by location: urban hospitals are defined as located in a county that is part of a metropolitan statistical area (MSA), a community of more than 50,000 inhabitants, and a total population of 100,000. As of 2007 there were 2,926 urban community hospitals. By contrast, rural hospitals are located in a county that is not part of an MSA. As of 2007 there were 2,001 rural community hospitals in the U.S. Classification by size: small (less than 100 beds), medium (from 100 to under 500 beds), and large (more than 500 beds). Other types of hospitals include teaching and academic medical center hospitals that are affiliated with a medical, public health, and/or nursing school, critical access hospitals in rural areas with an undersupply of health professionals, and doctor-owned specialty hospitals. This latter group of institutions is controversial because critics believe that they capture the most profitable specialty procedures away from non-profit community hospitals. These institutions remain controversial and are targeted by their critics as promoting unnecessary procedures that unnecessarily run up the cost of healthcare for the nation. Finally, a healthcare system consists of multiple hospitals that owned, leased, sponsored, or contract managed by a central administrative organization. As of 2007 there were 2,755 community hospitals affiliated with a healthcare system.

By contrast, a healthcare network is an affiliated group of hospitals, physicians, other providers, insurers, and community agencies that collaborate to provide a broad range of healthcare services to a given community.

2 Verderber, Stephen and David J.Fine (2000) *Healthcare Architecture in an Era of Radical Transformation*, New Haven: Yale University Press, p. 177.

3 Duany, Andres, Elizabeth Plater-Zyberk, and Jeff Speck (2001) *Suburban Nation: The Rise of Sprawl and the Decline of the American Dream*, Boston: North Point Press.

4 McHarg, Ian (1995) *Design With Nature*, New York: John Wiley & Sons.

5 Farr, Douglas (2008) *Sustainable Urbanism: Design With Nature*, New York: John Wiley & Sons.

6 Verderber and Fine, pp. 156–7.

7 Guenther, Robin and Gail Vittori (2008) *Sustainable Healthcare Architecture*, New York: McGraw-Hill, pp. 208–10.

8 Chinese News Service (2008) 'Automobiles increasing in China'. Online. Available at http://www.news.xinhuanet.com/english/2008-10/18/content_10213769.htm (accessed 10 May 2009).

9 Guenther and Vittori, p. 127.

10 Ibid., p. 380.

11 Anon (2008) 'Potential of offshore wind energy', *The Scottish Government*. Online. Available at http://www.scotland.gov.uk/News/Releases/2008.html (accessed 13 May 2009). Fourteen developers had applied to the Crown Estate for 23 potential widely distributed sites. Scotland, in particular, has 25 percent of Europe's wind potential and there is much interest in developing this resource in shallower territorial waters off the coast. The Crown Estate currently owns the seabed out to 12 nautical miles.

12 Anon (2001) 'Great River Medical Center', *Modern Healthcare*, 8 October, 30.

13 Guenther and Vittori, p. 44, and Guenther, Robin (2009) 'The Zero Waste Hospital', *Presentation at the 3rd Epidaurus Condense*, National Defense Medical Center, Bethesda, Maryland.

14 Guenther and Vittori, pp. 381–2.

15 Verderber and Fine, pp. 184–5.

16 Ibid., pp. 182–3.

17 Landmarks Preservation Council of Illinois (2003) *A Reuse Plan for Cook County Hospital*, Springfield: Landmarks Preservation Council of Illinois. Online. Available at http://www.landmarks.org/images/cook_county%20Hospital.pdf (accessed 10 May 2009).

18 Landmarks Council of Chicago (2008) 'Mies Van Der Rohe', *Landmarks Council of Chicago*. Online. Available at http:www.cityofchicago.org/landmarks/c/crownhall.html (accessed 11 May 2009).

19 Verderber and Fine, pp. 120–9.

20 Anon (2009) 'VitalArts'. Online. Available at http://www.vitalarts.org.uk/commissions/vital-arts-past.html (accessed 12 May 2009).

21 Author's notes from workshop on 'Art in the Hospital Environment' at the Third Epidaurus Conference, National Defense Medical Center, Bethesda, Maryland, April 2009.

22 Verderber and Fine, pp. 199–200.

23 Goldin, Grace (1994) *Work of Mercy: A Picture History of Hospitals*, Toronto: Boston Mills Press, p. 47.

24 Verderber and Fine, pp. 126–8.

25 Anon (2006) 'Orange City (Iowa) Area Health System', *Modern Healthcare*, 25 September, 32.

26 Yanni, Carla (2007) *The Architecture of Madness: Insane Asylums in the United States*. Minneapolis: University of Minnesota Press, pp. 56–9.

27 Goldin, pp. 52–5.

28 Threadkell, Simon (2009) 'Sustainability does not mean compromise, now or ever', *FX Magazine*. Online. Available at http://www.fxmagazine.co.uk/story.asp?sectioncode=87&storycode=2399.html (accessed 12 May 2009).

29 Appleton, Jay (1975) *The Experience of Landscape*, London: John Wiley & Sons.

30 Joseph, Anjali and L. Fritz (2006) 'Ceiling lifts reduce patient handling injuries', *Healthcare Design*, 6(1), 10–13.

31 Malkin, Jain (2008) *A Visual Reference for Evidence-based Design*, Concord: CA: The Center for Health Design, p. 26.

32 Cahnman, Sheila F. (2008) 'The changing face of critical care', *Healthcare Design*, 11(8). Online. Available at http://www.healthcaredesignmagazine.com/ME2/Segments/Publications/print.asp.html (accessed 12 May 2009). Also see O'Connell, N.H. and H. Humphreys (2000) 'Intensive care unit design and environmental factors in the acquisition of infection', *Journal of Hospital Infection*, 45:11, 255–62. Also Taraska, Julie (2008) 'Amenity hospital', *Metropolis*, 23:2, 24–8.

33 Anon (2009) 'Mary Sharp Birch Hospital for Women: Labor and delivery'. Online. Available at http://www.sharp.com/mary-birch/labor-delivery.cfm (accessed 10 May 2009). Also see McFadden, Kathleen L. (1996) 'Hospital policy changes in obstetric patient movement', *International Journal of Operations & Production Management*, 16:3, 28–41.

34 Levin, Aaron (2007) 'Psychiatric hospital design reflects treatment trends', *Psychiatric News*. Online. Available at http://pn.psychiatryonline.org/cgi/content/full/42/2/9.html (accessed 15 May 2009). Also see Gamble, Leslie, David Fowler, Don Duncan, and Tanis Evans (2008) 'Designing for safety in an adolescent psychiatric unit', *Healthcare Design*. Online. Available at http//:www.healthcaredesignmagazine.com/ME2/Segments/Publications.html (accessed 5 May 2009).

35 Oberlin, John (2009) 'HGA completes largest rehab center in Sacramento region', *Healthcare Design*. Online. Available at http://www.healthdesignmagazine.com/ME2/Segments.html (accessed 10 May 2009). Also see Herr, Beau (2007) 'Tokyo Bay Rehabilitation Hospital: design collaboration across the Pacific', *Healthcare Design*. Online. Available at http://www.healthdesignmagazine.com/ME2/Segments.

html (accessed 15 May 2009). Also Peck, Richard L. (2008) 'Rehab by design', *Healthcare Design*, 8:12, 51–8.

36 Verderber, Stephen and Ben J. Refuerzo (2005) *Innovations in Hospice Architecture*, London: Taylor & Francis, pp. 112–21.

37 Gordon, Douglas (2007) 'Pre-op, PACU, and Stage 2 recovery', *Healthcare Design*. Online. Available at http://wwwhealthdesignmagazine.org/ME2/Segments.html (accessed 10 May 2009).

38 Rodriguez, Havidán and Aguirre, Benigno E. (2006) 'Hurricane Katrina and the healthcare infrastructure: a focus on disaster preparedness, response and resiliency', *Frontiers of Health Services Management*, 23(1), 13–25.

39 Branigan, William and William Booth (2009) 'CDC: Swine Flu outbreak signs encouraging', *The Washington Post*. Online. Available at http://www.washingtonpost.com/wp-dyn/content/article/2009.html (accessed 4 May 2009).

40 Verderber and Fine, p. 48.

41 Anon (2009) 'Startracks custom mobile medical vehicles'. Online. Available at http://www.startracksmedical.com. (accessed 12 May 2009). Also see Anon (2009) 'LifeLine mobile'. Online. Available at http://www.lifelinemobile.com. (accessed 12 May 2009).

42 Anon (2005) 'Changi General Hospital', *The Greenroof Projects Database*. Online. Available at http://www.greenroofs.com/projects. (accessed 10 May 2009). Also see Levenston, Michael (2008) 'Urban growers go high-tech to feed city dwellers', *City Farmer News*. Online. Available at http://www.cityfarmer.info. (accessed 12 May 2009).

43 Cooper Marcus, Clare (2007) 'Healing gardens in hospitals', *Interdisciplinary Design and Research e-Journal*, 1(1), 1–27. Online. Available at http://www.idrp.wsu.edu/html (accessed 14 February 2009).

44 Ulrich, Roger (1999) 'Effects of gardens on health outcomes: theory and research'. In Cooper Marcus, Clare, and Mimi Barnes, *Healing Gardens: Therapeutic Benefits and Design Recommendations*, New York: John Wiley & Sons, pp. 27–86.

45 United States Green Building Council (2009) 'Green building facts', *U.S. Green Building Council*. Online. Available at http://www.usgbc.org. (accessed 12 May 2009).

46 Guenther and Vittori, pp. 210–13.

47 Klevins, R.M., J.R. Edwards, C.L. Richards, T.C. Horan, R.P. Gaynes, D.A. Pollock, *et al.* (2007) 'Estimating health care-associated infections and deaths in U.S. hospitals', *Public Health Reports*, 122(2), 160–6.

48 Ulrich *et al.* (2008). Also see American Hospital Association (2005) *The Costs of Caring: Sources of Growth in Spending for Hospital Care*. Washington, D.C.; American Hospital Association and J. Weinstein (1998) 'Nosocomial infection update', *Emerging Infectious Diseases*, 4(3), 416–20.

49 Guenther and Vittori, pp. 13–15.

50 Sackett, D.L., W. Rosenberg, J.A.M. Gray, R.N. Haynes, and W.S. Richardson (1996) 'Evidenced-based medicine: what it is and what it is not', *British Medical Journal*, 312: 71–2.

51 The Center for Health Design (2008) *EDAC Study Guides 1–3*, Concord, California: The Center for Health Design.

52 U.S. Government Accounting Office (2006) 'Health information technology: HHS is continuing efforts to define its national strategy', *Southern California Evidence Based Practice Center*. Online. Available at http://www.research.microsoft.com/towards2020science (accessed 12 April 2009).

53 Kurlantzick, Joshua (2007) 'Mixing pleasure and health for low-cost, high-quality care', *The New York Times*. Online. Available at http://www.livemint.com/articles.html (accessed 5 May 2009). Also see Leung, Rebecca (2005) 'Vacation, adventure and surgery?' *60 Minutes*. Online. Available at http://www.cbsnews.com/stories/2005.html (accessed 13 May 2009).

54 Author's email correspondence with Gary W. Collins, 16 May 2009. In 2009 there were 18,000 IFMA members organized into one of 16 IFMA councils, one of which is the Healthcare Council.

Index

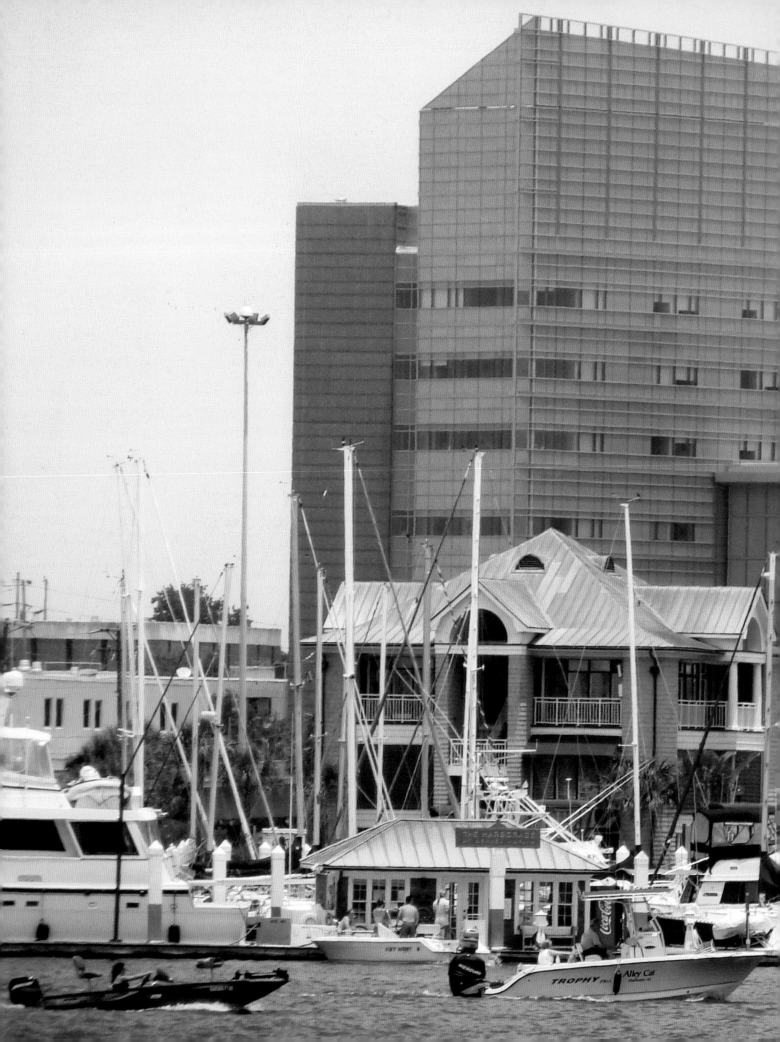

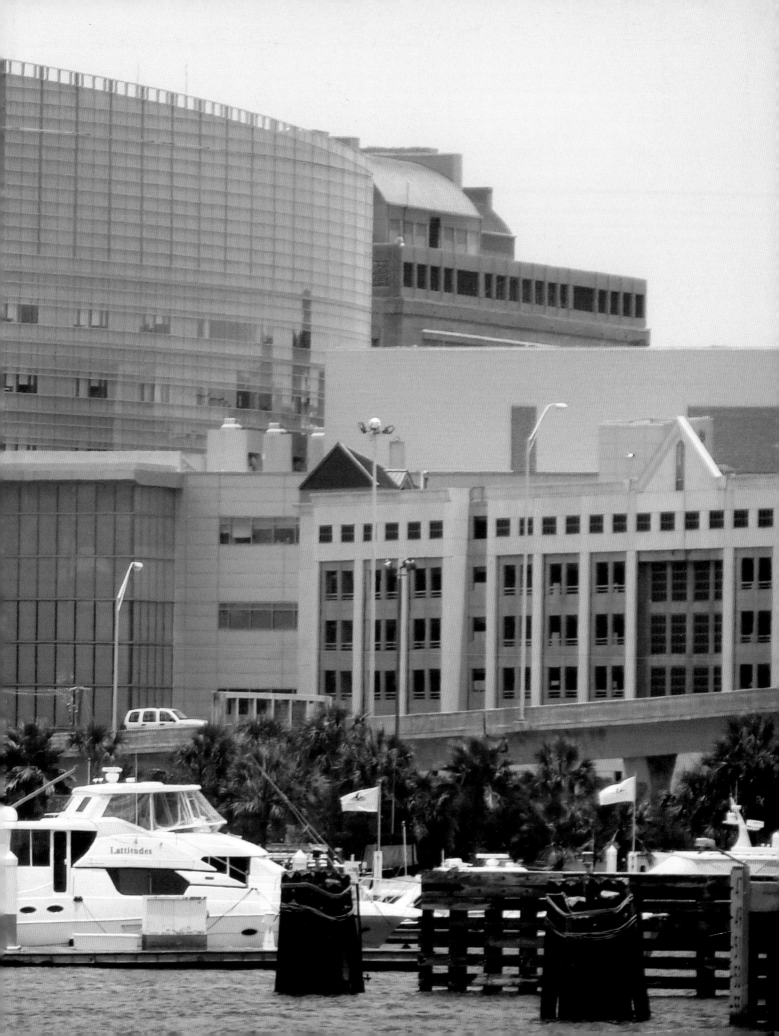